THE YELLOW EMPEROR'S CLASSIC OF MEDICINE

Essential Questions

Translation of
Huangdi Neijing Suwen

Other Related Titles from World Scientific

A History of Medicine in Chinese Culture
In 2 Volumes
by Boying Ma
ISBN: 978-981-3237-96-4 (set)
ISBN: 978-981-3237-97-1 (Vol. 1)
ISBN: 978-981-3237-98-8 (Vol. 2)

Traditional Chinese Medicine Is an Intangible Science
by Boxin Guo
ISBN: 978-981-3239-29-6

Tu Youyou's Journey in the Search for Artemisinin
by Wenhu Zhang, Yiran Shao, Dan Li and Manyuan Wang
translated by Junxian Yu
ISBN: 978-981-3207-63-9
ISBN: 978-981-3207-64-6 (pbk)

Cancer Management with Chinese Medicine: Prevention and Complementary Treatments
Revised Edition
by Rencun Yu and Hong Hai
ISBN: 978-981-3203-88-4
ISBN: 978-981-3231-85-6 (pbk)

Anecdotes of Traditional Chinese Medicine
by Lifang Qu
edited by Mary Garvey
ISBN: 978-1-938134-99-9
ISBN: 978-1-945552-02-1 (pbk)

THE YELLOW EMPEROR'S CLASSIC OF MEDICINE

Essential Questions

Translation of Huangdi Neijing Suwen

Edited by

Jinghua Fu

China Academy of Chinese Medical Sciences, China

Translated by

Mingshan Yang

Shanghai University of Traditional Chinese Medicine, China

World Scientific

NEW JERSEY • LONDON • SINGAPORE • BEIJING • SHANGHAI • HONG KONG • TAIPEI • CHENNAI • TOKYO

Published by

World Scientific Publishing Co. Pte. Ltd.

5 Toh Tuck Link, Singapore 596224

USA office: 27 Warren Street, Suite 401-402, Hackensack, NJ 07601

UK office: 57 Shelton Street, Covent Garden, London WC2H 9HE

Library of Congress Cataloging-in-Publication Data
Names: Fu, Jinghua, author.
Title: The Yellow Emperor's Classic of medicine — essential questions :
translation of Huangdi neijing suwen / edited by Jinghua Fu ; translated by Mingshan Yang.
Other titles: Huangdi nei jing su wen yi zhu. English | Su wen. English
Description: New Jersey : World Scientific, 2019. | This translated book is based
on the Chinese version annotated and edited by Jinghua Fu and his team,
published by China Renmin University Press in 2010.
Identifiers: LCCN 2018031834 | ISBN 9789813273573 (hardcover : alk. paper)
Subjects: | MESH: Su wen. | Medicine, Chinese Traditional | China
Classification: LCC R601 | NLM WZ 294 | DDC 610.951--dc23
LC record available at https://lccn.loc.gov/2018031834

British Library Cataloguing-in-Publication Data
A catalogue record for this book is available from the British Library.

《黄帝内经素问译注》
Originally published in Chinese by China Renmin University Press

For any available supplementary material, please visit
https://www.worldscientific.com/worldscibooks/10.1142/11080#t=suppl

This book is supported by the B&R Book Program.

Typeset by Stallion Press
Email: enquiries@stallionpress.com

Contents

Translator's Preface		xi
Chapter 1	The Art of Health Cultivation in Ancient Times	1
Chapter 2	Great Theory on Spirit Regulation in Four Seasons	6
Chapter 3	Generative Qi Communicating with Nature	10
Chapter 4	Distinctive Words in the Golden Chest	15
Chapter 5	Great Theory on Yin–Yang Corresponding to Nature	20
Chapter 6	Separation and Combination of Yin and Yang	30
Chapter 7	Distinctive Theory on Yin and Yang	33
Chapter 8	Secret Canon Stored in Numinous Orchid Chamber	37
Chapter 9	Six-Sixty System and Visceral Manifestations	39
Chapter 10	Comprehensive Generation of Five Solid Viscera	45
Chapter 11	Additional Theory on Five Solid Viscera	50

Chapter 12	Proper Therapies for Different Diseases Geographically	52
Chapter 13	Transferring Essence and Changing Qi	54
Chapter 14	Thin and Thick Medical Wine	58
Chapter 15	Fundamental Theory Inscribed in Jade	61
Chapter 16	Diagnostic Essentials and Manifestations of Twelve-Meridian Exhaustion	64
Chapter 17	Diagnosis for Pulse-Taking and Pulse Subtlety	69
Chapter 18	Pulse-Qi Conditions of Healthy Person	78
Chapter 19	Vital Theory on Critical Visceral Pulses Inscribed in Jade	85
Chapter 20	Three Regions and Nine Positions of Pulse	95
Chapter 21	Distinctive Theory on Meridians and Diseased Pulses	101
Chapter 22	Transference of Solid Visceral Qi Following Regularity of Four Seasons	104
Chapter 23	Clarification of Five-Visceral Qi	110
Chapter 24	Blood, Qi, Body and Emotions	113
Chapter 25	Cherishing the Life and Guarding the Body	115
Chapter 26	Eight Solar Terms and Medical Perspective	119
Chapter 27	Separation and Combination of Genuine Qi and Evil Qi	124
Chapter 28	Comprehensive Theory on Deficiency and Excess	129
Chapter 29	Taiyin and Yangming Meridians	135

Chapter 30	Explanation on Yangming Meridian	138
Chapter 31	Heat Disease	140
Chapter 32	Treatment of Heat Disease with Acupuncture	144
Chapter 33	Commentary on Heat Disease	149
Chapter 34	Disharmony of Diseases	153
Chapter 35	On Malaria	156
Chapter 36	Theory on Acupuncture for Malaria	163
Chapter 37	Qi Reversal	167
Chapter 38	Cough	169
Chapter 39	Listing and Analyzing Pain-Disease	172
Chapter 40	Abdominal Disorders	177
Chapter 41	Treatment of Lumbago with Acupuncture	181
Chapter 42	Wind Evil	186
Chapter 43	Impediment Syndrome	190
Chapter 44	Flaccidity Syndrome	195
Chapter 45	Reversal Syndrome	198
Chapter 46	Manifestations of Seven Diseases	202
Chapter 47	Uncommon Diseases	206
Chapter 48	Extraordinary Diseases	210
Chapter 49	Explanations of Twelve Meridians	214
Chapter 50	Keys of Needling	219
Chapter 51	Restrictions of Needling	221
Chapter 52	Contraindications of Acupuncture	223
Chapter 53	Notes of Needling	226
Chapter 54	Explanations of Needling	228
Chapter 55	Extension of Needling Manipulation	232
Chapter 56	Skin Regions	235
Chapter 57	Meridians and Collaterals	238
Chapter 58	Qi-Acupoint	239

Chapter 59	Qi-House	244
Chapter 60	Bony Foramen	249
Chapter 61	The Acupoints for Water-Disease and Heat-Disease	255
Chapter 62	Regulation of Meridians	259
Chapter 63	Contralateral Needling	269
Chapter 64	Needling for Reversing or Complying with the Changes in Four Seasons	277
Chapter 65	Branch–Root and Transmission of Diseases	281
Chapter 66	Great Theory on Law of Primordial Qi in Nature	285
Chapter 67	Great Theory on Movement of Five Phases	291
Chapter 68	Great Theory on Movement of Six-Qi	300
Chapter 69	Great Theory on Shifting and Interaction of Qi	310
Chapter 70	Great Theory on Routine Functions of Five Phases	325
Chapter 71	Great Theory on Normality of Six-Qi	346
Chapter 72	Acupuncture Therapy for Abnormal Qi-Phase	404
Chapter 73	Root of Diseases	405
Chapter 74	Great Theory on Crucial Principles	406
Chapter 75	Elucidation of Perfect Teaching	443
Chapter 76	Administration of Reasonable Analysis	446
Chapter 77	Listing and Analysis of Five Diagnostic Errors	450
Chapter 78	Precautions for Four Diagnostic Faults	455
Chapter 79	Categorization of Yin and Yang	458

Chapter 80 Measurement of Exuberance and Exhaustion 463
Chapter 81 Explanation of Subtleties of Essence 467

Appendix A Acupuncture Therapy for Abnormal Qi-Phase 471
Appendix B Root of Diseases 487

About the Editor 505
List of Translators 506

Translator's Preface

There are many human races in the world and different races may show different skin colors, yet there are no significant differences in physical and visceral functions. Since ancient times, people living in the eastern and western hemispheres have explored various medical herbs and methods for the treatment of human diseases. It is not hard to see that the object of the ancient medicinal service is no alien beings from outer space but human beings in the world, which is just the common basis of ancient eastern and western medicine.

It can be said that the ancient Greeks started western medicine with *Hippocratic Corpus*, while ancient Chinese people established the foundation of oriental medicine with *Huang Di Nei Jing* (*The Yellow Emperor's Classic of Medicine*). As the medical giants of western and oriental medicine in ancient times, how could they obtain the scientific instruments for medical research as we do today? The great contributions they made for the human medicine all came from their extraordinary intelligence to observe the images of life and to summarize the experiences of preventing and treating diseases, so as to establish the respective medical systems, by which the medical masterpieces came out admirably.

Before Qin (221–207 BCE) and Han (206 BCE–220 CE) Dynasties, ancient Chinese medical books were simply written with a concise but comprehensive structure. Linguistically, Traditional Chinese Medicine (TCM) and western medicine are quite different from each other. "Formal Equivalence" by Eugene Nida is generally adopted to solve most problems in my translation accordingly. As for the selection of English words or terms in translation, etymology of the original Anglo-Saxon language was referred. The sentence pattern and word order should follow the style of Chinese classical literary works. This is the principle and technique employed in my translation.

"Any explanation of a Chinese character means a cultural history in detail," the Titan of Chinese studies, Mr. Chen Yinque remarked. Could the academic notion be used for translation of *The Yellow Emperor's Classic of Medicine*? The answer is positive. Nevertheless, it needs to be humbly suggested that the *Yellow Emperor* is too great to comprehend in its every detail. Thus, not every source of each character in the course is equally and accordingly traced. Hence, I conducted a linguistic research project on the main terms and characters according to the method of "Textual Research of Integrating Chinese with Western Literature" designed by myself. Nearly two hundred TCM words have been textual-researched and nearly two hundred articles have been written abiding by the model of "One character requires one detailed document compiled". There are no fewer than thirty kinds of TCM English dictionaries (based on word phrase of TCM) but I often failed to select suitable English words from those dictionaries when translating *The Yellow Emperor's Classic of Medicine*. Following the idea of Mr. Chen Yinque, I specifically compiled the *Essential Chinese–English*

TCM Dictionary (based on single Chinese character), which was published by Fudan University Press in 2013. In fact, *Essential Chinese–English TCM Dictionary* was especially compiled for the translation of *The Yellow Emperor's Classic of Medicine — Essential Questions*, and readers may consequently categorize the *Dictionary* as a reference book for the translation of TCM classics. Whenever there is any difference between TCM terminologies in this book and the versions of other scholars, it can be discussed based on the *Essential Chinese–English TCM Dictionary*.

The translated text mainly refers to the *Huang Di Nei Jing Su Wen Yi Zhu* (*Translation and Annotation of the Essential Questions in Yellow Emperor's Inner Canon*) published by China Renmin University Press in 2010, which is based on the Chinese version of *Essential Questions in Yellow Emperor's Inner Canon* (Gu Congde version in Ming Dynasty) published by China Renmin University Press in 1963.

All in all, though I am a pediatrician of western medicine, I admire TCM so much that I could spare no effort in translating the book. I would like to express my deep appreciation to all those who are committed to translating and publishing the book.

Mingshan Yang
June 2018

Chapter 1

The Art of Health Cultivation in Ancient Times

The Yellow Emperor lived in ancient China. He was born with high intelligence; as a toddler, he was able to talk well; as a child, he was quick in understanding of things; later, in his younger days, he was honest and nimble; finally, in his adulthood, he was accomplished and became the Emperor.

The Emperor asked Master Qibo: I've heard that people in ancient times could live to about one hundred years without decline in action, but today I see people doddering much earlier from the age of fifty! Is it due to the change in era or the loss of health cultivation?

Qibo answered: People in ancient times knew the way to cultivate their health and followed the rules of Yin and Yang; they kept fit with exercises, moderate eating and drinking, led a routine daily life, and avoided overstrain or sexual intemperance. Thus, this helped them integrate their soul and body and enjoy a natural life span, and meet their peaceful end at the age of about one hundred. Today, people behave oppositely. They drink wine as though it were water, regard indulgence as normal and seek sexual pleasure after being drunk, so their essence of life is exhausted and the genuine Qi is dissipated. They don't know how to maintain maximum health or control their minds; they do whatever they like while violating the tenets of life, and live an irregular daily life; they appear to be aging much faster, and visible signs of aging are seen as early as in their fifties.

When teaching people in ancient times, the sages will mention that all deficient evil and sinister wind should be avoided in time, and people should cultivate a quiet mind against any distractions, which can thus help soothe the genuine Qi and guard their spirits intact. Thus how can any diseases develop? Therefore, people can live a peaceful life with fewer desires, make their mind stable with no anxiety, and perform physical labor without much fatigue, so that their Qi can flow smoothly such that they can meet their satisfaction according to their proper wishes. Then people can enjoy whatever food they eat, feel ease with whatever clothes they wear, enjoy themselves in their customs, and never make upward social comparison; they were really plain honest people. Therefore, no addiction can distract their attention, and no lust can disturb their mind. Whether being intelligent or ignorant, and moral or unworthy, they are not anxious about materialistic living and can attain the status prescribed in ancient laws. The reason why people in ancient times lived up to one hundred years without any aging in action was that they mastered the way of health cultivation beyond illness.

Emperor: Elderly people are unable to give birth to any child. Is it due to the exhaustion of the essence or the natural law of physiology?

Qibo: For a female, her kidney Qi becomes exuberant at the age of seven when permanent teeth erupt and hair starts growing long. Menarche occurs at the age of fourteen when the Conception meridian starts opening up, followed by the exuberance of the Thoroughfare meridian resulting in regular menstruation cycle; the woman thus becomes fit to conceive a child. She has plentiful kidney Qi at the age of twenty-one, when her wisdom teeth erupt leading to permanent dentition. At the age of twenty-eight, her sinews and bones become firm, the hair grows long enough and the physique attains peak condition. At the age of thirty-five, her Yangming meridian starts to decline, her face begins to wither and hair starts to fall. At the age of forty-two, there is deficiency in triple-Yang meridians from upward while the face withers completely and the hair turns white. At the age of forty-nine, there is deficiency in both Conception and Thoroughfare meridians, menopause occurs leading to exhaustion in the reproductive essence, so that her body looks shapeless and loses the ability to bear a child.

For a male, his kidney Qi starts getting enriched at the age of eight when hair starts to grow and permanent teeth erupt. At the age of sixteen, his kidney Qi is exuberant signaling the arrival of the reproductive essence, and his spermatic essence too overflows. If Yin and Yang are harmonized, a male is able to bear a child. At the age of twenty-four, his kidney Qi is plentiful and he has firm sinews and bones, the wisdom teeth erupt leading to permanent dentition. At the age of thirty-two, his sinews and bones become stout and muscles become strong. At the age of forty, his kidney Qi falls into a decline, with hair loss and withering teeth. At the age of forty-eight, his Yang Qi declines from upward when his complexion withers and the hair on the temples turns white. At the age of fifty-six, his liver Qi declines further and the sinews become rigid while the reproductive essence is exhausted with less spermatic essence due to kidney Qi decline; his physique and body functions deteriorate. At the age of sixty-four, his teeth and hair are gone. The kidney governs water, receives and stores the essence from five solid and six hollow viscera, and discharges the excess when five solid viscera are substantially full. These five solid viscera degenerate when the sinews and bones become flaccid, and the reproductive essence is exhausted. So his earlock turns white, the body becomes clumsy, the walking develops a doddering pattern and he is therefore unable to bear a child.

Emperor: But some elderly people are still able to conceive a child. How do you explain this phenomenon?
Qibo: This is because they have a robust natural constitution, the circulation of both Qi and blood is always smooth and their kidney Qi is richer. Nevertheless, the age for a male to have a child is no more than sixty-four, and for a female, no more than forty-nine, beyond which the essence Qi of Yin and Yang is completely exhausted.

Emperor: Those who have complied with the law of health cultivation live over one hundred years. Can they bear a child?
Qibo: Those who have complied with the rule of health cultivation can delay aging and keep fit; although aged, they can still bear a child.

Yellow Emperor: I'm told that in ancient times there were Immortals, who could adapt to the changes of nature, comply with the law of Yin–Yang, inhale 'vital air', guard their spirits independently and keep their muscular structure integrated, so they could live with heaven and earth having endless span, and this is the outcome of living according to the way of life. In the middle ancient times, there were Perfect Men, who had superior moral values and mastered health cultivation, harmonized their Yin–Yang, adapted themselves to four seasons, abandoned worldly interests, and concentrated their spirits, as if they could travel between the heaven and the earth and see or hear beyond eight directions. This was their way to extend life span, become stronger and attain immortal status. Next, there were Sages, who lived in the harmony of the heaven and the earth and followed the rules of eight winds. They moderated their interests and desires in the secular world and freed themselves from anger and complaints. They had no intention to separate themselves from common life; even though they wore common clothes, they never followed the behavior of ordinary people. Physically, they didn't exhaust themselves and spiritually they didn't worry themselves; they regarded peace and happiness as their life goals and self-gratification as the accomplishment. As a result, their bodies weren't susceptible to decline and their spirits did not dissipate. Therefore, they were able to live to about one hundred years. Finally, there existed Virtue Men, who maintained their health in accordance with the laws of the heaven and the earth, with changes of the sun or moon and shifting of the stars; they complied with the alteration of Yin–Yang and four seasons such that they could prolong the life as long as possible.

Chapter 2

Great Theory on Spirit Regulation in Four Seasons

The three months of spring is the period for growing the new, instead of the old, when the heavens and the earth are resuscitating and all the living things are flourishing. People will sleep late at night and get up early in the morning to walk in the courtyard with hair untied and body relaxed, so as to refresh their spirit. In this period, one should prefer growing to killing, promotion to punishment and giving to depriving, which is just the adaptation to spring Qi and also the rule of health cultivation for generating Qi. Reversing the rule impairs liver, which will lead to excessive cold diseases in summer due to insufficient supply for growth.

The three months of summer is the period for prosperity when heavenly Qi and earthly Qi are mingling and all the living things are in fruitful blossom. In this period, people sleep late at night and get up early in the morning without being tired of long daytime, avoid angry mood as if being in floral exuberance to make Qi communication smooth and enjoy the outer world. This is just the adaptation to summer Qi and also the rule of health cultivation for growing Qi. Reversing the rule impairs heart, which will lead to malaria in autumn due to insufficient supply for collection and the exacerbation in winter.

The three months of autumn is the period for peace and maturation when the wind is strong and the air over the earth is clear and bright. People sleep early at night and get up early in the morning when hearing the crow of a rooster, to keep the spirit calm for separating oneself from the conquering sough of autumn, to astringe the spirit and energy internally for balancing the autumn Qi, and to guard the mind against anxiety for clearing lung Qi. This is just the adaptation to autumn Qi and also the rule of health cultivation for collecting Qi. Reversing the rule impairs lung, which will lead to diarrhea after indigestion in winter due to insufficient supply of Qi for storage.

The three months of winter is the period for closure and storage when the water freezes and the earth cracks. People should not disturb Yang Qi, and go to bed early at night and get up late in the morning to wait for the rising sunlight and to make the spirit hidden or concealed as if having the privacy or keeping it for one's own. They should dispel cold and keep warm, avoid discharge from the skin and exhaustion of Qi. This is just the adaptation to winter Qi and also the rules of health cultivation for storing Qi. Reversing the rule impairs kidney, which will lead to loss of vigour in spring due to insufficient supply of Qi for generation.

Heavenly Qi is clear and bright, which can embrace the natural power ceaselessly so that all the living things won't subside. If the heavens are too brilliant, the sun and moon will seem dim and evils will attack the hollow orifices. If Yang Qi is blocked, earthly Qi glooms while the cloud and mist cannot obtain the essence, so the corresponding dew upward won't fall. If the heavens and the earth fail to communicate with each other, all the living things will lose their vitality, in which even precious trees will die mostly. If bad Qi isn't dispelled, the wind and rain cannot be regulated and the dew cannot fall, because of which grasses and trees will wither. The evil wind attacks frequently and rainstorm often sweeps in which the heavens and the earth as well as four seasons lose their orders to reverse the law of nature and even lead to early death. Only the sages can follow the law of nature, so they won't contract any rare diseases. Similarly, if all the living things follow the law, their vitality will never be exhausted.

If spring Qi is reversed, Shaoyang Qi fails to be born and then liver Qi will be changed abnormally and internally. If summer Qi is reversed, Taiyang Qi will fail to develop and then heart Qi will become empty internally. If autumn Qi is reversed, then Taiyin Qi fails to be astringed, leading to dryness and feverish distension of lung Qi. If winter Qi is reversed, then Shaoyin Qi fails to be stored, leading to sinking of kidney Qi alone.

The change of Yin and Yang in four seasons is the root of all the living things in nature. The sages can cultivate Yang energy in spring and summer while nourishing Yin energy in autumn and winter to comply with the root of the nature, so that they can live with the rule of all the living things. If one reverses the law, the root of life will be felled and the primordial Qi will be destroyed. Therefore, the change of Yin and Yang in four seasons is fundamental to all the things in nature and is the root of birth and death. The reversal will cause disasters while compliance will lead to no disorder, which is known as enlightenment of law. The law of health cultivation will be followed by the sages but the foolish will violate.

Compliance with the law of Yin and Yang will protect life, while reversing it will cause death; compliance with the law will bring about peace, while reversing it will cause disorders. Reversing the common law is known as internal rejection. Therefore, the sages will not always focus on the treatment of the developed disease but will emphasize treating the pre-disease state; they will not focus on the treatment of the developed disorder but will emphasize treating the pre-disorder state. After the disease has been developed, it is given medication, or after the disorder has been formed, it is given treatment; this is just like digging a well when one feels thirst, or making weapons when a war is breaking out. Isn't it too late?

Chapter 3

Generative Qi Communicating with Nature

Yellow Emperor: The communication with heavenly Qi has been considered to be fundamental to life since ancient times, which is in turn based on Yin and Yang. Between the heavens and the earth, or within six directions of the universe, Qi exists in nine states, in nine orifices, five solid viscera and twelve joints of the body, all of which communicate with heavenly Qi. Yin–Yang generates five elements, which in turn correspond to triple-Yin and triple-Yang. If people frequently violate the rule, evil Qi will impair their bodies, which is the root of long life.

If heavenly Qi is fresh and clear, people can maintain a peaceful mind and comply with it to strengthen Yang Qi. Even the evil around cannot impair the body, which is due to adaption to the seasonal order. Therefore, the sages can keep the essence of Yin and Yang to comply with heavenly Qi, and thus are able to communicate with the deities. If this is reversed, the evil will block the nine orifices internally and congest muscles externally, leading to dispersion of the defensive Qi, which is called self-impairment with Qi damaged.

Yang Qi is just like the sun in the heavens, and if the essential sun is lost, it will lead to reduction of life and insufficient vitality. Therefore, the normal movement of the heavens depends on the brightness of the sun. So, Yang Qi will be ascending, which can defend the body against external evils.

Affected by cold, the desire is like a running pivot, and if there is much unease in daily life, the spirit Qi will float. Affected by summer heat, the body sweats with vexation and the person pants loudly even while speaking and at rest. When the body develops high fever as if being a burning coal, the stagnated heat can be dissipated with perspiration. Affected by damp, the head will have a feeling of being wrapped. If the damp heat isn't dispelled, the large sinew will become short while the small one will become loose, the former displaying a constricted pattern and the latter a flaccid pattern. Affected by wind, swelling will develop while four evils will attack four limbs alternatively, leading to exhaustion of Yang Qi.

Yang Qi will be hyperactive during vexation or overworking, and essence Qi will be exhausted when the disease is lingering in summer, which may bring out the hot reversal.

The blind loses sight and the deaf loses hearing, just like the raging torrent through a breached dyke, which is impossible to be checked.

Yang Qi will divorce the physique Qi in a rage, while blood will stagnate in the upper region, resulting in sudden syncope. If impaired, the sinew will become flaccid and disabled, and if not held, there will be sweating over half of the body, leading to hemiparalysis. If sweating is complicated by the invasion of damp, it will cause boils or prickly heat. Too much fatty and refined food tends to cause big boils on foot, which is just like putting something in the empty. When the body is attacked by wind when working with sweat, cold evil will invade the skin to cause roughness and stagnation, leading to acne.

With the nourishment of Yang Qi, the spirit can be nourished by its essence and the sinew can be nourished by its gentle part. With abnormal opening and closing of interstitial striae, the cold evil will invade and result in humpback. The intrusion into vessels will result in fistula, which has lingered between the muscle and interstitial striae. Cold Qi invading through acupoints will attack the viscera in transmission, which may cause susceptible fear and fright. If the nutrient Qi fails to flow normally and stagnates in the muscular interstices, it will result in carbuncle and swelling. When evaporation of Yin-sweat isn't enough, the physique will be weak and Qi will be exhausted while acupoints will be closed, leading to wind-malaria. Therefore, wind is the leading cause of various diseases. However, only if people can keep a quiet mind and moderate workload, the muscular striae can be closed and even the violent wind or toxin cannot cause damage, which is in compliance with the seasonal changes.

So, prolonged diseases tend to transmit and change. Then, when the upper and the lower cannot communicate, even a good doctor can do nothing about it. Therefore, the accumulation of Yang Qi will lead to disorder and even death while Yang Qi has been blocked. The blocked Yang Qi should be purged. If the treatment cannot be given immediately and properly, the patient will die. So, Yang Qi governs the exterior in the daytime. Yang Qi begins to emerge at the crack of dawn, grows into exuberance at noon and becomes feeble at dusk, thus closing the sweat pores. Hence, at dusk, Yang Qi is astringed, during which time the sinews and bones shouldn't be disturbed, and the body should avoid being exposed to fog and dew. Any violation in the three sequences can encumber the physique.

Qibo: Yin can keep the essence inside, which can play a vital role, and Yang can protect the exterior and consolidate it. If Yin is dominated by Yang, the pulse will be strenuous and rapid, leading to drastic diseases. If Yang is dominated by Yin, Qi of five solid viscera will conflict one after another so as to block the nine orifices. Hence, the sages can balance Yin and Yang to harmonize the sinews and vessels, strengthen the bone and marrow, and smoothen Qi and blood flow. Thus, the internal and the external can be harmonized and the evil cannot impair the body, so that people can maintain good sight and hearing and Qi can circulate normally as usual. With wind invading and Qi disturbed, the evil will impair liver when Yin essence has been exhausted. So, overeating will make sinews and vessels flaccid, which will cause dysentery and hemorrhoids. So, overdrinking will cause Qi to flow reversely. Overexertion or excessive intercourse will impair kidney Qi and even injure the lumbar spine.

The fundamental of Yin and Yang is that only when Yang is compact can Yin be consolidated. If there is no harmony between Yin and Yang, it is as if there were spring but no autumn, or winter but no summer in a year. It is the rule of the sages to harmonize Yin and Yang. So, if Yang Qi is too hyperactive to be secluded, Yin Qi will be exhausted. If Yin is peaceful and Yang is secluded, the spirit will be flourishing. If Yin and Yang are separate from each other, the essence Qi will be exhausted. If attacked by dew and wind, one will develop chill and fever. Hence, the evil Qi will linger to cause acute watery diarrhea when the wind attacks in spring. The evil Qi will lead to malaria in autumn when the summer heat attacks in summer. Evil Qi will ascend reversely to cause cough, leading to flaccid reversal when the damp attacks in autumn. Evil Qi will cause the warm disease in spring when the cold attacks in winter. Evil Qi in four seasons can impair five solid viscera alternately.

Yin is transformed from five flavors, while five solid viscera where Yin is stored will be conversely impaired by excess of five flavors. So, taking the sour excessively will make liver Qi hyperactive, which will in turn make spleen Qi exhausted. Taking salt excessively will impair the large bone, shrink muscle and restrain heart Qi. Taking sweets excessively will cause hyperactive heart Qi, panting and distending with black complexion and unbalanced kidney Qi. Taking bitters excessively will make spleen Qi lose moistness and stomach Qi be excessively dry. Taking pungent foods excessively will make sinews and vessels flaccid and spirit collapse. Hence, the harmony among the five flavors can make bones strong, sinews soft, Qi and blood flow smoothly, and interstitial striae tight by which the bone can obtain the essence Qi and people can even live a much longer life if they follow this regimen carefully.

Chapter 4

Distinctive Words in the Golden Chest

Yellow Emperor: There are eight winds in the heavens while there are five winds in the meridians. Why is this so?

Qibo: If eight winds rise as the evils, they turn into meridian winds involving five solid viscera to cause diseases. The so-called predominance of four seasons is that spring dominates late summer, which in turn dominates winter, which dominates summer, which dominates autumn, that in turn dominates spring; this is the dominance of four seasons.

The east wind rises in spring, reflecting the diseases in liver and the acupoints in the neck; the south wind rises in summer, reflecting the diseases in heart and the acupoints in the chest and libs; the west wind rises in autumn, reflecting the diseases in lung and the acupoints in the shoulders and back; the north wind rises in winter, reflecting the diseases in kidney and the acupoints in the waist and thigh; and, the central wind corresponds to earth, reflecting the diseases in spleen and the acupoints in the spine. So, the spring Qi reflects the diseases in the head. The summer Qi reflects the diseases in solid viscera. The autumn Qi reflects the diseases in the shoulders and back.

The winter Qi reflects the diseases in four limbs. Thus, nosebleed tends to develop in spring, the diseases of the chest and hypochondria in middle summer, watery diarrhea and interior cold in late summer, wind-generated malaria in autumn, and impediment and stroke in winter. If having not been disturbed by pressing and stepping, one cannot have nosebleed or diseases in the neck in spring, diseases in the chest and hypochondria in the middle summer, diarrhea and interior cold in the late summer, wind-generated malaria in autumn, and impedimental reversal as well as diarrhea after indigestion with sweating. The essence is the root of the human body. So, when essence is hidden, one cannot suffer from warm diseases in spring. If there is no sweating in hot summer, one will have the accumulative disease of wind-generated malaria in autumn. These are the rules of pathogenesis among ordinary people.

It's believed that there is Yin in Yin and Yang in Yang. From early morning to noon, Yang in the heavens is the Yang in Yang. From noon to dusk, Yang in the heavens is the Yin in Yang. From night to dawn, Yin in the heavens is the Yin in Yin. From dawn to early morning, Yin in the heavens is the Yang in Yin. Therefore, the human body has a similar regularity.

As far as Yin and Yang of human body are concerned, the exterior corresponds to Yang while the interior corresponds to Yin. As far as Yin and Yang of the trunk are concerned, the back corresponds to Yang while the abdomen corresponds to Yin. As far as Yin and Yang of viscera are concerned, solid viscera corresponds to Yin while hollow viscera corresponds to Yang. The five solid viscera, that is liver, heart, spleen, lung and kidney, are categorized as Yin while six hollow viscera, that is gallbladder, stomach, large intestine, small intestine, bladder and triple-Jiao, are all categorized as Yang. Therefore, it should be known that there is Yin in Yin and Yang in Yang — why? It is because the diseases in winter are associated with Yin, the diseases in summer are associated with Yang, the diseases in spring are associated with Yin, and the diseases in autumn are associated with Yang. All the aspects of Yin or Yang should be analyzed in order to determine the acupuncture therapy with stone needles. Moreover, the back corresponds to Yang, and Yang in Yang is associated with heart. The back corresponds to Yang, and Yin in Yang is associated with lung. The abdomen corresponds to Yin, and Yin in Yin is associated with kidney. The abdomen corresponds to Yin, and Yang in Yin is associated with liver and the abdomen corresponds to Yin, and the extreme Yin in Yin is associated with spleen. All these are examples of the relationship between Yin and Yang, exterior and interior, internal and external as well as female and male, which correspond to Yin and Yang in the heavens.

Yellow Emperor: In addition to five solid viscera corresponding to four seasons, are there any practical actions like reception and awarding, respectively?

Qibo: Yes, there are. The east corresponds to green, communicates with liver, opens orifices to eyes and hides essence in liver. Then it reflects fear and fright in diseases, sour in flavors, wood and grass in five elements, chicken in animals, wheat in grains and spring in four seasons. It corresponds to Wood Star (Jupiter) in the sky and then spring Qi is above the head; and it reflects Jue in musical scales and eight in numbers. Therefore, it is known that the disease reflected is in tendons with the foul smell in odors.

The south corresponds to red, communicates with heart, opens orifices to ears and hides essence in heart. Then it reflects the disease in five solid viscera. It reflects bitterness in flavors, fire in elements, sheep in animals, millet in grains and summer in four seasons. It corresponds to Fire Star (Mars) in the sky. Therefore, it is known that the disease reflected is in vessels; and it reflects Zhi in musical scales, seven in numbers and burnt smell in odors.

The center corresponds to yellow, communicates with spleen, opens orifices to mouth and hides essence in spleen. Then it reflects the disease in the root of the tongue. It reflects sweet in flavors, earth in five elements, cattle in animals, glutinous millet in grains and later summer in four seasons. It corresponds to Earth Star (Saturn) in the sky. Therefore, it is known that the disease reflected is in muscle; and it reflects Gong in musical scales, five in numbers and aromatic smell in odors.

The west corresponds to white, communicates with lung, opens orifices to nose and hides essence in lung and then it reflects the disease on the back. It reflects pungency in flavors, metal in five elements, horses in animals, rice in grains and autumn in four seasons. It corresponds to Metal Star (Venus) in the sky. Therefore, it is known that the disease reflected is in skin and hair, and it reflects Shang in musical scales, nine in numbers and fishy smell in odors.

The north corresponds to black, communicates with kidney, opens orifices to anal and genital orifices and hides essence in kidney and then it reflects the disease on the knee. It reflects salty in flavors, water in five elements, pigs in animals, bean in grains, and winter in four seasons. It corresponds to Water Star (Mercury) in the sky. Therefore, it is known that the disease reflected is in bone, and it reflects Yu in musical scales, six in numbers and smell in odors.

Hence the doctor good at pulse-taking will observe five solid viscera and six hollow viscera and their compliance and reversal, and categorize Yin and Yang, exterior and interior, as well as male and female, which is kept in mind integrated with wisdom. These fundamental theories cannot be instructed to those who are not qualified or not devoted to learning, which is the correct academic attitude.

Chapter 5

Great Theory on Yin–Yang Corresponding to Nature

Yellow Emperor: Yin–Yang is the law of the heavens and the earth, the rules of all creatures, the parent cause of changes and alterations, the origin of life and death, and the house of spirit. The treatment of diseases should follow nothing but the root, Yin–Yang.

So, the accumulation of primordial Yang is converted into heavens and the primordial Yin into earth. Yin is static while Yang is dynamic. Yang governs growth while Yin governs development, and Yang is associated with consumption while Yin is associated with storage. Yang can be transformed into Qi while Yin can be transformed into shape. Extreme cold generates heat and extreme heat generates cold. Cold Qi generates the turbid and heat Qi generates the clear. Clear Qi descending will cause diarrhea after indigestion, and turbid Qi ascending will cause severe distention. These are the alterable movements of Yin and Yang and the reversal and compliance of diseases.

Therefore, clear Yang becomes the heavens while turbid Yin becomes the earth. Earthly Qi ascends to form clouds while heavenly Qi descends to form rains. Rain originates from earthly Qi while clouds originate from heavenly Qi. Therefore, clear Yang goes out of the upper orifices while turbid Yin emits out of the lower orifices. Clear Yang is distributed into interstitial striae and turbid Yin runs through five solid viscera. Clear Yang fills four limbs and turbid Yin returns to six hollow viscera.

Water corresponds to Yin and fire corresponds to Yang; Yang can manifest in Qi while Yin manifests in flavor. Flavors contribute to the physique that contributes to Qi. Qi in turn contributes to the essence that contributes to the transformation of primordial Qi. Then, the essence is nourished by Qi while the physique is nourished by flavors, and transformation of primordial Qi leads to essence, which is transformed into physique. Excessive flavors damage the physique and excessive Qi damages the essence; the essence can be transformed into Qi, which can be damaged by excessive flavors. Yin flavor emits out of the lower orifices while Yang Qi emits out of the upper orifices. Thick flavors correspond to Yin and while thin flavors correspond to Yang in Yin. Thick Qi corresponds to Yang while thin Qi corresponds to Yin in Yang. Thick flavors tend to discharge while thin flavors tend to dredge. Thin Qi tends to disperse while thick Qi tends to heat up. Strong fire reduces Qi while moderate fire strengthens Qi. Strong fire consumes Qi while moderate fire warms Qi. Strong fire disperses Qi while moderate fire supplements Qi. In terms of flavors, the pungent and sweet flavors induce dispersion that corresponds to Yang, while the sour and bitter flavors induce vomiting and discharge that correspond to Yin.

Predominance of Yin causes Yang diseases while predominance of Yang causes Yin diseases. Predominance of Yang generates heat while predominance of Yin generates cold. Extreme cold is transformed into heat while extreme heat is transformed into cold. Cold damages the physique and heat damages Qi. Qi damage causes pain and the physique damage leads to swelling. So, the pain that precedes swelling indicates Qi damaging the physique. Swelling preceding the pain indicates physique damaging Qi. Predominance of wind leads to stirring, predominance of heat leads to swelling, predominance of dryness leads to withering, predominance of cold leads to edema, and predominance of damp leads to watery diarrhea.

In nature, there are shifts of four seasons and five elements, which manifest in the generation, growth, harvest and storage as well as in cold, heat, dryness, damp and wind. In the human body, there are five solid viscera that are associated with five types of Qi, which are responsible for five emotions of joy, anger, grief, anxiety and fear. So, over-joy and anger damage Qi while over-cold and summer heat damage the physique. Violent rage damages Yin and violent joy damages Yang. When reversal Qi is flowing upwards, meridians will be packaged and the body will be out of shape. Uncontrolled joy and anger as well as excessive cold and summer heat can endanger the life. Thus, extreme Yin must be converted into Yang while extreme Yang must be converted into Yin.

It's believed that if there is damage by cold in winter, there must be a warm disease in spring. If there is damage by wind in spring, there is diarrhea after indigestion in summer. If there is damage by summer heat in summer, then there is malaria in autumn. And if there is damage by damp in autumn, there is cough in winter.

Yellow Emperor continued: I'm told that sages in ancient times illustrated the structures of the human body, distinguished solid and hollow viscera and their functions, identified the distribution of meridians, and connected the six communications following their own routes. Acupoint Qi emerging from the foci has a special nomenclature. Intermuscular septum together with the bone has its starting acupoints. The reversal and compliance of the subordinate parts have their respective regulations. The change of four seasons and Yin–Yang has its rule. The external and internal environment correspond with each other in an interior–exterior relationship. Are they all reasonable?

Qibo: In the east, the wind springs up and vitalizes the wood; the wood brews the sour flavor; the sour flavor moistens liver. The liver governs sinews that boost heart and liver determines the eyes. Such wonderful variations are manifested in the cosmology of the heavens, the law among human beings, and transformation on the earth. By such transformation, five flavors are generated; by evolution of the law, the wisdom emerges; and, by cosmology, the spirit arrives. The spirit embodies wind in the heavens, wood on the earth, sinews in the body, liver among solid viscera, dark green in colors, Jue in scales, calling in sounds, grasp in motion, eyes in orifices, sour in flavors, and anger in emotions. Anger damages liver while sorrow dominates anger, wind damages sinews while dryness dominates wind, and sour damages sinews while pungency dominates sour.

The heat rises up in the south to make a fire. Fire causes the bitter flavor that strengthens heart; heart generates blood; blood replenishes spleen, and heart determines the conditions of tongue. Such wonderful variations are manifested in the heat in the heavens, fire on the earth, blood vessels in the human body, heart among five solid viscera, red in colors, Zhi in scales, laugh in sounds, anxiety in morbid changes, tongue in orifices, bitterness among flavors, and joy in emotions. Over-joy damages heart while fear dominates joy. Heat damages Qi while cold dominates heat; bitter flavor damages Qi while saltiness dominates bitterness.

The damp spreads in the center to fertilize the earth, which generates the sweet that nourishes spleen. The spleen strengthens muscles that ensure the function of lung, and spleen determines the conditions of the mouth. Such wonderful variations are manifested in the dampness in the heavens, soil in the earth, muscles in the body, spleen in the solid viscera, yellow in colors, Gong in scales, singing in sounds, spitting in actions, the mouth in orifices, sweet in flavors and thinking in emotions. Excessive contemplation impairs spleen, while anger dominates over contemplation. Excessive dampness impairs muscles, while wind dominates over damp; excessive sweet impairs muscles, while the sour dominates over sweetness.

There exists dryness in the west which contains metal; metal bears a pungent flavor that nourishes lung. Lung functions together with skin and hair, which have an effect on kidney; and, lung governs nose. The variation in the west is manifested as dryness in the heavens, metal under the earth, skin and hair in the body, lung among solid viscera, white in colors, Shang in scales, cry in the sounds, cough in morbid changes, nose in orifices, pungency in flavors and anxiety in emotions. Anxiety damages lung while joy dominates anxiety; heat damages the skin and hair while cold dominates heat; pungency damages the skin and hair while bitterness dominates pungency.

There exists the cold source in the north which turns into water; water contains a salty flavor that boosts kidney. Kidney produces bone and marrow that nourishes liver, and kidney governs the ears. Such wonderful variation in the north is manifested as cold in the heavens, water on the earth, bone in body, kidney among solid viscera, black in colors, Yu in scales, groan in sounds, shivering in morbid changes, ears in orifices, saltiness in flavors, and fear in emotions. Fear impairs kidney while over-thinking dominates fear. Cold damages blood while dryness dominates cold; saltiness damages blood while sweetness dominates saltiness.

It's believed that the heavens and the earth are the spaces between the upper and the lower where all creatures live in. Yin and Yang embody the unity of opposites of blood and Qi. The left and the right are the routes of Yin and Yang. Water and fire are the signs of Yin and Yang. Yin and Yang are the source of all creatures. It's believed that Yin resides inside to support Yang while Yang acts outside to embody Yin.

Emperor: How should one apply the principle of Yin and Yang?

Qibo: If Yang predominates Yin, there will develop fever, closure of interstitial striae, shortness of breath while propping up or sitting upright, fever with no sweating, dryness of teeth with dysphoria and severe abdominal distension, indicating that death is approaching, in which the patient can live through winter but not summer. If Yin dominates Yang, there will be fearing cold, sweating, feeling cold, frequent trembling with chillness and further Qi reversal, and then severe abdominal distention, indicating that death is approaching, in which the patient can live through summer but not winter. These denote the alternative predominance of Yin and Yang, which is reflected in manifestations and mechanisms of diseases.

Emperor: How should one regulate Yin and Yang properly?
Qibo: If seven disadvantages and eight benefits of physiological rules are understood, Yin and Yang can be regulated; otherwise, it will lead to early aging. At the age of forty, Yin Qi declines by half, leading to deterioration of daily life. At the age of fifty, the body becomes heavy and the eyes and ears are also no longer acute. At the age of sixty, impotence appears, Qi greatly declines and the nine orifices are blocked, leading to deficiency in the lower and excess in the upper along with sniveling and tears dripping frequently. It's believed that knowing the regulation of Yin and Yang leads to strong health, while not knowing it leads to early aging. For this reason, the people with the same constitution originally will have different outcomes of health. A wise man is good at identifying the common sense for health while a stupid person only observes the different health status from the healthy one. Such a stupid person is in the status of insufficiency while a wise man is in the status of sufficiency. A man with sufficient essence has acute ears and eyes as well as a strong and smart body. The elderly can be revitalized and the strong can gain the perfect physique. Hence, the sages do nothing against nature, enjoy themselves in peaceful and plain life, and find pleasures in indifference to fame and gain, so that they can maintain their life long enough together with the heavens and the earth, which is the way for sages to cultivate their health.

The heavens have their insufficiency in the northwest which then corresponds to Yin, and accordingly the ears and eyes on the right are not as acute as that on the left. The earth has its insufficiency in the southeast which then corresponds to Yang and accordingly the hand and foot on the left are not as strong as that on the right.

Emperor: Why is it so?

Qibo: The east corresponds to Yang that gathers the essence in the upper so that there is bright health but deficiency in the lower, and accordingly ears and eyes are sharp while hands and feet aren't nimble. The west corresponds to Yin that gathers its essence in the lower body so that there is exuberance in the lower but deficiency in the upper, and accordingly ears and eyes aren't sharp while hands and feet are nimble. So, when both sides are invaded by evil, the right side is more severe in the upper while the left side is more severe in the lower. It is just because Yin and Yang between the heavens and the earth cannot be perfect that evil can take advantage to reside.

So, the heavens have the Qi essence while the earth has its formation. The heavens have eight recording marks while the earth has five elements, which will be the parents of all creatures. The clear Yang ascends to the heavens while the turbid Yin descends to the earth. Hence, the heavens and the earth are moving or resting based on the principle of the deity, and the cycle of birth, growth, harvest and storage can run round and again. Only a wise man can nourish the head in the upper body like treating the heavens, in the lower strengthen the feet like treating the earth and in the middle replenish five solid viscera like treating human affairs. Qi in the heavens communicates with lung, Qi on the earth communicates with throat, wind Qi communicates with the liver, thunder Qi with the heart, grain Qi with the spleen and rain Qi communicates with the kidney. The six meridians function like river, intestine and stomach like sea and nine orifices are acupoints for fluid Qi to infuse into the body. If the heavens and the earth are compared to Yin and Yang, the sweat from Yang is named as the rain in the nature and Qi from Yang as the swift wind between the heavens and the earth. The rage of a man is like the rolling of thunder and reversal Qi is like Yang. Thus, the treatment given, neither according to the principle of the heavens nor the rules of the earth, will result in disasters immediately.

So, the evil wind comes as swiftly as the heavy rain and wind. So, a doctor at the top level can treat diseases that invade the skin and hair; at the second level, the doctor will treat diseases in the skin and muscles; at the third level, he will treat the sinew and vessels; at the fourth level, treat diseases in six hollow viscera; at the lowest level, he will treat the diseases in five solid viscera. When the disease is treated after invading into five solid viscera, the survival rate of the patient is reduced by half.

Thus, if evil Qi from the heavens invades the body, five solid viscera will be damaged; if the cold and heat evil from water and grain invade the body, six hollow viscera will be damaged; and if the damp Qi invades the body, the skin, muscle, sinews and vessels will be damaged.

Therefore, a doctor good at acupuncture can induce Yang from Yin or induce Yin from Yang, treat the right side for the disease on the left or treat the left for the disease on the right, observe himself to know others or observe the exterior to know the interior, analyze the mechanism of the excess or insufficiency to identify the subtle abnormality, which never fails.

Any doctor good at diagnosis, when inspecting complexion and palpating pulses, firstly differentiates Yin or Yang of diseases, analyzes its clarity or turbidity to know its focus, observes the respiration and listens to the sound to know the suffering of patients, observes the complexion and pulses related with four seasons to know the organs involved, and feels Chi-Chun to identify the floating, sunken, slippery and unsmooth pulse to know the causes of the diseases. If there is no error in diagnosis, there is no error in treatment.

It's believed that when the disease occurs at the beginning, acupuncture can be applied to cure it. When the disease is at its peak, acupuncture can be delayed till the disease subsides. Therefore, for moderate diseases, dispersion therapy can be applied; for severe diseases, reduction therapy can be applied; and for declining diseases, supporting therapy can be applied. For the case with insufficient physique, warm therapy can be applied to invigorate Qi. For the case with insufficient essence, supplement therapy can be applied to give thick flavors. For the disease at the top, vomiting therapy can be used; for the disease at the bottom, guiding therapy can be used; for the distension in the middle, purging therapy can be applied internally; for the disease with evil hidden, soaking therapy can be applied to induce sweating; for the skin diseases, sweating therapy can be applied to disperse it; for the drastic diseases, inhibiting therapy can be applied to control it; for the excessive disease, dispersing therapy can be applied to purge it. After analyzing the diseases concerned with Yin or Yang and differentiating between moderate and fulminant diseases, Yin aspect will be treated for Yang disease while Yang aspect will be treated for Yin disease. After identifying the disease concerned with the aspect of blood or Qi and controlling the original focus in the respective origin, the disease with excessive blood is purged and the disease with deficient Qi is guided and supplemented.

Chapter 6

Separation and Combination of Yin and Yang

Yellow Emperor: I was told that the heavens correspond to Yang while the earth to Yin, and the sun corresponds to Yang while the moon to Yin. There are 365 days in a year divided into greater or lesser months. Humans also share the same correspondence. However, at present, triple-Yin or triple-Yang are not consistent in number with single Yin or Yang in general, why is it so?

Qibo: Yin and Yang can be inferred from one to ten, from ten to one hundred, from one hundred to one thousand, from one thousand to ten thousand and from ten thousand to infinity, all of which share the unity of Yin and Yang.

Under the heavens and upon the earth, there are all living things in birth, in which the one under earth is called Yin origin and known as Yin in Yin, and the one breaking through earth is known as Yang in Yin. Yang endows creatures with vitality while Yin endows them with the substantial form. Therefore, all living things grow in spring, develop in summer, are harvested in autumn and stored in winter. If the life rhythm is out of order, there is obstruction of four seasonal variations in the heavens and on the earth. Such rhythm variation of Yin and Yang, which can be expressed in the human body, can also be inferred in numbers similarly.

Emperor: I'd like to learn the individual and combinative conditions of triple-Yin and triple-Yang.
Qibo: When a sage stands facing the south, the front is termed grand-bright and the back is termed Taichong meridian. The route where Taichong runs is termed Shaoyin meridian. The route above Shaoyin is termed Taiyang meridian. Taiyang meridian starts from acupoint Zhiyin (BL67)* and terminates at acupoint Mingmen (Jingming, BL1), which is known as Yang in Yin.

The upper region of the body is called grand-bright, the region below grand-bright is termed Taiyin meridian, and the region in front of Taiyin is termed Yangming meridian. Yangming meridian starts from acupoint Lidui (ST45), which is known as Yang in Yin. The exterior of Jueyin is termed Shaoyang meridian, starting from acupoint Zuqiaoyin (GB44), which is termed Shaoyang in Yin. As to the individual and combinative conditions of triple-Yang, Taiyang meridian is associated with opening, Yangming meridian is associated with closing and Shaoyang meridian with pivoting. These three Yang meridians shouldn't be separated from one another. If their pulses beat with no floating, then they are collectively oneness of Yang.

Emperor: I'd like to learn the individual and combinative conditions of triple-Yin.

---

*The acupuncture points are referred to by their traditional names in *Huangdi Neijing*. The meridians and numbers are added by the translator.

Qibo: The external body corresponds to Yang. The internal body corresponds to Yin below which is the Thoroughfare meridian termed Taiyin meridian. Taiyin meridian starts from acupoint Yinbai (SP01), known as Yin in Yin. Behind Taiyin is Shaoyin meridian, starting from acupoint Yongquan, which is known as Shaoyin in Yin. In front of Shaoyin is Jueyin meridian, starting from acupoint Dadun (LB01), which is known as extreme Yin in Yin. As to the individual and combinative conditions of the triple-Yin meridians, Taiyin is associated with opening, Jueyin with closing and Shaoyin with pivoting. These three Yin meridians shouldn't be separated from one another, and if their pulses beat with no sinking, they are collectively called oneness of Yin. Yin and Yang cycle unceasingly daily around the whole body, and thus Qi circulates interiorly and physique stands exteriorly, which leads to the formation of their integrated relationship.

Chapter 7

Distinctive Theory on Yin and Yang

Yellow Emperor: There are four seasonal pulses and twelve meridians in the body. What are they?
Qibo: Four seasonal pulses comply with four seasons and twelve meridians with twelve months.

The pulses have divisions of Yin and Yang, and knowing Yang is to know Yin while knowing Yin is to know Yang. Yang pulses have five seasonal types, and each type has five sub-types of solid-viscera-pulse, totally with twenty-five Yang pulses. The so-called Yin pulse is the critical one which has no stomach Qi, and when felt, it indicates the deterioration that indicates the doomed death. The so-called Yang pulse is the one which has Yang Qi in stomach. If the Yang pulses can be differentiated, the disease can be located. If the Yin pulses can be differentiated, the death date and survival time can be predicted. The changes of three Yang meridians are reflected in head while the changes of three Yin meridians are reflected in hand, whose conditions constitute oneness of Yang. When Yang pulses can be differentiated, the unfavorable or favorable timing of disease can be predicted. When Yin pulses can be differentiated, the death date and survival time can be predicted. Yin or Yang of pulses should be carefully and skillfully differentiated so that it's unnecessary to follow others blindly. The so-called Yin or Yang of pulse is as follows: Going corresponds to Yin while coming to Yang; stillness to Yin while movement to Yang; and slow to Yin while rapid to Yang.

Anyone who has the critical pulse, showing that liver pulse with stomach Qi exhausted critically, will die in eighteen days; those, showing that heart pulse with stomach Qi exhausted critically, will die in nine days; those, showing that lung pulse with stomach Qi exhausted critically, will die in twelve days; those, showing that kidney pulse with stomach Qi exhausted critically, will die in seven days; and those showing that spleen pulse with stomach Qi exhausted critically, will die in four days.

It's believed that the second Yang meridians (Yangming) have diseases in heart and spleen, with a urinary and fecal retention or irregular menstruation for a female. For long, it can be transmitted as wind-consuming diseases or lung amassment, indicating an incurable disease. It's believed that the third meridian (Taiyang) has diseases of chill and fever, carbuncle and swelling in the lower region or having flaccid knees and feet as well as sour calf. For long, it can be transmitted as dry and rough skin or as Yin hernia. It's believed that the first Shaoyang meridians have diseases with less breath, frequent cough and diarrhea. For long, it can be transmitted as dragging pain in heart and dysphagia. Both Yangming and Jueyin meridians have diseases chiefly manifesting in fear and fright, backache, frequent belching and yawning, termed wind reversal. Both Shaoyin and Shaoyang meridians have diseases with frequent abdominal distension and fullness below heart and frequent sighs. Both Taiyang and Taiyin meridians have diseases of hemiplegia, flaccid knees and tetraplegia.

The pulse beating with sole Yang is termed hooky pulse, that beating with sole Yin is termed furry pulse, that beating with Yang dominance and urgency is termed stringy pulse, that beating with Yang dominance but faint tactility is termed stony pulse, and that beating with Yin and Yang balance is termed slippery pulse.

When Yin is struggling inside and Yang is disturbed outside, Yin-sweat cannot be hidden and four limbs are reversely cold, which ascends to fumigate lung and results in panting and wheezing. Yin is generated endlessly, which is associated with the balance of Yin and Yang, termed harmony. Therefore, if the hard is supplemented with the hard, Yang Qi will be broken and Yin Qi will be exhausted; if it is mired, the hard and the soft are out of balance, so that meridian Qi will be depleted.

The patient with dead Yin will die in three days. The patient with generative Yang will recover in no more than four days. As for generative Yang and dead Yin, liver wood Qi is compliantly transmitted into heart fire Qi, termed generative Yang; heart fire Qi is reversely transmitted into kidney water Qi, termed dead Yin; lung metal Qi is transmitted into kidney water Qi, termed double Yin; and kidney water Qi is transmitted into spleen earth Qi, termed extreme Yin, and the latter three are incurable diseases.

Yang meridians are stagnated with evil, leading to edema of four limbs; Yin meridians are stagnated with evil, leading to hematochezia with one liter of blood; when stagnated twice, with two liters of blood; when stagnated thrice, with three liters of blood; if both Yin and Yang meridians are stagnated with evil with Yin dominance, there will be more Yin and less Yang, termed stony water with water retention in lower abdomen. The second Yang (Yangming) meridian stagnated by evil causes consumptive diseases, the third Yang (Taiyang) meridian stagnated by evil causes dysphagia, the third Yin (Taiyin) meridian stagnated by evil causes ascites, and the first Yin (Jueyin) and Yang (Shaoyang) meridians stagnated by evil cause throat impediment.

When Yin pulses are throbbing, being different from Yang pulses, it indicates pregnancy. When both Yin and Yang pulses are deficient, it indicates approaching death from dysentery. Yang pulses more exuberant than Yin cause sweating. When Yin pulses are weak and Yang pulses are throbbing, it indicates metrorrhagia. When both of third Yin (liver and spleen) pulses are throbbing, the patient will die at midnight in twenty days. When both of second Yin (heart and kidney) pulses are throbbing, the patient will die at dusk in thirteen days. When both of first Yin (pericardium and liver) pulses are throbbing, the patient will die in ten days. When all of third Yang (bladder and small intestine) pulses are throbbing forcefully, the patient will die in three days. When third Yin pulses and third Yang pulses are throbbing together, the patient will have heart fullness, abdominal distension, exhausted Yang distribution and excretory retention, and will die in five days. When both of second Yang pulses are throbbing, the patient will suffer from incurable warm diseases and die in no more than ten days.

Chapter 8

Secret Canon Stored in Numinous Orchid Chamber

Yellow Emperor: Will you please tell me the collaboration of the twelve organs and their major and minor statuses?
Qibo: What an elaborate question! Please allow me to explain it. Heart is the organ serving as the monarch, from whom the spirit comes out. Lung is the organ serving as the prime minister, who governs the administration of the body. Liver is the organ serving as the general, from whom the strategy comes out. Gallbladder is the organ serving as the official of justice, from whom judgment comes out. Pericardium is the organ serving as the chamberlain, from whom emotions come out. Spleen and stomach are the organs of food granary, from where the five flavors come out. Large intestine is the organ serving as the official of transportation, from whom the transformation comes out. Small intestine is the organ in charge of reception, from which the digestion comes out. Kidney is the organ serving as the official of powerful action, from whom the elaborate functions come out. Triple-Jiao is the official in charge of dredging watercourse, who can regulate water transportation. Bladder is the official in charge of water gathering,

where body fluid is stored and processed by Qi transformation before excretion. All the twelve organs shouldn't lose their collaboration. If the monarch is wise, the subordinates will be peaceful, by which one can cultivate health with a long life and avoid drastic diseases all his life. Under this condition, all the states will be prosperous. If the monarch is muddle-headed, all the twelve organs will be in danger, lose their normal functions because of blocked Qi course and have their physique impaired, as a result of which one can't cultivate health, leading to life crisis. Under this condition, all the states will suffer from disasters, for which alerts should be sounded again and again.

The greatest theory lies in the least world, which is endlessly changeable. And who can know its origin? How difficult is it? Though the learners are struggling to observe it, who can know its key points? They are profound and subtle, and which one is the ingenious? Infinitesimal substance originates from tiny things, which can be measured definitively. When tiny things were multiplied thousand- and million-fold, the creatures are formed after expanding progressively.

Yellow Emperor: Great! I have heard the incisive and enlightening rule of health cultivation, which clarifies how to become a sage, and I cannot accept it without total abstinence and selection of an auspicious day.

Then Yellow Emperor selected an auspicious day when the canons were kept in the royal library full of elegance and fragrance for preservation for generations to come.

Chapter 9

Six-Sixty System and Visceral Manifestations

Yellow Emperor: I have heard that the six-sixty system of the heavens makes one year while the nine-orifice and nine-viscera systems of the human body matches the system of the heavens, and there are also 365 acupoints for man to correspond to the heavens and the earth. It has lasted for long. However, I don't know what the theory is.

Qibo: What a concise question! Please allow me to explain it. The six-sixty system and the corresponding nine-nine system are used to define the degrees of the heavens and Qi numbers of solar terms, respectively. The heavenly degrees are used to measure the movement of the sun and the moon while Qi numbers of solar terms are used to record the growth and changes of all the living things in nature. The heavens correspond to Yang while the earth corresponds to Yin; the sun corresponds to Yang while the moon corresponds to Yin. They move in certain orders and along certain orbits. Since the sun moves one degree and the moon thirteen or more degrees daily, greater months and lesser months altogether make a year with three hundred and sixty-five days and the remainder of solar terms make a leap month. The first thing is to decide the beginning of a year, then adjust the solar terms by sundial, and calculate the remainder of the solar terms till the end of a year. Thus, the degrees of the heavens can be worked out.

Emperor: I have known the degrees of the heavens, and now I'd like to know how the solar terms match the degrees of the heavens.
Qibo: There is a six-sixty system for the heavens to be measured and a nine-nine system for the earth to correspond to the heavens. In the former measurement, for the heavenly system, ten-day times six making sixty (threescore) days and sixty-day times six making a year just refer to the calculation of the three hundred and sixty days in a year. Since ancient times, it has been known that anything communicating with the heavens is the root of life and is rooted in Yin and Yang, in which the nine states and nine orifices all communicated with heavenly Qi. So, Yin and Yang generate five elements and are divided into triple-Yin Qi and triple-Yang Qi, in which the three make up the heavens, the three the earth and the three the man. Three times three is nine, which refer to the nine administrative regions for the earth and nine viscera for a human being. Thus, there are four viscera-storing substances and five viscera-storing spirits in human body summed into nine viscera matching heavenly Qi.

Emperor: I have understood the theory of six-sixty system which matches nine-nine system. You, Master, have mentioned that the remainder of solar terms make the leap month. I'd like to know what Qi is. Please enlighten me on this, Master.
Qibo: This is the theory that the Supreme God has kept in secret and my ancient teachers have taught me.

Emperor: Please explain it to me.
Qibo: Five days make a pentad and three pentads make a solar term while six solar terms make a season and four seasons make a year, each of which should follow phases of five elements in compliance with main rule, respectively. Five elements move in regular phases matching the respective season in a year, each of which dominates the season alternately. The evolution goes around and begins again at the start of a year; the seasonal variation and solar terms are distributed endlessly in the same rhythm and so does the pentad. It's believed that without knowing the superposing of year movement, exuberance and decline of Qi, and the cause of deficiency and excess, it's impossible to become a good doctor.

Emperor: The five elements cycle and begin again with no end. What will happen if it goes excessively or deficiently?
Qibo: The cycle of five elements evolves in turn and dominates, respectively, in which the alteration of exuberance and deficiency is a normal phenomenon.

Emperor: What is the normal solar term?
Qibo: It is not in excess or insufficiency.

Emperor: How about the excess and insufficiency?
Qibo: It has been discussed in the medical classics.

Emperor: What does it mean by dominating?
Qibo: Spring dominates late summer that dominates winter that dominates summer that dominates autumn that dominates spring. It refers to the so-called domination of five elements in due season and solid viscera are named by the characteristic of Qi, respectively.

Emperor: How do we know its domination?
Qibo: It is in waiting for arrivals, which is all from spring; the season that shouldn't have come but has come is called excess. While meeting the undominating, the excessive arrival can overrestrain it, which is called Qi excess. If the solar term that should have come hasn't come, it is called deficiency. The dominating Qi will move frantically and the generated Qi will be damaged, so that undominating Qi can attack it, which is called Qi oppression. The so-called obtaining of Qi arrival is achieved by calculating the time of solar term arrival. By carefully observing its time, solar term arrival can be predicted. If Qi does not correspond to due time of the solar term, the Qi dominance of five elements cannot be differentiated and the evils are bred internally, for which physicians can do nothing for the treatment and prevention.

Emperor: Is there any case for the five elements not to move regularly?
Qibo: The Qi of the five elements in nature cannot move without regular rule. If Qi doesn't succeed in regular order, it is called abnormality, which can lead to disorders.

Emperor: What will happen if there is an abnormal succession?
Qibo: Abnormal movement of the five elements will cause diseases. The dominating Qi in due season can only cause mild diseases, otherwise it can cause severe ones. When attacked by additional evil in the meantime, it can cause death. Therefore, when abnormal climate is not in due time, it will cause mild diseases; otherwise, it can cause severe ones.

Emperor: Good! I have known that the Qi integration configures all creatures while all creatures are named according to

their changes of configuration. Both the movement of the heaven–earth and the changes of Yin–Yang are important for all creatures, and there is more or less significance of their influence. Shall I know about it?
Qibo: What a concise question! The heavens are too vast to be measured and the earth is too boundless to be surveyed. Since you have raised such a profound question, please allow me to explain it. The grass has five colors, whose variation is hard to be observed fully, while the grass has five flavors, whose deliciousness is hard to be tasted extremely. People have different likings for different things and their preferences are accordingly different. The heavens provide human beings with five kinds of Qi and the earth provides human beings with five kinds of flavors. The five kinds of Qi are inhaled through the nose and stored in heart and lung, which tend to ascend to make five kinds of colors bright and the voice sonorous. The five kinds of flavors are taken in through the mouth and stored in intestines and stomach, which can have a reserved place and then their essence can nourish the five kinds of Qi. They are harmonized to ensure vitality, and with the assistance of fluid and liquid, the spirit Qi will be naturally produced.

Emperor: How about viscera and their manifestations?
Qibo: Heart is the root of life and the place of spiritual variation. Its luster appears on the face and its fulfillment is in the blood and vessel. Heart is Taiyang of Yang which communicates with summer Qi. Lung is the root of Qi and the location of Yin-soul. Its luster appears on the body hair and its fulfillment is on the skin. It is Taiying of Yang, which communicates with autumn Qi. Kidney, which governs sealing, is the root of storage and the location of essence. Its luster appears on the

hair and its fulfillment is in the bone. It is Shaoyin of Yin, which communicates with winter Qi. Liver is the root of fatigue resistance and the house of Yang-soul. Its luster appears on the nails and its fulfillment exhibits through the sinews, which can produce blood and Qi. Liver corresponds to the sour flavor and green complexion. It is Shaoyang of Yang, which communicates with spring Qi. Spleen, stomach, large and small intestines, triple-Jiao and bladder are the root of storage and digestion, and the place of nutrition Qi; they are called the containers in that they can transport the dross and transform the essence into five flavors; their luster appears on all sides of the lips and their fulfillment is in the muscle; they correspond to sweet flavor and yellow complexion; they are of the extreme Yin, which communicate with earthly Qi. All eleven viscera are influenced by gallbladder.

If Renying pulse is one degree greater than normal, the disease is in Shaoyang; if the pulse is two degrees greater than normal, it is in Taiyang; if the pulse is three degrees greater than normal, it is in Yangming; if the pulse is over four degrees greater than normal, it causes the closure of Yang. If the Cunkou pulse is one degree greater than normal, the disease is in Jueyin; if the pulse is two degrees greater than normal, it is in Shaoyin; if the pulse is three degrees greater than normal, it is in Taiyin; if the pulse is over four degrees greater than normal, it causes the closure of Yin. If both Renying and Cunkou pulses are over four degrees greater than normal, it will cause closure rejection, which is characterized by the exuberant Yin and Yang that cannot communicate with the essence Qi of the heavens and the earth, indicating death.

Chapter 10

Comprehensive Generation of Five Solid Viscera

Heart corresponds to the vessel, its luster is reflected on complexion and it is restrained by kidney. Lung corresponds to the skin, its luster is reflected on body hair and it is restrained by heart. Liver corresponds to the sinew, its luster is reflected on the nails and it is restrained by lung. Spleen corresponds to the muscle, its luster is reflected on the lips and it is restrained by liver. Kidney corresponds to the bone, its luster is reflected on the hair and it is restrained by spleen.

Hence, excessive intake of salty food will lead to vessel damping and complexion change; excessive intake of bitter food will lead to dry skin and body hair loss; excessive intake of pungent food will lead to sinew spasm and withering nails; excessive intake of sour food will lead to tough and shrinking muscle, and chapped lips; excessive intake of sweet food will lead to bone pain and hair loss; all the above are the damages caused by excessive intake of five flavors. So, heart has an affinity for the bitter, lung has an affinity for the pungent, liver has an affinity for the sour, spleen has an affinity for the sweet and kidney has an affinity for the salty; these are the respective correspondences between five flavors and five solid viscera.

The correspondences between five complexions and five solid viscera are as follows: If the complexion is as green as withered grass, as yellow as trifoliate orange fruit, as black as soot, as red as stagnated blood or as white as dry bone, they are all the signs of death. All these five complexions indicate approaching death. Accordingly, if the complexion is as green as the feather of kingfisher, as red as the cockscomb, as yellow as crab's abdomen, as white as lard or as black as crow's feather, they are all the signs of life, and all these five complexions indicate life. The color originating from the vital heart is like the cinnabar wrapped in thin white silk; the color originating from the vital lung is like the dark purple wrapped in thin white silk; the color originating from the vital liver is like the red wrapped in thin white silk; the color originating from the vital spleen is like the kirilowii seed wrapped in thin white silk; the color originating from the vital kidney is like the purple wrapped in thin white silk. All the above are the external lusters of the five solid viscera.

Five colors and five flavors correspond to five solid viscera, respectively: The white as well as the pungent correspond to lung; the red as well as the bitter correspond to heart; the green as well as the sour correspond to liver; the yellow as well as the sweet correspond to spleen; the black as well as the salty correspond to kidney. Thus, the white corresponds to the skin, the red corresponds to the vessel, the green corresponds to the sinews, the yellow corresponds to the muscle, and the black corresponds to the bone.

All the meridians belong to the eyes, all the marrow belong to the brain, all the sinews belong to the joint, all the blood belong to the heart, and all the Qi belong to the lung; all the Qi and blood in four limbs and eight joints are riding day and night.

So, when the body is sleeping, the blood flows into liver. Nourished by the blood, the eyes can see, the feet can walk, the palms can hold, and the fingers can take. Being attacked by wind evil outdoor immediately after sleeping will lead to blood stagnation; the blood stagnation in the skin will lead to impediment syndrome; the blood stagnation in vessels will lead to damping; the blood stagnation in feet will lead to reversal syndrome; all these three conditions are caused by the blood failing to flow in and out through acupoints, which leads to the impediment and reversal syndromes. In the human body, there are twelve major joints, and three hundred and fifty-four acupoints (enthesis), excluding twelve back transport (Shu) acupoints. These are all the places where defensive Qi lingers and evil Qi often invades. Stone needling these acupoints can dispel these evils.

At the beginning of the diagnosis of disease, the five formulas should be taken as principle. In order to know the cause of a disease, the viscera involved have to be identified. The so-called five-formula principle helps in differentiating the five pulse conditions.

Therefore, headache and other vertex diseases are associated with deficiency in the lower region and excess in the upper region, where the disorder rests in the foot-Shaoyin and foot-Taiyang meridians, and severe diseases will be transmitted internally to the kidney. Vertigo with head shaking, blurred vision or deafness are associated with excess in the lower region and deficiency in the upper region, where the disorder rests in the foot-Shaoyang and foot-Jueyin meridians, and severe diseases will be transmitted internally to the liver. Abdominal fullness and distension, sticking feeing in diaphragm, armpit and hypochondria are associated with Qi reversal in the lower region and dizziness in the upper region, where the disorder rests in the foot-Taiyin and foot-Yangming meridians. Cough and ascending Qi are associated with Qi reversal in the chest, where the disorder rests in the hand-Yangming and hand-Taiyin meridians. Dysphoria and headache are associated with the illness in the diaphragm, where the disorder rests in the hand-Taiyang and hand-Shaoyin meridians.

The small, large, slippery, unsmooth, floating and sunken pulses can be differentiated by the doctor's fingers. The manifestations of five solid viscera can be inferred by analogy. The five scales corresponding to five solid viscera can be sensed by doctor's perceptions. The subtle changes in five complexions can be inspected by doctor's eyes. If the pulse conditions are integrated with the complexions, the diagnosis will be perfect. The pulse resulting with red complexion appears to be rapid and firm, indicating evil Qi accumulating in the middle region with frequent interference in digestion, which is termed heart impediment. It is usually contracted by the invasion of external evil as a result of heart Qi deficiency due to excessive thinking. The pulse resulting with white complexion appears to be panting and floating, reflecting upper deficiency and lower excess as well as frequent fright, indicating evil Qi accumulating in the chest with panting and lung deficiency, which is termed lung impediment. There will be chill and fever triggered by sex indulgence after being drunk. The pulse resulting with green complexion appears to be long and flickering on the left and the right, indicating evil Qi accumulating below the heart propping the armpits, which is termed liver impediment and is usually caused by the invasion of cold-damp. It shares the same mechanism with hernia, including lumbago, cold feet and headache. The pulse resulting with the yellow complexion appears to be large and weak, indicating Qi accumulating in the abdomen, termed reversal hernia if there is Qi reversal. It is usually caused by the invasion of wind evil when limbs are sweating due to strenuous movement. It is also seen in women. The pulse resulting with the black complexion appears to be firm and large, indicating evil Qi accumulating in the lower abdomen and the external genitalia, which is termed kidney impediment and is usually caused by a common cold caught while sleeping after a cold bath.

While the five complexions not resulting with the due pulse are inspected, if yellow complexion appears with blue eyes, with red eyes, with white eyes or with black eyes, none of these are the signs of death. If blue complexion appears with red eyes, red complexion appears with white eyes, blue complexion appears with black eyes, black complexion appears with white eyes or red complexion appears with blue eyes, all of these are the signs of death.

Chapter 11

Additional Theory on Five Solid Viscera

Yellow Emperor: I have heard that some alchemists take brain and marrow as solid viscera and some others take intestines and stomach as solid viscera, while some even take all of them as hollow viscera. If questioned with contrary opinions, they all insist that their own views are correct. I don't know which one is correct and I'd like to know your explanation.

Qibo: The six organs, brain, marrow, bones, vessels, gallbladder and womb, are all developed with earthly Qi, and all contain Yin inside just like the earth, and are for storage but not discharge and are termed extraordinary hollow viscera. The five organs, stomach, large intestine, small intestine, triple-Jiao and bladder, are developed with the heavenly Qi and their Qi is like the heavens, which are for discharge but not storage. They receive turbid Qi passed from five solid viscera and are termed the house of transportation and transformation, which cannot be retained for long and have to be discharged properly. The anus also functions as discharging organ for five solid viscera, and then water and grain cannot be retained for long. The so-called five solid viscera have the function of storing essence Qi but not discharge, which can be in full but not in replete status. The so-called six hollow viscera have the function of transportation and transformation but not storage, which can be in replete but not permanently full status. The reason is that, after water and grain are taken into the mouth, stomach will be replete, while intestine is then empty, and in turn, when the food enters intestine, intestine will be replete while stomach is then empty. It's believed that six hollow viscera are characterized by repletion but not fullness while five solid viscera are characterized by fullness but not repletion.

Emperor: Why can Qikou alone reflect the conditions of five solid viscera?
Qibo: Stomach is the sea of water and grain and the great source of six hollow viscera. After being taken into the mouth, five flavors are received in stomach and digested into Qi to nourish five solid viscera, and therefore Qikou pulse also corresponds to Taiyin meridian. Hence, all Qi and flavors of five solid and six hollow viscera come from stomach, whose variations can be reflected in Qikou. Thus, the five odors are taken in through the nose and received into lung, and when there is a morbid change in heart or lung, the nose must be obstructed. While treating any diseases, the general conditions should be carefully observed, pulses should be palpated properly, and the emotional and mental statuses should be inspected in order to ensure the cure of the disease.

For those patients believing in ghosts and superstitions, it's futile to tell them about the medical theories. For those patients disliking acupuncture and stone therapy, it's futile to tell them about the technical skills. For those patients reluctant to be treated, it's futile to treat their disease, as otherwise it will be in vain.

Chapter 12

Proper Therapies for Different Diseases Geographically

Yellow Emperor: In treatment, different doctors use different therapies for the same disease, which can be cured anyhow. Why is this so?
Qibo: It is just associated with different geographical environments. The east region, where Qi of the heavens and the earth grows, teems with salt and fish, and is adjacent to seashores and ocean. The local people are accustomed to eating fish and salty food, and live in peace there. They enjoy fish food, which tends to facilitate heat accumulation in the body. Since the salt tends to dominate in blood, the local people look dark in skin and loose in muscle, and also tend to suffer from carbuncles and ulceration, which are suitable to be treated by stone needles. So, the therapy with stone needles comes from the east.

The west region teems with metals and jades, and there is sand and stone everywhere, where the creatures between the heavens and the earth contract. The local people live in the windy hills with hard water and soil, pay less attention to garments with rough clothes, and sleep on straws, and are accustomed to eating plenty of fat food. Thus, the evil cannot damage their physique, and they tend to suffer from diseases in the interior, which are suitable to be treated with drugs. So, the drug therapy comes from the west.

The north is the region where the heavens and the earth are closed and all things are stored; there are high mountains, where people live in sweep of cold wind and icy sleets. The local people are accustomed to wild nomadic life and drinking milk, so they tend to accumulate cold inside and suffer from diseases with interior distension, which are suitable to be treated by moxibustion and roasting. So, the moxibustion therapy comes from the north.

The south is the region where everything between the heavens and the earth develop and flourish, and Yang Qi is exuberant; it's characterized by low altitude, soft water and soil, as well as fog and dew gathering. The local people are accustomed to eating sour food and fermented bean curd, so they look fine and reddish in skin, and tend to suffer from diseases with spasm and arthralgia, which are suitable to be treated with fine needles. So, the therapy with nine kinds of needles comes from the south.

The center, with plain land and moist air, is the region where all creatures are living. The local people are accustomed to eating miscellaneous food and living an easy life, and tend to suffer from the diseases of flaccidity, Qi reversal, chill and fever, which are suitable to be treated with limb exercises and Chinese massage. So, the therapies of limb exercise and Chinese massage come from the center.

Therefore, the sages can integrate the comprehensive methods to treat similar diseases. The reason why the similar diseases with different manifestations can be cured is that they can obtain complete information and catch the general principle.

Chapter 13

Transferring Essence and Changing Qi

Yellow Emperor: I have heard that in ancient times the treatments for diseases were only for transferring the essence and changing Qi, which can be completed by the witch doctor. Nowadays, drugs are used to treat the internal diseases, and stone needles and acupuncture are used to treat the external diseases, some of which are cured but some are not. Why is this so?
Qibo: The people in remote antiquity lived with the birds and beasts, protected themselves from cold through physical movement and stayed in the shade to avoid summer heat. They were free from any avaricious burden inward and from the struggle for fame and gain outward. Evil cannot invade deeply into people living such a peaceful and quiet life. Thus, neither drugs can be used to treat internal diseases nor can stone needles and acupuncture be used to treat external diseases, but diseases can be cured simply through the transfer of the spirit and severing of the source by the witch doctor. Nowadays, the world is so different that people are not only internally affected by anxiety and suffering, and externally injured by toil and moil, but also affected by the reversal of the changes in four

seasons. Moreover, theft wind frequently attacks and the deficient evil arrives day and night, which internally invade the five solid viscera as well as the bone and marrow, and externally hurt the orifices, skin and muscle. As a result, minor illness will certainly become worse and serious illness will definitely lead to death, which is far beyond the witch doctor's ability to treat and cure.

Emperor: Good! While approaching a patient, I want to predict life or death, and solve the refractory and complicated issues, for which the keys have to be mastered clearly as sunshine or moonlight. Shall I know about them?
Qibo: The examination of complexion and pulse is the key that the Supreme God cherishes and is handed down from ancient teachers. In ancient times, Doctor Jiu Daiji was ordered to study complexion and pulse to communicate with the deity and integrate them with metal, wood, water, fire and earth, eight winds and six directions. Through never deviating from the regular principles and noticing the dynamic variations, one can observe the mystery and catch the key; in order to catch the key, one must observe nothing but complexion and pulse conditions. The variations in complexion correspond to the sun and the variations in pulse correspond to the moon. It is just the key for the practice to master the essentials. The variations in complexion correspond to the changes in pulse in four seasons, which the Supreme God cherishes and is in conformity with the Deity. In this way, one can help patients survive and keep death away. Those who can make patients live a long life in this way are called the Great Sages. In the middle ancient times, treatment is given as soon as the disease occurs. If rice juice is given for ten days, eight winds and five impediments

will be removed. If not, herbal leaves and roots will be applied, and through the treatment with priority for root and branch, evil Qi can be eliminated. However, the later generations of doctors treat diseases in an irrational way. Those doctors aren't able to follow the variations of four seasons to understand the corresponding relationship between the sun and the moon and to judge the reversal and compliance of complexion and pulse. As a result, only when diseases have already been formed do they begin to use small needles for external illness and rice juice for internal illness. The unqualified doctor flatters himself on offensive therapy, but unexpectedly a new disease occurs while the old one hasn't been cured.

Emperor: I'd like to know the essentials.
Qibo: The crucial thing to treat the disease is not to misjudge complexion and pulse; applying them correctly is the leading principle for the treatment. If the reversal or compliance of disease cannot be distinguished, and the syndromes of the branch or the root cannot be balanced, it will result in loss of spirit when treating a patient, similar to the destruction of a country when governing it. So, only by bringing forth the new from the old can a doctor reach the level of the Immortals.

Emperor: I have heard the essentials from you, and you emphasized the significance of complexion and pulse, which I've already known.
Qibo: All treatment can be summed up into one key.

Emperor: What is meant by "one key"?
Qibo: It refers to the diagnosis based on inquiry.

Emperor: How to inquire?

Qibo: Closing the doors and windows, and communicating with the patients, you carefully inquire about their sufferings while expecting the desire of patients. Keeping spirit means life while losing spirit means death.

Emperor: Good.

Chapter 14

Thin and Thick Medical Wine

Yellow Emperor: How can one make thin and thick medical wine with five grains?
Qibo: Rice should be used as material and rice straw as fuel just because rice has the perfect essence and rice straw is tough enough to make a fire.

Emperor: Why is it so?
Qibo: The rice grows in the harmonization of the heavens and the earth and in proper altitude, so it can obtain the perfect Qi. When harvested in autumn, the rice stalk is extremely firm.

Emperor: In remote ancient times, though, the sages prepared thin and thick medical wine, why didn't they use them medically?
Qibo: In remote ancient times, the sages prepared thin and thick medical wine only for contingency, and thus, they could prepare these medications, but these were not for routine medication. Till the middle ancient times, social morality and health status had declined gradually, and though the evil Qi was attacking frequently, the disease can be cured by taking the medical wine.

Emperor: Why can't the patients get rid of their diseases with the medication at the present time?
Qibo: At the present time, people have to use many drugs to treat internal diseases and sharp stone needles, acupuncture and moxibustion to treat external diseases.

Emperor: Why are these medications ineffective when the body is withered and blood is exhausted?
Qibo: It is just because of the spirit failure.

Emperor: What is meant by "spirit failure"?
Qibo: The stone acupuncture is associated with this principle. For anyone without spirit endowment or mind regulation, the disease is difficult to be cured. Today, the patient's essence is damaged and his spirit is separated, so nutrition Qi and defense Qi can no longer recover. Why? It is because of the excessive indulgence and endless anxiety about suffering that leads to the dysfunction of essence Qi, damping of the nutrition Qi and diminishing of the defense Qi. Spirit is separated and then the disease cannot be cured.

Emperor: So, the onset of the disease is insidious and subtle, and the evil enters and lingers in the skin. Today, all the good doctors hold the view that the disease having formed is referred to as the reversal, for which neither acupuncture nor good medicine is effective. Though now all good doctors know the principle and follow the methods in treatment, the close kin or the distant relatives look after the patient and the patient's voice and complexion can be inspected at any time, the disease still cannot be cured. How can it be said that the disease wasn't treated as early as possible?
Qibo: The patient is root while the physician is branch. If the patient and the physician cannot cooperate with each other, the

evil Qi is impossible to be eliminated. This provides the information concerned.

Emperor: Some diseases don't arise from the skin and hair but from Qi exhaustion of five solid viscera. Thus, body fluid floods over the surface, Yin-soul exists alone, essence is isolated internally, and Qi is exhausted externally, so that the clothes don't fit the body. There is urgent swelling of the four extremities because it affects middle Qi that is repelled from inside and body bulges outside. How can this be treated?
Qibo: In order to give the comprehensive treatment and to remove stale water and waste material, the patient should be instructed to move his extremities moderately, wear warm clothes, and receive contralateral needling on the focus, by which the original physique can be restored. Five Yang can be distributed to clear five solid viscera by opening the ghost gate, cleaning the bladder and administration at the proper time. Thus, naturally, the essence Qi is produced, the physique becomes strong spontaneously, the bones and muscles collaborate with each other and the great Qi is then normalized.

Emperor: Good.

Chapter 15

Fundamental Theory Inscribed in Jade

Yellow Emperor: I have heard of the classics of *The Measurement and Judgment* and *The Extraordinary and Ordinary Diseases*, which are different in content. How can one apply them?

Qibo: *The Measurement and Judgment* focuses on how to judge the different severities of the diseases. *The Extraordinary and Ordinary Diseases* focuses on how to state the uncommon disorders. Please allow me to introduce the extreme law. Though the variations in *Five complexions* and *Five pulses*, described in *The Measurement and Judgment* and *The Extraordinary and Ordinary Diseases,* are different in content, their fundamentals share the same oneness. The spirit of human body moves with no reversal, and if there is spirit reversal, there is no movement of spirit and then the human body will lose its vitality. The key of extreme law is very important in that the feasible examination can disclose the subtle changes in the spirit movement, which is carved in jade and referred to as *Jade Confidential*.

The variation in complexion manifests in the upper or lower region as well the left or right region, which can indicate the corresponding disease, respectively. If the ill complexion is seen as the shallow one, thin medical wine should be mainly used to treat the disease, which can be cured in ten days. If the ill complexion is seen as the deep one, the drug concerned should be mainly used to treat the disease, which can be cured in twenty one days. If the ill complexion is seen as the deepest one, the thick medical wine should be mainly used to treat the disease, which can be cured in one hundred days. The withered complexion and macerated face indicate that the disease is incurable, and the patient will die in one hundred days. The short pulse and the depleted Yang Qi indicate the death syndrome, so does the warm disease with severe deficient Qi.

The shift in complexion manifests in the upper or lower as well as the left or right region, which should be inspected for the corresponding disease, respectively. The complexion shifting from the lower to the upper region is regarded as reversal and conversely, the complexion shifting from the upper to the lower region is regarded as the compliance. For female, the ill complexion on the right indicates reversal and the ill complexion on the left indicates compliance. For male, the ill complexion on the left indicates reversal and the ill complexion on the right indicates compliance. Additionally, the double Yang indicates death for male, while the double Yin indicates death for female. If Yin or Yang manifests oppositely, the conditions should be comprehended for balance, and it is high time *The Measurement and Judgment* and *The Extraordinary and Ordinary Diseases* should be applied.

The surging pulse with impeded limbs indicates that both cold and heat evils have invaded the body. The sole pulse indicates exhaustion of primordial Qi while deficient pulse with diarrhea indicates the depletion of blood. The sole pulse indicates reversal while feeble pulse indicates compliance. Application of *The Extraordinary and Ordinary Diseases* should start from the Cunkou on Taiyin meridian. The pulse beats in undominating condition, which is called as reversal dominance and indicates death. The pulse beats in dominating condition, which is called as compliance and indicates survival. The dominance of eight winds and four seasons goes around and again, and if there is a reversal abnormality, the norm cannot be applied in the same way, which is beyond the fundamental principles of the two above-mentioned books.

Chapter 16

Diagnostic Essentials and Manifestations of Twelve-Meridian Exhaustion

Yellow Emperor: What are the essentials of diagnosis?
Qibo: In the first and second lunar months, heavenly Qi is about to spread, earthly Qi begins to emerge and human Qi becomes active in liver. In the third and fourth lunar months, heavenly Qi spreads, earthly Qi rises and human Qi becomes active in the spleen. In the fifth and sixth lunar months, heavenly Qi is in exuberance, earthly Qi rises high and human Qi becomes active in the head. In the seventh and eighth lunar months, Yin Qi begins to conquer and human Qi becomes active in lung. In the ninth and tenth lunar months, Yin Qi begins to freeze, earthly Qi begins to close and human Qi becomes active in heart. In the eleventh and twelfth lunar months, the ice covers the land, earthly Qi begins to be sealed and human Qi becomes active in kidney.

So, in spring, the acupoints on meridians are needled to reach the inter-muscle till bleeding; the needle isn't withdrawn till Qi is transmitted for the severe case or while Qi at acupoint is around acupoint for the moderate case. In summer, the acupoints on collaterals are needled till bleeding. After the evil Qi is dispelled and the pinhole is blocked for a Qi circus, the pain will be relieved. In autumn, the skin is needled along the interstitial striaes and the same manipulation can be applied for both the upper and lower regions. The acupuncture has to be stopped as soon as the complexion is changed. In winter, the acupoints are needled deep into the inter-muscle. For the severe case, the direct manipulation is applied and for the moderate case, the four-direction manipulation is applied. There are different manipulations for spring, summer, autumn and winter seasons according to the different foci. In spring, wrong needling of the acupoints corresponding to summer will cause pulse disturbance with faint Qi and evil Qi invading deep into bone marrow, so the disease cannot be cured, which makes the patient lose appetite with less Qi. In spring, wrong needling of the acupoints corresponding to autumn will cause sinew spasm and cough induced by reversing Qi circulation in lung, so the disease cannot be cured, which makes the patient get frightened frequently and cry. In spring, wrong needling of the acupoints corresponding to winter will cause evil Qi hiding in viscera with distension, so the disease cannot be cured, which makes the patient talk excessively.

In summer, wrongly needling the acupoints corresponding to spring will cause the disease not to be cured, which makes the patient weary. In summer, wrongly needling the acupoints corresponding to autumn will cause the disease not to be cured, which makes the patient have no desire to speak and feel scared as if one is going to be arrested. In summer, wrongly needling the acupoints corresponding to winter will cause the disease not to be cured, which makes the patient have less Qi and get frequently angry.

In autumn, wrongly needling the acupoints corresponding to spring will cause the disease not to be cured, which makes the patient feel restless to do something but forget it when rising. In autumn, wrongly needling the acupoints corresponding to summer will cause the disease not to be cured, which makes the patient feel somnolent and dream frequently. In autumn, wrongly needling the acupoints corresponding to winter will cause the disease not to be cured, which makes the patient feel chilly continuously.

In winter, wrongly needling the acupoints corresponding to spring will cause the disease not to be cured, which makes the patient fail to fall asleep or dream of something even during sleeping. In winter, wrongly needling the acupoints corresponding to summer will cause the disease not to be cured, which makes the patient have Qi ascending and then triggers various impediment syndromes. In winter, wrongly needling the acupoints corresponding to autumn will cause the disease not to be cured, which makes the patient feel thirsty frequently.

While pricking over the chest and abdomen, five solid viscera proper should be avoided. The patients with heart punctured will die instantly; those with spleen punctured will die in five days; those with kidney punctured will die in seven days; those with lung punctured will die in five days; those with diaphragm punctured will have nothing but internal injuries, and even though the injuries are healed, the patient shall die in one year. In order to avoid needling five solid viscera, one should know the concepts of 'complying and reversing'. The so-called 'complying' means clarifying the respective positions of diaphragm, spleen and kidney, and otherwise, it's called 'reversing'. When needling the chest and abdomen, one should use a cloth to cover them and then prick through the cloth; if not cured, needle again. While needling, one should keep a concentrated manner. While needling the swelling, the needles should be shaken, and while needling the meridians, needles should not be shaken, which is the rule of acupuncture.

Emperor: I'd like to know what the Qi exhaustion of twelve meridians means?
Qibo: The Qi exhaustion of Taiyang meridian is characterized by fixed glassy eyes, opisthotonus, convulsion, pale complexion and expiry sweating. If the patient develops expiry sweating, it indicates the approaching death. The Qi exhaustion of Shaoyang is characterized by deafness, flaccidity of all the joints, and the patient will open eyes wide with lost Qi; if the eyes lose Qi, the patient will die in one and a half days; the complexion appears greenish and then turns white while the patient is dying. The Qi exhaustion of Yangming is characterized by twisted mouth and eyes, frequent fear, confused speech, and sallow complexion. When both the upper and lower meridians are exuberant, the patient will develop general numbness, indicating the approaching death. The Qi exhaustion of Shaoyin is characterized by black, long and dirty teeth, and abdominal distention and blockage; no communication between the upper and the lower indicates approaching death. The Qi exhaustion of Taiyin is characterized by abdominal distension with difficult breathing, frequent sighing and vomiting. Qi reversal will develop after vomiting and red complexion will develop after Qi reversal. If there is no communication between the upper and lower Qi with no reversal, black complexion and withered skin and hair will appear, indicating the approaching death. The Qi

exhaustion of Jueyin is characterized by heat in the middle, dry throat, frequent urination, heart vexation, even curled tongue and retracted testicles, indicating the approaching death. These are the statuses of the deterioration of twelve meridians.

Chapter 17

Diagnosis for Pulse-Taking and Pulse Subtlety

Yellow Emperor: What are the methods of pulse-taking?
Qibo: Pulse-taking is usually done at dawn, when Yin Qi hasn't been stirred, Yang Qi hasn't been dispersed, food hasn't been consumed, meridians haven't been hyper-activated with harmonized collaterals and Qi-blood hasn't been disturbed, so that the abnormal pulses can be detected.

While taking the dynamic and static pulses, eye essence and spirit should be inspected, five-complexion should be observed, and insufficiency or excess of five solid viscera, the strength or the weakness of the hollow viscera and the exuberance or decline of physique should be analyzed, by which all these factors are integrated in order to predict death or survival.

The vessel is the house of blood. The long pulse indicates Qi harmonization, the short pulse indicates Qi disorder, the rapid pulse indicates heart irritation, the large pulse indicates the progress of disease, the upper exuberant pulse indicates Qi ascending, the lower exuberant pulse indicates Qi distension, the regularly intermittent pulse indicates Qi decline, the thin pulse indicates Qi insufficiency and the unsmooth pulse indicates heart pain. The strong and acute pulse like gushing spring indicates a worsening disease with deteriorated complexion, and the faint pulse like a breaking string indicates dying.

The essence and spirit of eyes and five-complexion indicate the bloom of Qi. The reddish color should appear like cinnabar wrapped in white silk instead of like ochre. The white color should appear like goose feathers instead of like salt. The green color should appear like jade luster instead of like pure blue. The yellow color should appear like realgar wrapped in gauze instead of like loess. The black color should appear like lacquer instead of like charcoal. If the critical essence of five-complexion is seen, then life will not exist for long. The spiritual vigor of eyes functions to see all the things, to distinguish the white from the black, and to differentiate the short from the long. If one takes long as short, or white as black, the spiritual vigor of eyes has already declined.

Five solid viscera guarantee the essence Qi in the middle. If the middle is exuberant and five solid viscera are full, Qi dominance will damage kidney with fright and the low and harsh voice as if speaking in an empty room, all of which are caused by damp Qi in the middle. Faint voice and repeating the words all day long indicate the depletion of Qi. Shamelessly wearing no clothing, obsessive or uncontrollable speech and failure to distinguish close or distant relatives, indicate disturbance of the mental spirit. Stomach and spleen fail to store water and grain because the anus fails to control. Urinary incontinence is seen because bladder fails to store water. Guaranteeing visceral Qi means life, while losing visceral Qi means death.

Five solid viscera are the basis of a strong and healthy body. The head is the house of spiritual vigor, so drooped head and sunken eyes with dim eyesight indicate that the spirit is about to be depleted. The back is the house of the chest, so when curved back with drooping shoulders appears, it indicates that chest Qi is about to deteriorate. The waist is the house of kidney, so when the waist cannot turn around, it indicates that kidney Qi is about to be exhausted. The knees are the house of sinews, so when they cannot flex or extend and walk with humpback, it indicates that sinews are about to be exhausted. The bones are the house of marrow, so when one cannot stand for long or shakes while walking, it indicates that the bones are about to be exhausted. Therefore, obtaining the vital Qi means the life while losing it means the death.

Qibo: If pulse Qi reverses four seasons, the excess is referred to as aggression while the insufficiency is referred to as consumption. If the correspondence is excessive, its insufficiency is referred to as aggression, while if the correspondence is insufficient, its excess is referred to as consumption. Then if Yin and Yang cannot match each other, its resultant disease is called closure-rejection.

Emperor: How does the pulse vary with four seasons? How does one know the location of the disease? How does one know the variance of the disease? How does one know the sudden development of the disease internally? How does one know the sudden development of disease externally? I ask these five questions; shall I know their answers?

Qibo: Please allow me to explain the relationship between the variance of pulse and the grand movement in the heavens. In the surroundings of all creatures and within the six directions, the changes of the heavens and the earth correspond to the alteration of Yin–Yang. The warmth in spring turns into heat in summer, and similarly the cooling anxiety in autumn turns into cold rage in winter. Correspondingly, the dynamic changes of four seasons correspond to ups and downs of pulses. Thus, stringy pulse in spring is like a compass, full in summer like a ruler, floats in autumn like a scale and deep in winter like weight. Hence, during forty-five days from winter solstice, Yang is slightly ascending while Yin is slightly descending; during forty-five days from summer solstice, Yin is slightly ascending while Yang is slightly descending. The variance of Yin–Yang occurs in a regular time, to which the pulse condition should correspond. If the pulse condition cannot correspond to the due time, the focus of the disease can be detected and the course of the disease can be phased so that the date of death can be predicted. The subtle variation lies in the pulse, the detection of which should not be missed; this detection has its fundamentals which start from Yin and Yang as well as its principles of differentiation, while it can begin with the five elements as well as the rules of the generation and restriction. The detection is better when it is closely associated with the changes of four seasons and then in treatment, the supplement and purgation cannot lose their balance, just unified by the heaven–earth; thus, by integrating general information, life or death can be predicted. Therefore, the five sounds correspond to the five tones, the five colors to the five elements, and the pulse conditions to Yin and Yang.

Thus, the exuberance of Yin would lead to a dream of fright during wading across a river, while the exuberance of Yang would lead to a dream of being burnt in fire and exuberance of both Yin and Yang would lead to a dream of slaughtering each other; exuberance in the upper would lead to a dream of flying up while exuberance in the lower would lead to a dream of falling down; excessive fullness would lead to a dream of donating while excessive hunger would lead to a dream of reception; exuberant liver Qi would lead to a dream of getting angry while exuberant lung Qi would lead to a dream of crying; infestation with short worms would lead to a dream of gathering together while that with long worms would lead to a dream of fighting and injuring.

So, pulse-taking has its fundamentals and being quiet and peaceful guarantee the correct diagnosis. In spring, the pulse is felt floating like fish swimming upon a wave; in summer, the pulse is felt on the skin like all living things thriving; in autumn, the pulse is felt beneath the skin like the insects going into hibernation; and, in winter, the pulse is felt near the bone like insects in hibernation or people staying in the inner chamber. It's believed that to know the internal lies on the pulse condition concerned under pressure, while to know the external lies on the complete circus of meridians. These six points are the chief principles for pulse-taking.

When heart pulse is forceful, firm and long, it is associated with curled tongue and inability to speak; when it is soft and scattered, it is associated with consumptive disease which can recover spontaneously after Qi is restored. When lung pulse is forceful, firm and long, it is associated with disease having bloody sputum; when it is soft and loose, it is associated with disease having streaming sweating and shouldn't be treated by dispersing therapy. When liver pulse is forceful, firm and long with no greenish complexion, it is associated with fall with traumatic injury, leading to reversal panting due to blood stagnation under the hypochondria; when it is soft and scattered with lustrous complexion, it is associated with generalized edema due to excessive thirst and over drinking water that tends to overflow into the skin and muscles as well as outside the intestines and stomach. When stomach pulse is forceful, firm and long with reddish complexion, it is associated with breaking pain of thigh; when it is soft and scattered, it is associated with dyspepsia. When spleen pulse is forceful, firm and long with sallow complexion, it is associated with disease of less Qi; when it is soft and scattered with no lustrous complexion, it is associated with edema of shank as if being in water. When kidney pulse is forceful, firm and long with yellowish-reddish complexion, it is associated with the disease having breaking pain of the waist; when it is soft and scattered, it is associated with the disease having insufficient blood from which it is difficult to recover.

Emperor: If acute heart pulse is detected, what is the disease and what is the manifestation?
Qibo: The disease is termed heart hernia, in which there is a lump in the lower abdomen.

Emperor: What is the reason?
Qibo: Heart is Yang viscus while small intestine is its envoy, so the lower abdomen can have the lump.

Emperor: If stomach pulse is detected, what is the manifestation?
Qibo: Excessive stomach pulse indicates distension while deficiency indicates diarrhea.

Emperor: After the disease is formed, what are the changes of the disease?
Qibo: Wind can turn into cold-fever, fire-heat can turn into consumptive disease in the middle, reversal can turn into

vertex diseases, chronic wind can turn into diarrhea after indigestion, meridian wind can turn into leprosy; the variance of the diseases are beyond counting.

Emperor: As to all carbuncles, swelling, sinew spasm and bone pain, how do they develop?
Qibo: It's the accumulative swelling due to cold Qi and changes of eight-wind.

Emperor: How to treat them?
Qibo: These are the diseases caused by the partially dominating Qi in four seasons, which can be cured by applying the principle of sequential domination among five elements.

Emperor: The old disease triggered by evil from five solid viscera will damage the pulse and complexion, but how to know if the disease is old or new?
Qibo: What a detailed question! As a rule, findings of small pulse with unaltered complexion indicate a new disease, findings of unaltered pulse with altered complexion indicate the old disease, findings of altered pulse and complexion indicate the old disease, and findings of unaltered pulse and complexion indicate a new disease. When stringy liver-pulse and sunken kidney-pulse come together with dark green and reddish complexion, it is associated with traumatic injury without bleeding or if stringy liver-pulse and sunken kidney-pulse come together with bleeding, there will be dampness as if being in water.

Internal sides of the forearm-skin are examined to detect the conditions of hypochondria, the internal sides are examined to detect kidney and the middle sides are examined to detect abdomen. On the middle portion of the forearm-skin, the external side on the left forearm-skin is examined to detect liver and the internal side is examined to detect diaphragm; the external side on the right forearm-skin is examined to detect stomach and the internal side is examined to detect spleen. Toward the upper forearm gradually, the external side on the right forearm is examined to detect lung and the internal side is examined to detect the chest, while the external side on the left forearm is examined to detect heart and the internal side is examined to detect pericardium. Examination of the ventral region helps to detect chest and abdomen and that of the dorsal region to detect the back. The top on the upper portion is associated with the attacked conditions of the chest and throat, while the bottom of the lower portion is associated with the attacked conditions of lower abdomen, loin, thigh, knee, shank and foot.

The rough and large pulse indicates Yin insufficiency and Yang excess, leading to the internal heat diseases. The pulse coming rapidly and going slowly is associated with upper excess and lower deficiency, indicating reversal vertex disease. The pulse coming slowly and going rapidly is associated with the upper deficiency and lower excess, indicating evil wind. So, the disease attacked by evil wind is associated with Yang Qi attacked. The sunken, thin and rapid pulse indicates the reversal of Shaoyin. The sunken, thready, rapid and scattered pulse indicates chill and fever. The floating and scattered pulse indicates tumble due to vertigo. Floating and non-agitated pulses indicate diseases in three Yang meridians of the foot, leading to heat disease, while floating and rapid pulses indicate those of hand. Thin and sunken pulses indicate diseases in three Yin meridians of the hand, leading to bone pain, while thin, sunken and quiet pulses indicate those of the foot. Pulse with several beatings plus one intermittence indicates the disease in Yang meridians, leading to diarrhea with blood and pus. The abnormal conditions can be detected by pulse-taking in that unsmooth pulse indicates excess of Yang Qi, while slippery pulse indicates excess of Yin Qi. Excess of Yang Qi leads to fever with no sweating, while excess of Yin leads to profuse sweating and chill, and excess of both Yin and Yang leads to chill without sweating. By pressing exteriorly, the internal but no external conditions of the pulse can be felt, indicating the accumulative disease in heart and abdomen. By pressing interiorly, the external but not internal conditions of the pulse can be felt, indicating the heat inside the body. By pressing superiorly, the superior but not inferior conditions of the pulse can be felt, indicating the cold sensation in the waist and feet. By pressing inferiorly, the inferior but not superior conditions of the pulse can be felt, indicating the pain in the head and nape. When the pulse is felt heavily by touching the bone, it indicates insufficient Qi along with pain in the waist and spine as well as impediment in the body.

Chapter 18

Pulse-Qi Conditions of Healthy Person

Yellow Emperor: What is the pulse condition of a healthy person?

Qibo: The pulse beats twice within an exhalation and also twice within an inhalation; sometimes, the pulse beats the fifth time due to the longer interval between two respirations; this is the pulse condition of a healthy person. A healthy person is the one who has no illness. Usually, the healthy person's respiration is used to measure the patient's pulse. If a doctor is not ill, his resting respiration is also used to measure the patient's pulse, which is the rule concerned. If a person's pulse beats only once within an exhalation and also once within an inhalation, it indicates Qi insufficiency. If the pulse beats three times within an exhalation and also three times within an inhalation with agitated sense and with feverish sense on medial forearm skin, it indicates warm disease; if the pulse beats with no feverish sense on medial forearm but with slippery pulse, it indicates wind disease, and if it is unsmooth pulse, it indicates impediment syndrome. The pulse that beats over four times in an exhalation indicates death, the pulse that fails to come due to pulse Qi exhaustion indicates death, and the pulse that beats suddenly slow and suddenly rapid indicates death.

A healthy person obtains healthy pulse Qi from stomach, which is the normal Qi for a healthy person; if a person loses his stomach Qi, it is termed reversal sign, which indicates death.

In spring, the pulse with stomach Qi and slight stringy sense is normal, the pulse with more stringy sense and less stomach Qi indicates liver diseases, the pulse with only stringy sense and no stomach Qi indicates death, the pulse with stomach Qi and furry sense indicates diseases in autumn and the pulse with more furry sense indicates the current diseases. The visceral genuine Qi is distributed in liver and liver stores Qi for sinews and fascia. In summer, the pulse with stomach Qi but slight hooked sense is called a normal pulse, the pulse with more hooked sense and less stomach Qi indicates heart disease, the pulse with only hooked sense but no stomach Qi indicates death, the pulse with stomach Qi but stony sense indicates diseases in winter, and the pulse with an obviously stony sense indicates the current diseases. The visceral genuine Qi communicates to heart, and heart stores Qi for blood and vessels. In late summer, the slightly weak pulse with stomach Qi is normal, the obviously weak pulse with less stomach Qi indicates spleen disease, the only regular intermittent pulse with no stomach Qi indicates death, the soft and weak pulse with stony sense indicates diseases in winter and the obviously weak pulse indicates current diseases. The visceral genuine Qi nourishes spleen, and spleen stores Qi for muscles. In autumn, the pulse with stomach Qi and slight furry sense is normal, the pulse with more furry sense and less stomach Qi indicates lung disease, the pulse with only furry sense but no stomach Qi indicates death, the furry pulse with stringy sense indicates diseases in spring, and obviously stringy pulse indicates the current diseases. The visceral genuine Qi returns up to lung, which moves nutrition and defense Qi of Yin–Yang. In winter, the pulse with stomach Qi and slightly stony sense is normal; the pulse with more stony sense and less stomach Qi indicates kidney disease, the pulse with only stony sense but no stomach Qi indicates death, the pulse with stony and hooky senses indicates diseases in summer, and the obviously hooky pulse indicates current diseases. The visceral genuine Qi descends down to kidney, and kidney stores Qi for bones and marrow.

The large collateral of stomach is called Xuli (apex-beat), which passes through the diaphragm connecting the lung and turning out below the left breast, whose pulsation together with clothes can be inspected as the manifestation of pectoral Qi. If Xuli has rapid surging pulse with short pauses, it indicates the disease in the middle; tensed and transverse pulse indicates the accumulation; failure of the pulse to come due to exhaustion indicates death. Obvious pulsation under the breast together with the clothes is inspected, which indicates the leakage of pectoral Qi.

The excess and insufficiency of Cunkou pulse should be differentiated; when Cunkou pulse touching fingers appears short, it indicates headache. If Cunkou pulse touching fingers appears long, it indicates the pain in the foot and shank. If Cunkou pulse touching fingers appears short and surging up, it indicates the pain of shoulders and back. If Cunkou pulse appears sunken and firm, it indicates disease in the internal. If Cunkou pulse appears floating and surging, it indicates disease in the external. If Cunkou pulse appears sunken and weak, it indicates chill-fever and painful lump, and pain in the lower abdomen. If Cunkou pulse appears sunken and transverse, it indicates accumulation under hypochondria and transversely accumulative pain in abdomen. If Cunkou pulse appears sunken and rapid, it indicates chill-fever. If Cunkou pulse appears exuberant, slippery and firm, it indicates the disease in the external. If Cunkou pulse appears small, solid and firm, it indicates disease in the internal. If the pulse appears small, weak and unsmooth, it indicates the chronic diseases. If the pulse appears slippery, floating and swift, it indicates a new disease. The acute pulse indicates painful lump and pain in the lower abdomen. The slippery pulse indicates wind disease. The unsmooth pulse indicates impediment. The slow and slippery pulse indicates heat in the middle. The exuberant and tight pulse indicates distension. If the pulse complies with Yin–Yang, the disease is easy to be cured; if the pulse reverses Yin–Yang, the disease is difficult to be cured. If the pulse complies with four seasons, the disease will have no risk; if the pulse fails to comply with four seasons and has irregular transmission among viscera, the disease is difficult to be cured.

Too many blue vessels on the arms indicate blood depletion. Slow and unsmooth Chi pulse indicates lassitude. Exuberant pulse when sleeping indicates blood depletion. Unsmooth forearm-skin and slippery pulse indicate profuse sweating. Cold forearm-skin and thin pulse indicate diarrhea. Rough forearm-skin and usual feverish pulses indicate interior heat.

The appearance of critical liver pulse indicates the death on the seventh or eighth day; the appearance of critical heart pulse indicates the death on the ninth or tenth day; the appearance of critical spleen pulse indicates the death on the first or second day; the appearance of critical lung pulse indicates the death on the third or fourth day; the appearance of critical kidney pulse indicates the death on the fifth or sixth day; whatever critical visceral pulses appear, they all indicate death.

The rapid neck pulsation with panting and cough indicates water disease. The slightly swollen eyelids, like silkworms rising, indicates water disease. Yellow and red urine with sleepiness indicate jaundice. Hunger right after eating indicates stomach jaundice. Facial edema indicates wind disease. Edema of foot and shank indicates water disease. Yellow eyes indicate jaundice. Obvious pulsation on hand-Shaoyin meridian in women indicates pregnancy.

Pulse condition may reverse four seasons and have no corresponding condition in due season, such as thin pulse coming in spring and summer or floating and large pulse coming in autumn and winter, which are referred to as reversing four seasons. The wind-heat disease with calm pulse, diarrhea and blood depletion with excess pulse, disease in the internal with deficient pulse, and disease in the external with unsmooth and firm pulse, are difficult to treat. This mechanism is called reversing four seasons.

Since man lives on water and grain, the patient will die when deprived of water and grain, and also die when pulse is deprived of stomach Qi. The so-called pulse without stomach Qi refers to the pulse with only visceral genuine Qi but no stomach Qi. In the so-called pulse that is deprived of stomach Qi, liver pulse doesn't appear stringy or kidney pulse doesn't appear stony.

Taiyang pulse comes forcefully and largely with a long sense; Shaoyang pulse comes suddenly rapidly and suddenly slowly, or suddenly short and suddenly long; Yangming pulse comes floatingly and largely with short sense.

Normal heart pulse, coming like a string of pearls or feeling like a white pear-like stone, indicates a normal heart, and the pulse in summer is rooted in stomach Qi. Abnormal heart pulse comes acutely and continuously with slight hooky sense, which indicates heart diseases. Deadly heart pulse comes first with hooky sense and later with motionless sense, like feeling hooky pulse, which indicates dead heart pulse.

Normal lung pulse comes floatingly and lightly like elm legumens falling, which indicates a normal lung, and the pulse in autumn is rooted in stomach Qi. Abnormal lung pulse comes with neither ascending nor descending sense, like feeling chicken feathers, which indicates lung diseases. Deadly lung pulse comes like things floating on water or wind blowing hairs, which indicates dead lung pulse.

Normal liver pulse comes softly with long sense like holding long bamboo twig, which indicates a normal liver, and the pulse in spring is rooted in stomach Qi. Abnormal liver pulse comes fully and in a slippery manner like feeling a long bamboo, which indicates liver diseases. Deadly liver pulse comes acutely and vigorously like just drawing a full bow, which indicates dead liver pulse.

Normal spleen pulse comes softly and evenly like chicken keeping a claw on the ground, which indicates normal spleen, and the pulse in summer is rooted in stomach Qi. Abnormal spleen pulse comes excessively and rapidly like chicken raising its claw, which indicates spleen diseases. Deadly spleen pulse comes with a sense as sharp as the beak or claw of a bird, as irregular as roof leaking, or as rushing as flowing water, which indicates dead spleen pulse.

Normal kidney pulse comes acutely and continuously with hooky sense and appears firm under pressure, which indicates normal kidney, and the pulse in winter is rooted in stomach Qi. Abnormal kidney pulse comes like drawing a piece of vine and appears firmer under pressure, which indicates kidney diseases. Deadly kidney pulse comes like rope being broken or flicking a stone, which indicates dead kidney pulse.

Chapter 19

Vital Theory on Critical Visceral Pulses Inscribed in Jade

Yellow Emperor: The pulse in spring is like a string. What is a stringy pulse?
Qibo: Spring pulse corresponds to liver as well as the wood in the east, when all the things in nature begin to grow. Its Qi is soft, feeble, slippery, straight and long, termed stringy pulse. Its contrary condition indicates diseases.

Emperor: What is its contrary condition?
Qibo: The pulse Qi comes excessively and forcefully, called excess, and indicates external disease. The pulse Qi comes not excessively but weakly, called insufficiency, and indicates internal disease.

Emperor: If spring pulse is too excessive or deficient, what are the diseases concerned?
Qibo: If spring pulse is excessive, it makes the patient suffer from frequent amnesia, sudden vertigo with vexation; if it is insufficient, the patient will suffer from chest pain with referred back pain as well as fullness of rib cage.

Emperor: Good! The pulse in summer is like a hook, and what is hooked pulse?
Qibo: Summer pulse corresponds to heart as well as the fire in the south, when all the things in nature exuberate. Its Qi comes forcefully and goes weakly, termed hooked pulse. Its contrary condition indicates diseases.

Emperor: What is its contrary condition?
Qibo: The pulse Qi comes forcefully and also goes forcefully, called excess, and indicating the external disease. The pulse Qi comes not forcefully but goes forcefully, called insufficiency, and indicating the internal disease.

Emperor: If summer pulse is excessive or insufficient, what are the diseases concerned?
Qibo: If excessive, it makes the patient suffer from general fever, skin pain and acute eczema; if insufficient, it makes the patient have vexation, coughing in the upper region and Qi leakage in the lower region.

Emperor: Good! Autumn is floating. And what is a floating pulse?
Qibo: Autumn pulse corresponds to lung as well as the metal in the west, when all the things in nature are ripe and harvested. Its Qi comes lightly and floatingly, and comes acutely and goes dispersedly, termed floating pulse. Its contrary condition indicates diseases.

Emperor: What is its contrary condition?
Qibo: The pulse Qi comes floatingly like hairs with firmness in the middle and deficiency on both sides, called excess, and indicating the external disease. The pulse Qi comes floatingly

and feebly like hairs, called insufficiency, and indicating the internal disease.

Emperor: If autumn pulse is too excessive or insufficient, what are the diseases concerned?
Qibo: If excessive, it makes the patient suffer from reversal Qi and backache along with depression. If deficient, it makes the patient suffer from panting, shortness of breath and cough as well as ascending Qi with hemoptysis in the upper region and pathologic sound in the lower region.

Emperor: Good. The pulse in winter is like barracks. And what is the barracking pulse?
Qibo: Winter pulse corresponds to kidney as well as the water in the north, when all the things in nature are closed and stored. Its Qi comes steadily and is forcefully moist, termed barracking pulse. Its contrary condition indicates diseases.

Emperor: What is its contrary condition?
Qibo: The pulse Qi comes floatingly like a flicking stone, called excess, and indicating the external disease. The pulse Qi goes rapidly, called insufficiency, and indicating the internal disease.

Emperor: If winter pulse is excessive or insufficient, what are the diseases concerned?
Qibo: If excessive, it makes the patient suffer from limb flaccidity, spinal pain with shortness of breath and without any desire to speak. If insufficient, it makes the patient suffer from palpitation like overt hunger, coldness in the flank, spinal pain fullness in the lower abdomen and abnormal urination.

Emperor: Good.

Emperor: Pulses correspond to four seasons and differ in compliance and reversal. So, how does spleen pulse solely dominate?
Qibo: Spleen pulse, corresponding to the earth, is a solitary viscus that irrigates the other four solid viscera around.

Emperor: Can one feel whether or not spleen pulse is normal?
Qibo: A normal spleen pulse cannot be felt but the abnormal pulse can.

Emperor: How should one feel the abnormal spleen pulse?
Qibo: If the pulse comes like running water, called excess, it indicates external diseases; the pulse appearing like the beak of a bird, called insufficiency, indicates internal diseases.

Emperor: You, Master, have said that spleen is a solitary viscus in the center corresponding to the earth and irrigating the other four solid viscera. So, if spleen pulse is excessive or insufficient, what are the diseases concerned?
Qibo: If excessive, it makes the patient have inability of lifting four limbs. If insufficient, it makes the patient have obstruction of nine orifices, termed double rigidity.

Emperor stood up in surprise to bow and kowtow again, and said: Good. I've understood the fundamentals of the pulses and the extremely important rules in the world. The five complexion and pulse variations are observed as the abnormal or normal, which depend on spiritual unity point that operates without reversal. If reversed, the spirit won't operate and will lose its vitality. It is of top priority among extremely important rules and actually subtle. I'd like to engrave them in the jade plaque and store it in the royal repository for reading every morning, which is named as *Jade Confidential*.

Five solid viscera get Qi from the viscera they generate and transmit Qi to the viscera they dominate, respectively. Qi will linger in the viscera they generate but die in the viscera they cannot dominate. When the patient is dying, Qi must be transmitted to the viscera they cannot dominate, which then leads to death. It means Qi reversal causes the death. After liver gets morbid Qi from heart, it is then transmitted to spleen, lodged in kidney and finally to lung, leading to death. After heart gets morbid Qi from spleen, it is then transmitted to lung, lodged in liver and finally to kidney, leading to death. After spleen gets morbid Qi from lung, it is then transmitted to kidney, lodged in heart and finally to liver, leading to death. After lung gets morbid Qi from kidney, it is then transmitted to liver, lodged in spleen and finally to heart, leading to death. After kidney gets morbid Qi from liver, it is then transmitted to heart and lodged in spleen, leading to death. The deaths are all caused by Qi reversal. One day and one night are divided into five phases corresponding to five solid viscera, by which the time of death can be predicted.

Emperor: The five solid viscera communicate with one after another and the transmission of morbid Qi also has a regular order. If there is a disease in one of the five solid viscera, it will be transmitted to the viscus they dominate respectively. If not treated in proper time, in three or six months, or in three or six days, the disease will be transmitted to all five solid viscera, necessarily leading to death, which is the rule of transmission to the viscera they dominate. It is believed that one who can differentiate Yang knows where the disease comes from; while the one who can differentiate Yin knows the date of death. That is to say, the transmission of disease into the viscera where it cannot dominate will result in death.

Hence, the wind is the leading evil for all diseases. Now, if wind and cold invade the body, it makes vellus hair stand on end and closes the skin with fever. By this time, it can be dispelled with diaphoresis, or it will cause impediment, numbness, swelling and pain, and by this time, it can be dispelled with decoction, hot compression, moxibustion and acupuncture. Left untreated, the disease will lodge in lung, termed lung impediment, leading to cough and reversal ascending Qi. Left untreated, the disease will be transmitted to liver, termed liver impediment, also termed reversal syndrome, leading to hypochondriac pain and vomiting; by this time, it can be treated with Chinese massage and acupuncture. Left untreated, the disease will be transmitted from liver to spleen, termed spleen-wind, leading to jaundice, abdominal heat, vexation and dark urine. By this time, it can be treated with Chinese massage, medication or medicated bathing. Left untreated, the disease will be transmitted to kidney, where painful lump develops, leading to bleeding, depressive heat in the lower abdomen with pain, and cloudy urine, termed turbid urine; by this time, it can be treated with Chinese massage and medication. Left untreated, the disease will be transmitted from kidney to heart, leading to sinews and vessels drawing mutually with spasm, termed convulsion. By this time, it can be treated with moxibustion and medication. Left untreated, the patient is doomed to die in ten days. If the disease is transmitted from kidney to heart that is in turn transmitted to lung with cold and fever, the patient is doomed to die in three years. It is the transmission sequence of diseases.

However, for the disease that develops suddenly, it needn't be treated following the sequence of transmission; some diseases are not transmitted in sequence, including anxiety, fear, sorrow, joy and anger, which have no transmission sequence but can make the patient have major diseases. For instance, if the deficiency is due to great joy, kidney Qi will over-restrain heart; if the deficiency is due to anger, liver Qi will over-restrain spleen; if the deficiency is due to sorrow, lung Qi will over-restrain liver; if the deficiency is due to fear, spleen Qi will over-restrain kidney; and if it is due to anxiety, heart Qi will over-restrain lung, which is the rule for the no-transmission sequence. Hence, though five solid viscera have only five kinds of diseases, there are twenty-five changes with their transmission. The transmission is actually the term for over-restraining.

If withering of large bones, loss of major muscle, Qi fullness in the chest, panting and breathlessness, and shaking while breathing are seen, the patient is expected to die in six months; if the critical visceral pulse is found, the date of death can be predicted. If there appear withering of large bones, loss of major muscle, Qi fullness in the chest, panting and breathlessness, internal pain drawing shoulder and nape, the patient is expected to die in one month; if the critical visceral pulse is found, the date of death can be predicted. If there appear withering of large bones, loss of major muscle, Qi fullness in the chest, panting and breathlessness, internal pain drawing shoulder and nape, general fever, emaciation and ulceration, and the critical visceral pulse is found, the patient is expected to die in ten months. If there appear withering of large bones, loss of major muscle, internal consumption of shoulder marrow and increasingly slow motion with no critical visceral pulse found, the patient is expected to die in one month; if the critical visceral pulse is found, the date of death can be predicted. If there appear withering of large bones, loss of major muscle, Qi fullness in the chest, internal pain in abdomen, discomfort in the chest, fever in shoulders, nape and trunk, ulceration and emaciation, sunken eye socket, critical visceral pulse, loss of vision, the patient will die immediately; if left with some vision, the patient will die when the disease is transmitted to the solid viscera, its Qi cannot dominate.

If there is a sudden deficiency while the body is suddenly attacked by evil, there will appear blockage of five solid viscera, obstruction of vessels and paths, and loss of Qi circulation, as if falling and drowning, and the date of death cannot be predicted. If the pulse fails to come, or beats five to six times within a breath, even if there appears no emaciation and critical visceral pulse, the patient is still doomed to die.

If the critical liver pulse comes with sharp sense, interiorly or exteriorly, like feeling on the edge of knife or feeling like an instrument's string, green-white complexion with no luster as well as brittle hair, it indicates death. If the critical heart pulse comes firmly and forcefully, with cluster sense like feeling Job's tears, red-black complexion with no luster as well as brittle hair, it indicates death. If the critical lung pulse comes largely and feebly, with a sense like that of a feather touching human skin, white-red complexion with no luster as well as brittle hair, it indicates death. If the critical kidney pulse comes forcefully and critically, with a sense like that of a finger flicking a stone, black-yellow complexion with no luster as well as brittle hair, it indicates death. If the critical spleen pulse comes feebly and rapidly or slowly, with yellowish-greenish complexion and no luster as well as brittle hair, it indicates death. Whatever the critical visceral pulse appears, it indicates a fatal disease.

Emperor: There appears critical visceral pulse, it indicates death — why?
Qibo: Five solid viscera all obtain Qi from stomach, which is the root of five solid viscera. The visceral Qi cannot reach hand-Taiyin meridian alone and it has to do so with the aid of stomach Qi. Therefore, the Qi of all five viscera reaches hand-Taiyin meridian with its own pulse condition at its own proper time. If there appears evil domination, there will be decline of essence. Thus, for critical diseases, stomach Qi fails to reach hand-Taiyin meridian together with the visceral Qi so the critical visceral Qi appears alone, which indicates evil Qi dominating the visceral Qi and death.

Emperor: Good.

Emperor: When treating any disease, one should observe the physique, Qi, complexion with luster, exuberance and decline of pulse, and the new and the old diseases, so that one won't miss the proper opportunity for the treatment. If physique and Qi match mutually, the disease is treatable. If the complexion appears lustrous, the disease is easily cured. If the pulse complies with four seasons, the disease is treatable. If the pulse comes weakly and in a slippery manner, it indicates the existence of stomach Qi and the disease is easy to treat. All the diseases should be treated in proper time. If physique and Qi fail to match mutually, the disease is refractory. If the complexion has no luster, the disease is intractable. If the pulse comes excessively and firmly, the disease will worsen. If the pulse fails to comply with four seasons, the disease is incurable. The four difficult conditions should be examined carefully and explained clearly to the patient.

The so-called pulses reversing four seasons are that lung pulse appears in spring, kidney pulse appears in summer, heart pulse appears in autumn and spleen pulse appears in winter, and if all are being critically broken, sunken and unsmooth, they are termed pulse-reversing four seasons. If the pulse fails to express its visceral Qi in the appropriate season, for example, sunken and unsmooth pulse in spring and summer or floating and large pulse in autumn and winter, it is also termed pulse-reversing four seasons. There are quiet pulses in febrile diseases, large pulses in diarrhea, excessive pulses in massive bleeding, excessive and firm pulses in internal diseases, and weak and soft pulses in external diseases, all of which indicate the incurable diseases.

Emperor: I have heard that the excess and deficiency can determine death and survival; I'd like to know the reason.
Qibo: The five types of excess can cause death, and so do the five types of deficiency.

Emperor: I'd like to know the concrete conditions about the five kinds of excess or deficiency.
Qibo: Exuberant pulse, hot skin, severe abdominal distension, difficulty in urination and defecation, oppression and mental confusion are the five conditions of excess. Thin pulse, cold skin, dyspnea, diarrhea and incontinence, and anorexia are the five conditions of deficiency.

Emperor: The patient with these conditions may still survive, why is it so?
Qibo: After ingesting some thick fluid or porridge, if the severe diarrhea can be stopped, the patient with deficiency can survive, and if the patient can have sweating and smooth excretion, the patient with excess can also survive. This is the principle concerned.

Chapter 20

Three Regions and Nine Positions of Pulse

Yellow Emperor: I've heard of *Nine Kinds of Needles* from you with broad and profound scholarship beyond counting. Now, I'd like to know the key theory which can be known to my offspring and inherited for generations. I will learn them by heart and inscribe them in my memory. I swear a blood oath that I will receive the theory but will never reveal it, the theory will comply with the natural law and if not complied, reversal will happen. The theory can correspond to the daylight and stars upwards forever and to four seasons and five elements downwards. The theory, major and minor, alternates with Yin in winter and Yang in summer. How is their correspondence with the human body? I'd like to know.
Qibo: How careful your question is! It is the extreme law of the heavens and the earth.

Emperor: I'd like to know the extreme law which can correspond to human physique, blood and Qi, and predicate the death and life. What is the practice?
Qibo: The extreme number originates from one and terminates at nine. One represents the heavens, two represents the earth

and three represents the human being. Since each number has three subdivisions, three times three is nine corresponding to nine fields. So, the human being has three regions and each region has three locations so as to determine death and life, approach various diseases, regulate the deficiency and excess, and finally get rid of evil and diseases.

Emperor: What are the three regions?
Qibo: There are three regions, the lower, the middle and the upper. Each region has three locations, and the so-called three locations represent the heavens, the earth and the human being. Being instructed respectively, the theory can be regarded as the truth. At the heavens location of the upper region is the beating vessel on both sides of the forehead, at the earth location of the upper region is the beating vessel of the cheek, and at the human location of the upper region is the beating vessel anterior to ears. At the heavens location of the middle region is hand-Taiyin meridian. At the earth location of the middle is hand-Yangming meridian. At the human location of the middle is hand-Shaoyin meridian. At the heavens location of the lower region is foot-Jueyin meridian, at the earth location of the lower is foot-Shaoyin meridian, and at the human location of the lower is foot-Taiyin meridian. So, on the lower region, the heavens location indicates liver, the earth indicates kidney, and the human location indicates the Qi of spleen and stomach.

Emperor: How about the locations in the middle region?
Qibo: There are also the locations of the heavens, the earth and the human being. The heavens location indicates lung, the earth indicates the Qi in the chest, and the human location indicates heart.

Emperor: How about the indications of the upper region?
Qibo: There are also the locations of the heavens, the earth and the human. The location of the heavens indicates the Qi of the forehead, the earth indicates the Qi of mouth and teeth, and the human location indicates the Qi of ears and eyes. The three regions have the locations of the heavens, the earth and the human, respectively. The three locations consist of the heavens, the earth and the human, respectively. Three times three is nine. Nine divisions are nine fields which correspond to nine viscera. Then five spirit viscera and four physique viscera are combined as nine viscera. If the five solid viscera are deteriorated, their complexion must be faded, which indicates doomed death.

Emperor: How should one treat according to the indication?
Qibo: First, the doctor should distinguish the body between thinness or fatness and then regulate the deficiency and excess of the Qi, in which the excess should be purged and the deficiency should be supplemented. The removal of the excess blood and meridians should precede the regulation, and whatever the disease is, the goal for the treatment is harmony.

Emperor: How should one predict the death or life?
Qibo: Exuberant physique and thin pulse with less Qi and being out of breath indicate crisis; thin physique and large pulse with more Qi in the chest indicate death. Shape and Qi in harmony indicate life; irregular pulses indicate diseases; disharmony of three regions and nine locations indicate death; irregular pulses like pestle pounding, beating up and down, or left and right, indicate severe diseases; pulse beating irregularly up and down, or left and right beyond counting indicate

death; the location of the middle region in disharmony with other solid viscera, though regular on their own, indicates death; the location of the middle region in reduction indicates death; and sunken eyes indicate death.

Emperor: How should one define the focus of diseases?
Qibo: When observing the nine pulse positions, only one position with small pulsation indicates diseases, and so does the only position with large, with swift, with slow, with heat, with cold, or with sinking pulsations. The left hand is put on the foot five cun above the ankle which is then flicked by the right-hand finger. If the pulsation range is more than five cun with wriggling status, it indicates no disease. When Qi is coming swiftly, the heavy pulsation touching fingers indicates disease. The slow pulsation touching fingers indicates disease. The pulsation range less than five cun with no flicking response indicates death. Emaciation with difficult movement indicates death. Suddenly slow and suddenly rapid pulse indicates death. The regular intermittent pulse with hooky feeling reflects the disease in collateral. The correspondence of nine positions shows consistency up and down with no disharmony. One delayed position pulse indicates diseases; two delayed positions pulse indicates severe disease; three delayed positions pulse indicates crisis. The so-called delayed pulse means that the pulses of positions don't beat consistently. If combined with the observation of solid and hollow viscera, the date of death or life can be predicted. Knowing the normal meridian pulse should precede knowing the disease pulses. The observation of the critical pulse of solid viscera indicates death. The exhaustion of Taiyang Qi with inflexible feet indicates death with up-fixed glassy eyes.

Emperor: How about death or life concerned with Yin in winter and Yang in summer?
Qibo: The pulses at nine positions which are sunken, thin and critical expiry are all Yin pulses, which appear especially in winter and indicate death at midnight. The surging, agitated, hasty, and rapid pulses are all Yang pulses, which appear especially in summer, indicating death at noon. Hence, the patient with chill and fever will die at dawn. The patient with interior heat and fever will die at noon; the patient with wind will die at dusk. The patient with water diseases will die at midnight. Suddenly loose and suddenly dense pulse or suddenly slow and suddenly rapid pulses lead to death at four transient times in a day. If there is a disfigured body and emaciation, even if nine-position pulses are regulated, the patient cannot avoid death. If there is disease with seven findings but the nine-position pulses all cooperate, the patient can survive. The so-called survival refers to the diseases, such as the disorders due to wind and abnormal menstruation, which are similar to seven findings but are in fact not, so they do not indicate death. If there is the disease with seven findings, the pulse in deterioration indicates death with hiccups. The doctor should inquire the previous and current history of the patient, then feel the pulse along different vessels and observe the floating and sinking of the meridians and collaterals, up and down as well as reversal and compliance treatment. The rapid pulse indicates no diseases. The slow pulse indicates diseases. The pulse with no going and coming indicates death. The skin adhering to bones indicates death.

Emperor: How about their possible treatment?
Qibo: The disease involving the meridian is treated for the meridians; the disease involving minute collaterals is treated

for collateral blood. The disease involving blood with pain is treated for meridians and collaterals. If the disease involves extraordinary evil, the collaterals are needled on the contralateral sides. The disease with lingering evil is needled on the joints. The disease with upper excess and lower deficiency should be observed with the pulse-taking, and accord with the evil stagnated on the focus of the collaterals, which is needled till bleeding is seen. The upward vision indicates deficiency of Taiyang. Up-fixed glassy eyes indicate the exhaustion of Taiyang. These are keys to predict death and life, which cannot be ignored.

Chapter 21

Distinctive Theory on Meridians and Diseased Pulses

Yellow Emperor: Will the pulses change corresponding to the different housing conditions of the human beings, motion or stillness, and braveness or timidity?

Qibo: Any fear, fright, anger, labor, motion and stillness can become the variables. Therefore, the panting during night walk originates from kidney and its excessive Qi will affect lung; with fear, while falling, panting originates from liver and its excessive Qi will impair spleen; with fear and fright, panting originates from lung and its excessive Qi damages heart; with falling or tripping, while wading a river, panting originates from kidney and bones. On these occasions, the brave has good Qi regulation and respond normally while the timid has Qi stagnation, which is subjected to illness. It's believed that the principle for diagnosis is to observe the braveness and timidity as well as bones, muscles, and skin of a person in order to know the conditions and set these as the basis of the diagnosis.

So, for the over intake of a meal, sweating originates from stomach; for the fright with essence depleted, sweating originates from heart; for carrying heavy things for long distance, sweating originates from kidney; for rapid walk with fear, sweating originates from liver, and for strenuous physical labor, sweating comes from spleen. Thus, in spring, autumn, winter and summer seasons and in terms of Yin and Yang during the four seasons, the diseases are caused by overuse, which is the common etiology.

The food is taken into stomach and its essence Qi is transferred to liver and distributed along sinews. The food is taken into stomach and its turbid Qi returns to heart and is distributed along vessels. Vessel Qi flows through meridians and meridian Qi returns to lung, which is connected to hundreds of vessels, distributing essence over skin and hair. The essence and Qi of hair and vessels converge and run through hollow viscera. The essence of hollow viscera makes spirit Qi bright, which remains in four solid viscera, and all depend on the balance of Yin and Yang. Because of the balance, Qikou can be taken to predict life and death. Water is taken into stomach, which isolates essence Qi and transports it up to spleen. Spleen Qi can spread essence up to lung, which regulates water path and transports it down to bladder.

Water and essence are distributed all over the body and are in parallel to the five meridians to comply with four seasons, and Yin and Yang of five solid viscera, whose measurement is the norm of the human body.

If Taiyang pulse comes alone with critical panting due to reversal and deficient Qi, it reflects Yin deficiency and Yang excess. It should be purged from both exterior and interior meridians at the acupoints in foot meridian. If Yangming pulse comes alone due to combination of Yang Qi from Taiyang and Shaoyang, it should be purged for Yang and supplemented for

Yin at the acupoints in foot meridian. If Shaoyang pulse comes alone due to reversal Qi, with sudden exuberance pulse in front of Foot Yangqiao, the acupoints in foot meridian can be needled. Shaoyang pulse comes alone because of hyperactivity in the first Yang (Shaoyang) meridian. Taiyin pulse beats forcefully, for which the critical solid visceral pulse should be differentiated; if there is less Qi in five pulses and stomach Qi is uneven, indicating the hyperactivity in the third Yin (Taiyin) meridian, the acupoints in foot meridian should be needled for supplementing Yang and purging Yin. If the second Yin (Shaoyin) pulse surges alone due to Qi reversal of Shaoyin combined with kidney Yang, which makes pulses of four solid viscera vie with one another and Qi return to kidney, it should be treated in meridians and collaterals by purging Yang and supplementing Yin. The first Yin comes as a result of Jueyin hyperactivity and has critical Qi deficiency and heart pain due to lingering reversal Qi, leading to white sweating, which is regulated by dieting and medication or needled at the acupoints in foot meridian.

Emperor: What about the conditions of Taiyang pulse?
Qibo: This is similar to the third Yang (Taiyang) meridian with floating pulse.

Emperor: What about the conditions of Shaoyang pulse?
Qibo: This is similar to the first Yang (Shaoyang) meridian; the first Yang pulse is slippery with no excess.

Emperor: What about the conditions of Yangming pulse?
Qibo: This pulse is large and floating. Taiyin pulse beats forcefully like muffled drumming. The second Yin (Shaoyin) pulse comes, with kidney pulse being sunken but not floating.

Chapter 22

Transference of Solid Visceral Qi Following Regularity of Four Seasons

Yellow Emperor: In the view of human body, it should comply with the four seasons and five elements by which the treatment can be practiced; what is the compliance and what is the reversal? What are their advantages and disadvantages? I'd like to know these.

Qibo: Five elements are metal, wood, water, fire and earth. They dominate or are dominated among themselves alternatively, by which doctors can predict death and life and expect a prognosis; meanwhile, doctors can analyze Qi of five solid viscera, determine the timing of cure or progression and predict the date of death and life.

Emperor: I'd like to listen to it.

Qibo: Liver corresponds to spring, and its chief treatment is aimed at Jueyin and Shaoyang of foot. Its dominating day is the First–Second day. Its disease is characterized by the suffering of urgency, and sweet food is immediately ingested to relieve this. Heart corresponds to summer, and its chief treatment is aimed at Shaoyin and Taiyang of hand. Its dominating day is Third–Fourth day. Its disease is characterized by the suffering of moderation, and sour food is immediately ingested to astringe it. Spleen corresponds to late summer, and its related treatment is chiefly aimed at Taiyin and Yangming of foot. Its dominating day is Fifth–Sixth day. Its disease is characterized by the suffering of dampness, and bitter food is immediately ingested to dry it. Lung corresponds to autumn, and its chief treatment is aimed at Taiyin and Yangming of hand. Its dominating day is Seventh–Eighth day. Its disease is characterized by the suffering of upward reversal, and bitter food is immediately ingested to discharge it. Kidney corresponds to winter, and its chief treatment is aimed at Shaoyin and Taiyang of foot. Its dominating day is Ninth–Tenth day. Its disease is characterized by the suffering of dryness, and pungent food is immediately ingested to moisten it and open the interstitial striae for transporting fluid and Qi.

When the disease occurs in the liver, it will be cured in summer; if not cured in summer, the disease will be more severe in autumn; if the patient doesn't die in autumn, the disease will remain till winter and be cured in spring. The patient should avoid wind. Liver disease can be cured on the Third–Fourth day; if not cured on Third–Fourth, it will be more severe on the Seventh–Eighth day; if the patient doesn't die on the Seventh–Eighth day, the disease will remain till the Ninth–Tenth day and is cured on the First–Second day. Liver disease is relieved at dawn, more severe in the late afternoon and stable at midnight. Since liver tends to be dispersed, pungent food is immediately ingested to disperse it, and pungent food is used to supplement it and the sour to purge it.

When the disease occurs in heart, it will be cured in late summer; if not cured in late summer, the disease will be more severe in winter. If the patient doesn't die in winter, the disease will remain till the next spring and be cured in spring. The patient should avoid warm food and hot clothes. Heart disease can be cured on the Fifth–Sixth days; if not cured on the Fifth–Sixth, it will develop new manifestations on the Ninth–Tenth day; if the patient doesn't die on the Ninth–Tenth, the disease will remain till the First–Second day and is cured in the Third–Fourth. Heart disease is relieved at noon, more severe at midnight and stable at dawn. Since heart tends to be softened, salty food is immediately ingested to soften heart, and the salt is used to supplement it and the sweet to purge it.

When the disease occurs in spleen, it will be cured in autumn; if not cured in autumn, the disease will be more severe in spring; if the patient doesn't die in spring, the disease will last till summer and be cured in late summer. The patient should avoid warm food and overeating as well as staying in a humid field and wearing wet clothes. Spleen disease can be cured on the Seventh–Eighth day; if not cured on the Seventh–Eighth, it will develop new manifestations on the First–Second; if the patient doesn't die on the First–Second day, the disease will remain till the Third–fourth day and be cured on the Fifth–Sixth. Spleen disease is relieved in the early afternoon, more severe at sunset and stable in the late afternoon. Since spleen tends to be relieved, sweat food is immediately ingested to relieve spleen, and bitter medicinal is used to purge it and the sweet to supplement it.

When the disease occurs in lung, it will be cured in winter; if not cured in winter, the disease will be more severe in summer; if the patient doesn't die in summer, the disease will remain till late summer and be cured in autumn; the patient should avoid cold food and cold clothes. Lung disease can be cured on the Ninth–Tenth day; if not cured on the Ninth–Tenth, it will develop new manifestations on the Third–Fourth day; if the patient doesn't die on the Third–Fourth, the disease will remain till the Fifth–Sixth day and be cured on the Seventh–Eighth. Lung disease is relieved in the late afternoon, more severe at noon and stable at midnight. Since lung tends to be astringed, sour food is immediately ingested to astringe the lung, and the sour is used to supplement it and the pungent to purge it.

When the disease occurs in kidney, it will be cured in spring; if not cured in spring, the disease will be more severe in late summer; if the patient doesn't die in late summer, the disease will remain till autumn and be cured in winter; the patient should avoid extreme heating hot food and hot clothes. Kidney disease can be cured on the First–Second day; if not cured on the First–Second, it will be more severe on the Fifth–Sixth day; if the patient doesn't die on the Fifth–Sixth, the disease will remain till the Seventh–Eighth day and be cured on the Ninth–Tenth. Kidney disease is relieved at midnight, more severe at four transient times during a day and stable in late afternoon. Since kidney tends to be hardened, bitter food is immediately ingested to harden it, and the bitter is used to supplement it and the salt to purge it.

When evil Qi invades the human body, the dominating always overcomes the dominated. When evil comes into the visceral dominant phase, the disease will be cured; when it comes into the visceral non-dominant phase, the disease will be more severe; when in the visceral dominant phase, the disease will be stable; when in the visceral proper phase, the disease will be cured. After the pulses of five solid viscera are identified, the remission and progression of the disease can be predicted, as can the dates of death and life.

Liver diseases are characterized by pain in both hypochondria with referring pain to the lower abdomen as well as frequent anger. If deficient, the patient will have loss of vision and hearing and frequent fright as if being arrested. Meridians of Jueyin and Shaoyang are selected for acupuncture. If there is Qi reversal, there is headache, deafness and swollen cheek, for which needling till bleeding should be done.

Heart diseases are characterized by chest pain, sticking distension in hypochondria, hypochondriac pain, pain on the back and between the scapulae and pain on the inner side of both arms. If there is deficiency, big belly and bloating chest are seen, as is referred pain between hypochondria and waist. Meridians of Shaoyin and Taiyang with sublingual bleeding pricking are selected for acupuncture, with sublingual bleeding by needling. If the disease has changes, acupoint Xizhong (Weizhong, BL40*) can be needled till bleeding.

Spleen diseases are characterized by heavy body, frequent hunger, flaccid muscles, feet failing to raise, frequent spasm and foot sole pain. If there is deficiency, there is abdominal distension, rumbling, diarrhea after indigestion and dyspepsia. Meridians of Taiyin, Yangming and Shaoyin are selected for acupuncture; needling is applied till bleeding.

Lung diseases are characterized by panting, cough and reversal Qi, shoulder and back pain, sweating, and pain in buttocks, genitals, thighs, knees, hip, calf, shin and feet. If there is deficiency, there is less Qi, shortness of breath, deafness and dry throat. Meridians of external Taiyin and Taiyang and

---

*The acupuncture points are referred to by their traditional names in *Huangdi Neijing*. The meridian and number are added by the translator.

internal Shaoyin are selected for acupuncture; needling is applied till bleeding.

Kidney diseases are characterized by bulging abdomen, swollen shank, panting, cough and heavy body, night sweating and fearing wind. If there is deficiency, there is chest pain, big belly, lower abdominal pain, and a feeling of cold and unhappiness. Meridians of Shaoyin and Taiyang are selected for acupuncture; needling is applied till bleeding.

Liver corresponds to green, and suitable food is sweet; non-glutinous rice, beef, dates and mallow are all kinds of sweet food. Heart corresponds to red, and suitable food is sour; adzuki bean, dog meat, plums, and leek are all kinds of sour food. Lung corresponds to white, and suitable food is bitter; wheat, lamb, apricot and shallot are all kinds of bitter food. Spleen corresponds to yellow, and suitable food is salty; soybeans, pork, chestnut and pulse leaves are all kinds of salty food. Kidney corresponds to black, and suitable food is pungent; millet, chicken, peach and scallion are all kinds of pungent food. The pungent is capable of dispersing, the sour of astringing, the sweet of moderating, the bitter of hardening, and the salty of softening.

Drug is capable of attacking evils. Five grains are used as main food, five fruits as supplementary food, five animal meats as beneficial food, and five vegetables as adjuvant food. The flavors are ingested collectively to supplement essence and benefit Qi. The five flavors include pungent, sour, sweet, bitter and salty, each with its advantages of dispersing, astringing, moderating, hasting, hardening or softening, respectively. In four seasons and to the five solid viscera, the disease is approached with the proper flavors.

Chapter 23

Clarification of Five-Visceral Qi

The entrances of five flavors into target viscera are as follows: The sour enters liver; the pungent enters lung; the bitter enters heart; the salty enters kidney; the sweet enters spleen.

The diseases of five Qi abnormalities are as follows: Qi disorder of heart leads to belching; that of lung leads to cough; that of liver leads to polyphrasia; that of spleen leads to acid regurgitation; that of kidney leads to yawning and sneezing; that of stomach leads to Qi reversal, hiccup and fear; that of large and small intestines leads to diarrhea; that of the lower Jiao overflow leads to edema; that of bladder in obstruction leads to urine retention or inability to control to urine incontinence; that of gallbladder leads to anger.

The stresses of five essences due to deficiencies are as follows: Stress of essence Qi in heart leads to overhappiness; that in lung leads to grief; that in liver leads to anxiety; that in spleen leads to fear; that in kidney leads to fright.

The aversions of five solid viscera are as follows: Heart dislikes heat; lung dislikes cold; liver dislikes wind; spleen dislikes damp; kidney dislikes dryness.

The liquid transformations from five solid viscera are as follows: Heart forms sweat; lung forms snivel; liver forms tears; spleen forms drooling; kidney forms spit.

The bans of five flavors are as follows: Since the pungent consumes Qi, the patient with Qi diseases shouldn't take in too much pungent food; since the salty consumes blood, the patient with blood diseases shouldn't take in too much salty food; since the bitter consumes bones, the patient with bone diseases shouldn't take in too much bitter food; since the sweet consumes muscle, the patient with muscular diseases shouldn't take in too much sweet food; since the sour consumes sinews, the patient with sinew diseases shouldn't take in too much sour food. These are the five bans for the food and accordingly the patients should take care not to be crapulent.

The origins of five kinds of diseases are as follows: Yin diseases originate from bones; Yang diseases originate from blood; Yin diseases originate from muscles. Yang diseases occur in winter, and Yin diseases occur in summer.

The disorders of five evils are as follows: The evil invading Yang causes mania; the evil invading Yin causes impediment; the evil struggling in Yang causes vertex diseases; the evil struggling in Yin causes aphonia. Yang into Yin causes stillness, and Yin out of Yang causes anger.

The signs of five evils are as follows: Autumn pulse appears in spring; winter pulse appears in summer; spring pulse appears in late summer; summer pulse appears in autumn; late summer pulse appears in winter. These are referred to as Yin out of Yang with frequent anger and is incurable. These signs of five evils have the same outcome, i.e. incurability and death.

The storages of five solid viscera are as follows: Heart stores spirit; lung stores Yin soul; liver stores Yang soul; spleen stores idea; kidney stores mind.

The governments of five solid viscera are as follows: Heart governs vessels; lung governs skin; liver governs sinews; spleen governs muscles; kidney governs bones.

The Injuries of five kinds of labor are as follows: Prolonged seeing injures blood; prolonged sleeping injures Qi; prolonged sitting injures muscles; prolonged standing injures bones; prolonged walking injures sinews.

The correspondence of the five pulses of five solid viscera are as follows: liver pulse is like string; heart pulse is like hook; spleen pulse is regularly intermittent; lung pulse is like fur; the kidney pulse is like stone.

Chapter 24

Blood, Qi, Body and Emotions

Under constant conditions in the human body, there is usually more blood and less Qi in Taiyin meridian, less blood and more Qi in Shaoyang, more Qi and more blood in Yangming, less blood and more Qi in Shaoyin, more blood and less Qi in Jueyin, and more Qi and less blood in Taiyin, which is also the norm seen in nature.

Foot-Taiyang meridian and foot-Shaoyin meridian are related as exterior and interior, as are Shaoyang and Jueyin as well as Yangming and Taiyin, which is the Yin–Yang relationship of foot meridians. Hand-Taiyang meridian and hand-Shaoyin meridian are related as exterior and interior, so are Shaoyang and Jueyin as well as Yangming and Taiyin, which is the Yin–Yang relationship of hand meridians. Once the suffering of Yin and Yang on foot or hand meridians is identified, the removal of excessive blood should precede the removal of the suffering in the treatment process and then the progression can be observed in order to purge the excess or supplement the deficiency.

In order to locate the back transport (Shu) acupoints, the length between two nipples is first measured with a straw that is then folded in half; another straw with the same length is cut in half and both halves are connected to form an equilateral triangle as the support. Then the triangle is put on the back, with top angle up to Dazhui (DU14)* on the spine and two bottom angles downwards; the acupoints that the two bottom angles direct are lung acupoints (BL13). When the angle is moved down one triangle-space, the top angle directs heart acupoint (BL15). When the angle is moved down one triangle-space, the two bottom acupoints direct liver acupoint (BL18) on the left and the spleen acupoint (BL20) on the right. When the triangle angle is moved down one triangle-space, the two bottom acupoints direct kidney acupoint (BL23). All the above are the transport acupoints of five solid vicera and the measurement for moxibustion and acupuncture.

Comfortable physique but uncomfortable emotion causes diseases in meridians, which can be treated with moxibustion and acupuncture. Comfortable physique and comfortable emotion cause diseases in muscle, which can be treated with stone needles therapy. Uncomfortable physique and comfortable emotion cause diseases in sinews, which can be treated with hot compression. Uncomfortable physique and uncomfortable emotion cause diseases in throat, which can be treated with various medicinals. Physique with frequent fear and fright with obstruction of meridians cause numbness diseases, which can be treated with Chinese massage and medicinal wine. These are the five classifications of physique and emotions.

Yangming meridian can be needled to remove excessive blood and Qi, Taiyang to remove excessive blood but not Qi, Shaoyang to remove excessive Qi but not blood, Taiyin to remove excessive Qi but not blood, Shaoyin to remove excessive Qi but not blood, and Jueyin to remove excessive blood but not Qi.

---

*The meridians and numbers in brackets are added by the translator.

Chapter 25

Cherishing the Life and Guarding the Body

Yellow Emperor: Under the heavens and upon the earth, there are all creatures great and small, and nothing is more valuable than human beings. People live on the Qi between the heavens and the earth, and depend on rules of four seasonal variations. From the monarch down to the people, all of them wish they could keep themselves physically fit, but they notice nothing when the disease is developing, so that the disease is lingering in the body and even goes into the bone morrow, which I am much concerned about. I want to relieve their sufferings with acupuncture; how to do this?

Qibo: For example, the salt has a salty taste, whose Qi makes water in the container effuse. The string is being broken with harsh sound. The tree is being perished due to the leaves fluttering down. The patient suffers from the severe disease with hiccup. There are the three conditions in any patient which indicate the deterioration of the viscera and no drug is curative and no short needle is effective for these conditions, all of which damage the skin and muscles and black out blood and Qi.

Emperor: I am concerned with these sufferings but puzzled about these conditions. They will be worse if given improper treatment, but there is no better therapy to replace them. From the viewpoint of ordinary people, it is regarded as cruel and rough behavior, so how can I do something for it?
Qibo: Human beings live on the earth and depend on the heavens, in which both heavenly Qi and earthly Qi are combined to make a creature termed human. Human beings can comply with four seasons in that the heavens and the earth are their parents; the one who knows the laws of all creatures is the Son of Heaven. So, nature has Yin and Yang while human body has twelve meridians; nature has cold and heat while human body has deficiency and excess. Those who can comply with the variations of Yin and Yang in nature cannot miss the rules of four seasons; those who know the mechanism of twelve meridians cannot be fooled by the sages and virtuous person; those who can master the changes of eight winds can gain normal predominance of five elements; those who can be familiar with the variations of deficiency and excess can act independently so that he is sharp-sighted enough to perceive a bird's fine hair in autumn, like subtle yawning or groaning.

Emperor: Human being has the physique shape that cannot exist without Yin and Yang. The combination of heavenly Qi and earthly Qi can be divided into nine fields or into four seasons; there are greater or lesser months and longer or shorter days. All creatures great and small exist in the world with innumerable changes. Deficiency and excess can be judged even according to subtle yawning or groaning. Excuse me, but can you tell me the method?

Qibo: Wood is cut when meeting metal, fire is put out when meeting water, earth is loose when meeting wood, metal is melted when meeting fire, and water is dried out when meeting earth. All creatures have such kinds of changes that are too numerous to list. Acupuncture applied to treat diseases everywhere has five keys, about which the ordinary people enjoying a full diet on their own have no interest. The first is to treat with concentrated mind, the second to know the way of culturing health, the third to differentiate the property of drugs, the fourth to prepare the stone needles with proper size and the fifth to understand the diagnostic methods to blood–Qi in viscera. All the five keys should be held, and it is more important to assign proper priority. When acupuncture is applied at present, a supplementing therapy is applied for deficiency and a purging method for the excess, which all the doctors have known. If according to the laws of the heavens and the earth and varying with the changed conditions, acupuncture has a therapeutic effect like resonance being a reflection of sound and shadow being a reflection of light, there is no secret ghost and the doctor can apply acupuncture independently.

Emperor: I'd like to learn the reason.
Qibo: The essentials of acupuncture include concentrating the mind firstly, defining the deficiency or excess of five solid viscera and mastering the nine positions before pricking with needles. When no other visceral exhaustion pulse is felt, no deterioration of five viscera is found, and the external and the internal is harmonized, not only depending on observing external physique conditions but being familiar with the ins and outs, acupuncture can be applied in patients. The patients are of two types: the deficient and the excessive. The doctor

shouldn't apply acupuncture when meeting five deficient syndromes, give up acupuncture when meeting five excessive syndromes, and catch the right timing to apply acupuncture without a moment's delay. Applying acupuncture is just like engaging in career, the needles are manipulated evenly. The doctor should keep calm to observe the change of the patient and the change of meridian Qi, which is shapeless and shadowless, like a flock of birds flying into or out of trees or crops growing exuberantly. The arrival and leaving of meridian Qi can be sensed like observing a flying bird without knowing what it is; retaining needles is like mounting a crossbow, and withdrawing needles is like shooting an arrow.

Emperor: How to treat the deficient and how to treat the excessive?
Qibo: For the case with deficiency, supplementing therapy should be applied; for the case with excess, purging therapy is applied. When the meridian Qi has arrived, the two therapies should be applied carefully and accordingly. No matter how deep or shallow it is, acupuncture techniques depend on reasonable judgement and, no matter how near or far, on consistent principle of application, as if being on the brink of a deep abyss or as if holding a tiger in your hands, it requires concentration of the mind without getting distracted.

Chapter 26

Eight Solar Terms and Medical Perspective

Yellow Emperor: There must be certain principles for the application of acupuncture; what are the methods and principles at present?
Qibo: The principle is to follow the laws of the heavens and the earth, combined with the movement of the sun, the moon and the stars.

Emperor: I'd like to know it.
Qibo: Whatever method is applied in acupuncture, it should be in accord with the Qi of the sun, the moon and the stars as well as four seasons and eight solar terms; the Qi should be peaceful before needling is performed. Thus, when weather is warm and sunny, the human blood is moist and distending, and defense Qi is floating, so that blood is easy to discharge and Qi can flow. When weather is cold and cloudy, the human blood congeals and defense Qi is sunken. During a new moon, blood Qi begins to be activated and defense Qi starts to flow; during a full moon, blood Qi is full and muscles are firm; during a hollow moon, muscles are loose, meridians are deficient, defense Qi leaves and physique exists alone. Therefore, blood

Qi should be regulated according to the natural time. Hence, there is no needling on a cold day, no slow needling on a warm day, no purging needling during a new moon, no supplement needling during a full moon, and no treatment during a hollow moon, which is called regulation according to the proper time. Similarly, based on the order in nature and time of exuberance or deficiency, light shifting is used to measure the time and the acupuncturist is standing and waiting for the treatment. It is believed that, purging needling during a new moon leads to deficiency of solid viscera; supplementing needling during a full moon leads to blood Qi overflowing and blood stagnation in collaterals, which is called as heavy excess; treating during a hollow moon leads to disordered meridians. As a result, Yin and Yang are identified oppositely, and the healthy or evil Qi cannot be differentiated, so that the disease can invade deeper and linger, with external deficiency and internal disorder, and excessive evil Qi rises.

Emperor: What about observation of the sun, the moon and stars as well as eight solar terms?
Qibo: Observation of stars is a means to measure the movement of the sun and the moon. Observation of the eight solar terms is a means to distinguish the deficiency and excess of winds from eight directions and their approaching time. Observation of four seasons is a means to identify the normal Qi position of spring, autumn, winter and summer for seasonal regulation and to avoid the attacking of deficient evil from eight solar terms. If there is a coincidence of deficiencies between the human body and nature, the double deficiencies affecting each other can invade bones, deep into five solid viscera. Then, doctors who know nature well can cure the disease and avoid the damage in time. It is believed that

it's impossible for doctors not to know the contraindication of nature.

Emperor: Good. I have heard that the principle following the rules of stars changes and I'd like to know how to learn it from the ancient.
Qibo: In order to follow the ancient principle, doctors should learn *Classic of Acupuncture* firstly. When proving ancient theory at the present time, doctors should first know the cold or warmth of the sun, waning or waxing of the moon and sinking or floating of seasonal Qi, so as to regulate the Qi of human body and obtain good therapeutic effect soon. So-called observing dim manifestation is that, though physique, Qi, nutrition and defense Qi haven't been exposed outside, a doctor can identify them by himself with comprehensive analysis of cold or warmth of the sun, waning or waxing of the moon, sinking or floating of four seasonal Qi and regulate it accordingly. Doctors can foresee something unexposed externally, which is believed to be the principle for observing dim manifestations. The extreme knowledge with broad sense can be passed down for generations, which is the difference from the common doctors. However physique Qi is not exposed outside and so cannot be seen, nor does it have forms when seeing and or flavors when tasting. That is called dim manifestation, just like a sprite.

Deficient evils are the Qi of deficient evils from eight solar terms. Excessive evil means that strenuous physical labor leads to sweating with opening interstitial striae and occasional contracting deficient wind. But though the excessive evil can attack the body, there is only mild morbid condition, the morbid condition is hard to be identified and the morbid manifestations are hard to be observed. If doctors want to save the patient with developing diseases, they should observe Qi of three regions and nine positions, and regulate the undeteriorated Qi to save the patient, so that they can be regarded as an excellent doctor. The poor doctor can treat the patient with developed diseases or with deteriorated diseases. Those who can treat the patient with developed diseases cannot know the harmony or disharmony of three regions and nine positions and let it worsen. In order to know the focus of diseases, doctors should identify the morbid pulse of three regions and nine positions to estimate the prognosis and then treat it, which is similar to guarding the defensive gate to know the internal evil trace without seeing its external manifestation.

Emperor: I've heard the therapies of supplement and purging but don't know their action.
Qibo: Application of purging therapy must be associated closely with a word 'Just'. The situations concerned with word 'Just' include Qi just in exuberance, the moon just in fullness, the sun just in warmness, the human body just in peace status, inserting needles just at the start of inhalation, rotating needles just at the start of the next inhalation, and withdrawing needles just at the start of exhalation. It is said that application of purging therapy must be associated closely with 'just' to ensure the normal Qi circulation. Application of supplementing therapy must be associated closely with the word 'Round'. The word 'Round' means circulation of Qi. The circulation means guiding Qi to the focus, so that the needles should be inserted at the acupoint for nutrition and be withdrawn during exhalation. Therefore, the words 'Round' and 'Just' do not refer to the needling instruments. Hence, those who want to culture spirit must know fatness or thinness of the body and exuberance or

decline of nutrition, defense, blood and Qi. Blood Qi is in fact the spirit of the human and everyone should emphasize nothing but a careful culturing spirit.

Emperor: What a wonderful elucidation! Human body is combined with Yin–Yang and four seasons with their deficiency and excess for observing the dim manifestation, for which nobody but you can master it. However you, the Master, have mentioned physique and spirit several times; what is the physique and what is the spirit? I'd like to know.
Qibo: Please allow me to introduce the physique. The so-called physique is something exposed outside that is sometimes hard to see. However, after inquiry about the case history and examination of meridians, it can be disclosed clearly. But if there is no sense with pulse-taking, there will be no more information about the disease, and this is called the physique.

Emperor: What is the spirit?
Qibo: Please allow me to introduce the spirit. The so-called spirit is something that isn't heard by ears but inspected by eyes and heart to have an appreciation, which a doctor can sense himself but cannot express linguistically. They can be seen by people but can only be perceived by a good doctor. No matter how complicated the case is, he can have an insight into the disease like wind blowing the cloud away, which is called spirit. If originating from three regions and nine positions, it's unnecessary to be tied up with the theory of nine needles.

Chapter 27

Separation and Combination of Genuine Qi and Evil Qi

Yellow Emperor: I've heard that Nine Needles has nine articles, and you have expanded it by nine times for each one, obtaining eighty-one articles, which I read over and understood. The symposium *Nine Needles* mentioned the exuberance and decline of Qi and their shift to the left and the right, regulation with the upper for the lower or with the left for the right, and excess and deficiency, for which purging or supplementing is applied at creek or stream acupoint. I already know it. All these changes are the shift of nutrition and defense and outcome of deficiency and excess, but not the invasion of evil into meridians from outside. I'd like to know, after evil invading the meridians, what are the manifestations of the patient and what are the treatments for it?

Qibo: When a sage is making the rules and measurements, he must comply with the laws of the heavens and the earth. Since the heavens have its orbits and the earth has its rivers, the human body has meridians. If the heavens and the earth are moderate, the meridian flow is peaceful. If the heavens are cold and the earth is frozen, the meridian flow is stagnant.

If the heavens and the earth are hot, the meridian flow is boiling. If there is sudden and violent windstorm, the meridian flow is characterized by roaring waves. After evil invades the meridian, the cold leads to blood congealing, while summer heat leads to Qi being smooth and moistening. The deficient evil invades meridians, as if the river were blown by a strong wind. The flow of the meridians is sometimes surging high at its arrival. It flows along the meridians in order and when it comes at Cunkou and is felt by hand, it can be large or small. The large is morbid and the small is normal. The evil Qi runs indefinitely, and it is difficult to measure whether it is in Yin or Yang, but it can be analyzed by palpitation on three regions and nine positions. As soon as the evil Qi is defined, it should be blocked as early as possible. At the start of inhalation, needles are inserted and Qi reversal should be prevented. At resting, needles are retained and evil Qi spreading should be prevented. At the start of inhalation, needles are rotated to wait for Qi arrival as a goal. During exhalation, needles are withdrawn slowly till the end of exhalation. Thus, the major evil is discharged outside, which is called as purging manipulation.

Emperor: How to apply supplementing therapy for the deficiency?

Qibo: The doctor should touch and search and feel the acupoint by hand, press and knead it, flick and expand it, pinch it and insert the needle, open it and then withdraw the needle, and block it to prevent Qi from leaking. At the start of exhalation, the needle is inserted, and at resting the needle is retained to wait for the Qi arrival as a goal. After inserting the needle, the doctor should wait for the arrival of Qi just like waiting for the guests, patiently no matter how long it takes. When Qi is arriving, it should be protected, and the needle can be withdrawn at the start of inhalation to avoid Qi leakage. At the proper place, the pinhole is closed to maintain its genuine Qi and retain the great meridian Qi, which is called as supplementing therapy.

Emperor: How to wait for diagnosis and treat evil Qi?
Qibo: When evil enters meridians from collaterals and lingers in blood vessels, the cold and heat are stirring up each other, like surging waves coming and going over the infinite places. So, when it is coming, the acupoint should be pressed, in order to stop the evil Qi; then the needle is inserted to purge it, but avoid needling against it. Genuine Qi is Qi in the meridians. If meridian Qi is too weak, purging therapy cannot be used at any time, which is the reason for this therapy. Therefore, when a doctor is waiting for evil Qi carelessly and major evil Qi has left elsewhere, the purging therapy will deplete genuine Qi, the genuine Qi is hard to recover and the evil will come again, which makes the disease more severe. That is to say, it's useless to trace the leaving evil. The crossbow shouldn't be hanged to delay drawing; when the evil comes, the needle should be inserted to purge the evil. If this application is too early or too late, blood and Qi will be depleted and the disease cannot be cured. Therefore, knowing the proper application of purging therapy is like drawing a crossbow, and not knowing the proper application is like using a wood mallet clumsily. Also, those who know the proper application shouldn't delay drawing a crossbow, and those who don't know the proper application will stop drawing a crossbow, which is the difference between them.

Emperor: How to apply the supplementing or purging therapy?
Qibo: It is associated with the therapy of attacking evil. The needle should be withdrawn rapidly to remove the excessive

blood to recover the genuine Qi; the new evil invades the body and has no definite focus, which will invade further if pushed and will stop if guided. If reverse needling is practiced, the blood will be stagnated, which should be needled till bleeding, and the disease can be cured immediately.

Emperor: Good! When the genuine Qi is mingled with the evil, there will be no pulse wave; how to palpate the patient?
Qibo: The excess and deficiency of three regions and nine positions should be carefully examined to regulate it. The pulses of inconsistency or loss, the left or the right, and up or down should be analyzed, in order to define the focus of the solid viscera and then needle it. If not knowing the three regions, a doctor cannot distinguish Yin and Yang and differentiate the heavens and the earth. The heavens part is judged based on pulse of the heavens region, the earth part based on pulse of the earth region, and the human part is based on pulse of human affairs region, which can confirm the conditions of three regions. It's believed that if not knowing the location of morbid pulses on three regions and nine positions, though the major disease comes in an obvious manner, the doctor still cannot inhibit it. It is regarded as the great mistake that the innocent part is inhibited or even killed, which disturbs the major meridians and makes genuine Qi not recover. Its causes include taking excess as deficiency, evil as genuine and unreasonable acupuncture to make Qi an evildoer that robs the body of the healthy Qi. As a result, the complying syndrome reverses, nutrition and defense Qi are disturbed, the genuine Qi is lost and only evil exists inside, which will shorten human's life span and lead to disaster. Those who don't know the positions of the three regions and nine pulses cannot work as a

good doctor for long term. Because he can't know the combination of four seasons and five elements, as well as the overlapping and domination, the doctor will release the evil and attack the healthy Qi, which will reduce the patient's life. When invading the body, the new evil has no definite target to attack. It will invade forward when using pushing needles, but stop if guided; the disease can be cured if it is purged against the evil flow.

Chapter 28

Comprehensive Theory on Deficiency and Excess

Emperor: What is deficiency and excess?
Qibo: Evil Qi being excessive is called the excess and essence Qi being depleted is called as deficiency.

Emperor: How about explaining deficiency and excess in details?
Qibo: An example of Qi deficiency is lung deficiency, while that of Qi reversal is foot coldness, which will not kill the patient when not in the due time but will kill the patient when the disease occurs in due time, so will the excess or deficiency of other solid viscera.

Emperor: What is double excess?
Qibo: The so-called double excess is, for example, great heat diseases with Qi heat and full pulse.

Emperor: How about the excess of both meridians and collaterals? How to treat it?
Qibo: The excess of both meridians and collaterals refers to acute Cun pulse and slow Chi pulse, both of which should be treated. It's believed that smooth pulse indicates compliance

while unsmooth pulse indicates reversal. Since the deficiency and excess of human body originate from living things in nature, respectively, the five solid viscera, bones and muscles reflect the smooth pulses, indicating the long life span.

Emperor: How about insufficient collaterals Qi and excessive meridian Qi?
Qibo: Insufficient collaterals Qi and excessive meridian Qi are characterized by heat Cun pulse and cold Chi pulse, which is regarded as reversal in autumn and winter and compliance in spring and summer, and the treatment should focus on the major disease.

Emperor: What are the conditions of deficient meridians and full collaterals?
Qibo: The deficient meridians and full collaterals are characterized by heat and full Chi pulse and cold and unsmooth Cun pulse, which indicates death in spring and summer and survival in autumn and winter.

Emperor: How to treat the two diseases?
Qibo: For full collaterals and deficient meridians, Yin meridians can be given moxibustion and Yang meridians can be needled; for full meridians and deficient collaterals, Yin meridians can be needled and Yang meridians can be given moxibustion.

Emperor: What is double deficiency?
Qibo: Pulse deficiency, Qi deficiency and Chi deficiency are collectively called double deficiency.

Emperor: How to differentiate it?
Qibo: Qi deficiency is characterized by intermittent speech in a low voice, Chi deficiency with feeble walking and pulse deficiency by non-Yin pulsation. Of them, the smooth pulse indicates survival and the unsmooth indicates death.

Emperor: Cold Qi is ascending violently and pulse is full and excessive, then what is the outcome?
Qibo: Excessive and slippery pulse indicates survival, while excessive and reversal pulse indicates death.

Emperor: Pulse is excessive and full with coldness of extremities and head heat, then what is the outcome?
Qibo: The disease occurring in spring and autumn leads to survival, while that in winter and summer leads to death. Pulse that is floating and unsmooth or unsmooth pulse with body heat indicates death.

Emperor: How about the outcome of generalized edema?
Qibo: Some patients have generalized edema as well as acute, large and firm pulse but their Chi pulse is unsmooth, which is inconsistent with each other. Under this condition, compliance indicates survival while reversal indicates death.

Emperor: What is the compliance for survival and reversal for death?
Qibo: The so-called compliance refers to warm hands and feet. The so-called reversal is cold hands and feet.

Emperor: Some breastfeeding women are ill with critical small pulse; what is the outcome?
Qibo: Warm hands and feet indicate survival and extremely cold hands and feet indicate death.

Emperor: Some breastfeeding patients are attacked by wind-heat and have wheezing and dyspnea with raised shoulders, so what are the pulse conditions?
Qibo: If the patient has wheezing and dyspnea with raised shoulders, the pulse is solid and large. Then, moderate pulse indicates survival and acute pulse indicates death.

Emperor: How about the dysentery with blood in stool?
Qibo: A hot body indicates death while an extremely cold body indicates survival.

Emperor: How about dysentery with white foam discharge?
Qibo: Sunken pulse indicates survival, while floating pulse indicates death.

Emperor: How about dysentery with white pus and blood?
Qibo: Critical expiry pulse indicates death while slippery and large pulse indicates survival.

Emperor: Some patients suffer from dysentery and the like without body heat and critical expiry pulse. What is the outcome?
Qibo: Slippery pulse indicates survival while critical unsmooth pulse indicates death, and this date of death can be inferred according the dominative date of solid viscera.

Emperor: How about the epilepsy?
Qibo: If pulse is large and slippery, the disease will be cured spontaneously after long time; if pulse is small, firm and acute, the disease will be incurable, leading to death.

Emperor: What about deficient and excessive pulse of epilepsy?
Qibo: Deficient pulse indicates a curable disease, while excessive pulse indicates death.

Emperor: What are the outcomes of deficient and excessive pulses concerned with consumptive thirst?
Qibo: Excessive and large pulse indicates a curable disease, while critical small and firm pulse indicates incurable disease.

Emperor: As to the degree of physique, bones, vessels and sinews, how to measure their degrees, respectively?

Emperor continued: In spring, the disease should be treated by needling acupoints on meridians and collaterals; in summer, the disease should be treated by needling acupoints on meridians; in autumn, the disease should be treated by needling acupoints of six hollow viscera; in winter, the disease is characterized by obstruction, which should be treated using medication more than needles and stone therapies. The so-called less usage of needles and stone therapies don't include carbuncles and gangrene, which should be treated by acupuncture without hesitation. If the location of carbuncle poison is vagous and impalpable, and pain is on and off, the acupoints of Qihu (ST13)* and Kufang (ST14) beside the hand-Taiyin meridian are needled three times and the acupoints of Shuitu (ST10) and Qishe (ST11) beside the neck are needled two times. For carbuncles in armpit, acupoints of Yuanye (GB22) and Zhejin (GB23) on Shaoyang of foot are needled five times. If the fever doesn't come down, the acupoint Tianchi (PC01) of Jueyin pericardium meridian of hand is needled three times, and acupoints of Lieque (LU07) on the hand-Taiyin meridian and acupoints of Jianzhen (SI09) on shoulder are needled three times, respectively. If there is acute pain, flaccid sinews, more pain with the progression of carbuncles and profuse sweating due to Qi deficiency of bladder meridian, the acupoints of the meridians concerned should be needled.

---

*The acupuncture points are referred to by their traditional names in *Huangdi Neijing*. The meridians and numbers are added by the translator.

If there is acute abdominal distension which cannot be pressed down, the acupoint on the hand-Taiyang meridian, i.e. the collection acupoint of stomach, and the acupoints of Zhishi (BL52), horizontal to Shenshu (BL23) and three cun away from the spine are needled with a round-sharp-tip needle. For cholera, the Zhishi (BL52) acupoints beside Shenshu (BL23) acupoints are needled five times and Weishu (BL21) acupoints and Weicang (BL50) acupoints beside foot-Yangming are needled three times. For epilepsy, the acupoints of five meridians are needled, including Jingqu (LU08) acupoints on hand-Taiyin meridian five times, Yanggu (ST15) acupoints of hand-Taiyang five times, Zhizheng (ST07) acupoints beside hand-Taiyang meridian one time, Jiexie (ST41) acupoints of foot-Yangming meridian, and Zhubing (KI19) acupoints five cun above the upper ankle three times.

The consumptive thirst, stroke, hemiplegia, flaccid paralysis and panting with reversal Qi are the diseases caused by greasy food, especially among those who are obese and rich men. Stuffy chest, obstructive respiration and loss of communication between the upper and the lower are caused by rage or depression. Sudden syncope with deafness, dysuria and constipation are caused by internal evil Qi violating the weak parts. Since some diseases are caused by external invasion instead of internal stirring, the wind evil lingers in the body leading to emaciation. Difficult and painful walking are caused by cold wind and damp.

Yellow Emperor: Jaundice, acute pain, epileptic disease and mania are caused by long-term invasion of evil. Disharmony of five solid viscera is caused by obstruction of six hollow viscera. Headache, tinnitus and obstruction of nine orifices are caused by gastrointestinal disease.

Chapter 29

Taiyin and Yangming Meridians

Yellow Emperor: Taiyin and Yangming are related as exterior and interior, i.e. spleen and stomach meridians. Why do these two meridians involve diseases with different manifestations?
Qibo: Yin and Yang meridians with different routes show deficiency or excess, reversal or compliance, and develop diseases from either the external or the internal factors alternatively, which results in different kinds of diseases.

Emperor: I'd like to know the different mechanisms.
Qibo: Yang, corresponding to heavenly Qi, governs the external defense, while Yin, corresponding to earthly Qi, governs the internal nourishment. So, Yang's property is associated with excess while Yin is with deficiency. When theft-wind and deficiency wind attack, Yang is affected, while when improper diet and irregular life occur, Yin is affected. After Yang is attacked, the evil invades six hollow viscera, while after Yin is attacked, the evil invades five solid viscera. Evil involving six hollow viscera leads to body fever, failure to sleep and panting due to surging Qi, while evil in five solid viscera leads to chest fullness, abdominal blockage, and diarrhea after indigestion, which progresses into dysentery in the long run. Then the

throat corresponds to heavenly Qi while the pharynx to earthly Qi. Moreover, Yang is exposed to wind evil while Yin to damp evil. Thus, Yin Qi ascends from feet to the head and descends along arms to finger tips, while Yang Qi ascends from hands to the head and descends to feet. It's believed that Yang diseases ascend to peak and then descend, while Yin diseases descend to peak and then ascend. Therefore in case of wind, the upper is affected first, while in case of damp, the lower is affected first.

Emperor: With spleen diseased, four limbs will be disabled, and why?

Qibo: Four limbs receive Qi from stomach, not directly through meridians but through spleen by which the limbs are endowed. If spleen is diseased and cannot directly transport fluid and liquid for stomach, four limbs cannot obtain Qi of water and grain and suffer from Qi declination day by day, so that the meridians are blocked and none of sinews, bones and muscles can be nourished, which leads to dysfunction of four limbs.

Emperor: Spleen does not correspond to one season alone, and why?

Qibo: Spleen corresponds to earth and governs the center, which nourishes the four solid viscera in four seasons, prospers to the peak taking the last eighteen days of every season and cannot correspond to sole season. Spleen embodies essence for stomach, like the earth generating all living things and following the rule of the heavens and the earth, so it can transport from the head to feet and cannot govern sole season.

Emperor: Spleen, connected with stomach by a membrane, can transport fluid and liquid for stomach, why?

Qibo: Foot-Taiyin meridian is the third Yin, which runs through stomach, belongs to spleen and is connected with pharynx, which transports Qi along all Yin meridians for stomach. Yangming meridian is the exterior of Taiyin and the sea of five solid and six hollow viscera, which can help transport Qi along triple-Yang meridians. The solid and hollow viscera receive Qi through spleen meridian from Yangming, so spleen transports fluid and liquid for stomach. Because four limbs cannot receive Qi of water and grain to be declined day by day, the Yin meridians are blocked, and sinews, bones and muscles cannot be nourished, which results in dysfunction of four limbs.

Chapter 30

Explanation on Yangming Meridian

Yellow Emperor: The patient ill with Yangming meridian disease is sick of seeing people and fire. He is frightened at hearing wood sound but not at hearing sound of bells or drums; why is he frightened at hearing wood sound? I'd like to know the reason.
Qibo: Yangming is the stomach meridian and corresponds to earth. The patient is frightened at hearing wood sound because earth fears wood.

Emperor: Good! Why does the patient fear fire?
Qibo: Yangming meridian governs muscles, which has exuberant blood–Qi, so invasion of evil will cause fever and high fever will lead to fearing fire.

Emperor: Why does the patient fear seeing people?
Qibo: Reversal Qi of Yangming meridian causes panting and even dyspnea, which leads to fear of seeing people.

Emperor: Some patients will die of panting and some will survive, what is the reason for this?
Qibo: Critical reversal Qi involving solid viscera will lead to death, while reversal Qi involving meridians leads to survival.

Emperor: Good! The patient with more severe disease will throw away the clothes to walk wildly and climb high to sing. Though he hasn't had food for several days, the patient can climb walls to the roof. He cannot do these deeds in usual days, but he can when suffering from this disease, why?
Qibo: Four limbs are the base of all Yang. Yang is exuberant and four limbs are in excess, which makes him climb high.

Emperor: Why does the patient throw away the clothes to walk wildly?
Qibo: Heat is exuberant in the body, which makes him throw away the clothes to walk wildly.

Emperor: The patient will scold and curse, fail to differentiate the close and the distant, and sing wildly. Why?
Qibo: Yang exuberance makes the patient scold and curse, fail to differentiate the close and the distant, and have no desire for food. No desire for food leads to walking wildly.

Chapter 31

Heat Disease

Yellow Emperor: Nowadays, febrile diseases are all categorized as cold damage, some of which are cured and some of which cause death; those who die have the disease course no more than six to seven days while those who survive have it for more than ten days, why? I don't know the cause, but would like to know the reason.
Qibo: Taiyang is the one that any other Yang meridians converge to. It is connected with acupoint Fengfu (DU16)*, so it can govern Qi for all Yang meridians. After being damaged by cold, the man will have febrile disease. Though with fever, the patient won't die. If two (exterior and interior) meridians are affected by cold and cause disease, the patient cannot avoid death.

Emperor: I'd like to know the manifestations.
Qibo: On the first day of cold damage course, Taiyang meridian is affected, leading to headache and nape pain as well as rigid waist and spine. On the second day of cold damage course, Yangming meridian is affected, which governs

---

*The acupuncture points are referred to by their traditional names in *Huangdi Neijing*. The meridians and numbers are added by the translator.

muscles, runs along both sides of the nose and is connected to eyes, so body fever, eye pain, dry nose and insomnia will develop. On the third day of cold damage course, Shaoyang meridian is affected, which governs gallbladder, and runs along hypochondria and is connected to ears, so there will develop chest pain, hypochondriac pain and deaf ears. If the three Yang meridians are all affected but not involved in viscera, the disease can be cured after sweating. On the fourth day of cold damage course, Taiyin meridian is affected, which is distributed over the stomach and is connected to pharynx, so abdominal fullness and dry pharynx will develop. On the fifth day of cold damage course, Shaoyin runs through kidney, which is connected to lung and linked with tongue root, so dry mouth and tongue with a feeling of thirst will develop. On the sixth day of cold damage course, Jueyin meridian is affected, which runs along genitals and is connected to liver, so vexation will develop, as will distention and dragging of testicles. If three Yin and three Yang meridians as well as five solid and six hollow viscera are all affected, nutrition and defensive aspects lose movement, and five solid viscera don't communicate, so the patient will die.

If two meridians are not affected by cold, on the seventh day the severity of Taiyang disease will be reduced and headache improved; on the eighth day, the severity of Yanming disease will be reduced and body fever decreased; on the ninth day, the severity of Shaoyang disease will be reduced and deafness improved; on the tenth day, the severity of Taiyin disease will be reduced and abdominal fullness will subside to normal with desire for food; on the eleventh day, the severity of Shaoyin disease will be reduced, there will be no thirst and no distention, and sneezing after tongue dryness; on twelfth day, the severity of Jueyin disease is reduced, so loose scrotum and lower abdomen will develop; when most of evil Qi has subsided, the disease can be cured in days to come.

Emperor: How to treat these diseases?
Qibo: The treatments are aimed at communication between the visceral meridians accordingly so that the disease severity will be reduced till it is cured. For disease course less than three days, sweating therapy can be applied to cure the disease; for disease course that spans three days or more, the purging therapy can be applied to cure the disease.

Emperor: Some febrile diseases have been cured in general, but there appears to be fever that still remains, why?
Qibo: Any remaining fever is caused by forcing feeding during the period of high fever, leading to the remaining fever. In such conditions, the disease severity is reduced, but the heat evil is hidden in the body. Influenced by grain Qi, two kinds of heat are combined to result in the remaining fever.

Emperor: Fine! How to treat the remaining fever?
Qibo: According to the deficiency and excess, purging and supplementing can be regulated so that the remaining fever can disappear.

Emperor: Is there any food contraindication for the patient with fever?
Qibo: When the severity of fever is reduced slightly, ingesting meat will make the disease recur and excessive dieting causes remaining fever, both of which are contraindicated.

Emperor: If two meridians concerned are both affected by cold, what is the correspondence between the meridians and the manifestation?
Qibo: If two meridians are both affected by cold evil, on the first day of the disease course, Taiyang and Shaoyin are both morbid, leading to headache, dry mouth, vexation and fullness; on the second day, Yangming and Taiyin are both morbid, leading to abdominal fullness, body fever, no desire for food, and ravings; on the third day, Shaoyang and Jueyin are both morbid, leading to deafness, dragging testes with severe chill, no desire for water and soup and unconsciousness; and the patient will die on the sixth day.

Emperor: Five solid viscera are damaged, six hollow viscera aren't communicating and the nutrition and defensive aspects lose movement. After this, the patient will die on the third day, why?
Qibo: Yangming meridian is the chief of the twelve meridians, whose blood Qi is the most exuberant, so the patient cannot recognize the acquaintance if it is damaged. In three days, its Qi is exhausted, indicating death. Among the diseases with cold damage that turn into warm disease, the one developing before the summer solstice is termed warm disease, while that which develops after summer solstice is termed summer-heat disease. Since summer heat should be expelled with sweating, its sweating cannot be inhibited.

Chapter 32

Treatment of Heat Disease with Acupuncture

The patient with febrile disease of liver first has yellow urine, followed by abdominal pain, sleepiness and body fever. When liver is struggling with heat evil, there will appear ravings even with fright, full and painful hypochondria, agitated hands and feet, and loss of sleep. During the Seventh–Eighth day, the manifestation is more severe; during the First–Second day, there is profuse sweating, and with Qi reversal the patient will die on the Seventh–Eighth day. For treatment, the acupoints on foot-Jueyin and foot-Shaoyang meridians can be needled. With reversal Qi, headache with vertigo will develop, due to heat evil surging to the head.

The patient with febrile disease of the heart first feels unhappy and then has fever lasting for several days; when the heart is struggling with heat evil, there will be sudden episodes of heart pain, vexation, frequent vomiting, headache, reddish face and no sweating; during the Ninth–Tenth day, the manifestation is more severe, and during the Third–Fourth day profuse sweating is observed; with Qi reversal, the patient will die on the Ninth–Tenth day; for treatment, acupoints on hand-Shaoyin and hand-Taiyang meridians can be needled.

The patient with febrile disease of spleen first has heavy head, cheek pain, vexation, green complexion, nausea and body fever. When spleen is struggling with heat evil, the patient cannot bow forward and lean backward due to lumbago, they also have abdominal fullness and diarrhea, and feel pain in both cheeks. In the First–Second day, the manifestation is more severe; in the Fifth–Sixth day profuse sweating will be seen, and with Qi reversal the patient will die in the First–Second day. For treatment, acupoints on foot-Taiyin and foot-Yangming meridians can be needled.

The patient with febrile disease of lung first has chill and feels cold, has erect hairs, fears wind and cold, and has a yellow tongue coating and body fever. When lung is struggling with heat evil, there will be panting with cough, wandering pain all over the chest and back, lack of deep breath, intolerant headache, and sweating with cold feeling. During the Third–Fourth day, the manifestation is more severe; on Seventh–Eighth day, there is profuse sweating, and with Qi reversal the patient will die in the Third–Fourth day; for treatment, acupoints on hand-Taiyin and hand-Yangming meridians can be needled. If there is bleeding with amount as much as big beans, it indicates that the disease is cured.

The patient with febrile disease of kidney first has lumbago, sour shanks, unbearable thirst with frequent drinking and body fever. When kidney is struggling with heat evil, signs such as painful and stiff nape, cold and sour shanks, sole heat and no desire to speak will appear. With reversal, there will be nape pain with vertigo and shaking. On the Fifth–Sixth day, the manifestation becomes more severe, during the Ninth–Tenth day there will be profuse sweating, and with Qi reversal the patient will die on the Fifth–Sixth day. For treatment, the acupoints on foot-Shaoyin and foot-Taiyang meridians can be needled. Any kind of sweating mentioned above appears in its dominating day and sweat is secreted.

In febrile disease of liver, the left cheek first appears reddish; in febrile disease of heart, the front head first appears reddish; in febrile disease of spleen, the nose first appears reddish; in febrile disease of lung, the right cheek first appears reddish; in febrile disease of kidney, the lower jaw first appears reddish; though not having developed, the disease can be treated with acupuncture whenever the reddish color appears, and this is called treating the pre-disease. If the febrile disease arises from its complexion region, it will be cured in the dominating day; if not given the right therapy, it will be cured after missing three dominating days. The severe Qi reversal indicates death. For any cases needing sweating therapy, perspiration can be induced on its dominating day to cure the disease.

In treating febrile diseases, the patient can drink cool water and then receive acupuncture; the patient should wear thin clothes and stay in a cool place so that the body can be cooled and the fever can subside. For febrile disease first with chest and hypochondriac pain as well as restless hands and feet, the acupoints on foot-Shaoyang meridian should be needled for dispersion and the acupoints on foot-Taiyin meridian should be needled for supplementation; for the more severe disease, manipulation of Fifty-Nine-Needling therapy should be administered. For the febrile disease starting with arm pain, the acupoints on hand-Yangming and hand-Taiyin meridians should be needled till sweating.

For the febrile disease starting from head, the acupoints on foot-Taiyang meridian should be needled till sweating. For the febrile disease starting from foot and shank, the acupoints of foot-Yangming meridian should be needled till sweating. For febrile disease starting with heavy body, bone pain, deafness and drowsiness, the acupoints on foot-Shaoyin meridian should be needled and for the more severe disease, Fifty-Nine-Needling manipulation therapy should be given. For the febrile disease first with vertigo and then fever, and fullness of the chest and hypochondria, the acupoints on foot-Shaoyin and foot-Shaoyang meridians should be needled.

For the disease of Taiyang meridian, a reddish color appears on the cheek bone, indicating febrile disease. If the reddish complexion does not lose its luster and sweating starts, it indicates the disease can be cured on its dominating day. If the change of Taiyin meridian is struggling with Jueyin, the patient will die in no more than three days, because the disease is associated with kidney, showing complexion of Shaoyang meridian. For the disease of Shaoyang meridian, the reddish complexion appears in the front of the cheek, indicating febrile disease. If the reddish complexion does not lose its luster and sweating appears then, it indicates the disease can be cured on its dominating day. If the change of meridian is struggling with Shaoyin meridian, the patient will die in no more than three days.

The Qi acupoints for febrile diseases are as follows: the acupoints at the interval below the third cervical vertebra is mainly for heat in the chest, below the fourth cervical vertebra mainly for heat in the diaphragm, below the fifth cervical vertebra mainly for heat in liver, below the sixth cervical vertebra mainly for heat in spleen, and below the seventh cervical vertebra mainly for heat in kidney; for the diseases in terms of the nutrition aspect, the acupoint needle is on the sacrum. On the nape, there are three vertebrae in the middle, of which the depression is Dazhui. The reddish complexion reversing from cheek to cheek bone indicates dysentery, to the lower jaw indicates abdominal fullness, to the back of the cheek bone indicates hypochondriac pain, and to upper part of the cheek indicates the disease above the diaphragm.

Chapter 33

Commentary on Heat Disease

Yellow Emperor: The patient with warm disease has fever again soon after sweating with an agitated swift pulse. The condition isn't relieved by sweating therapy and instead there appears delirium in speech and failure to eat, what is this term?
Qibo: It is termed Yin–Yang wrestle, which indicates approaching death.

Emperor: I'd like to know its explanation.
Qibo: Man can sweat in that sweat fluid originates from grains that originate from essence. Now the evil Qi is wrestling in bones and muscles leading to sweating, indicating that evil is expelled and the essence dominates. If essence can dominate, the patient can eat without fever relapse. Fever relapse indicates the existence of evil. Sweat embodies essence. Now when there is fever relapse soon after sweating, it indicates evil dominance. The patient cannot eat because the essence cannot be supplemented. The disease is lingering in the body and the patient is on the verge of death. Moreover it is said in *On Fever* that agitating exuberant pulse after sweating indicates death. Now the pulse doesn't correspond to sweating, which reflects the failure to overcome the disease, indicating approaching

death. Delirious speech reflects unconsciousness, which indicates the approaching death. Now there appears three indications of death with no indication of life, and though improved, the patient is doomed to die.

Emperor: Some patients with body fever have sweating, vexation and distention, and vexation and distention cannot be resolved by sweating therapy. What is this disease?
Qibo: Body fever after sweating is associated with wind, and vexation and distention unresolved after sweating are associated with reversal, both of which are termed as wind-reversal.

Emperor: I'd like to know its reason.
Qibo: Taiyang meridian governs Qi, so it is first affected by the evil. Shaoyin meridian is related with Taiyang through an interior and exterior relationship, so Shaoyin gets the heat to comply with Taiyang, which results in Qi reversal.

Emperor: How about its treatment?
Qibo: The acupoints of exterior and interior meridians can be needled and decoction can be medicated.

Emperor: What is overstraining with wind?
Qibo: Overstraining with wind manifests below the lung and reflects the disease with signs such as stiff nape, blurred vision, sputum like snivel, aversion to wind and shivering with cold.

Emperor: How about its treatment?
Qibo: To treat the obstruction in the chest, Taiyang meridian is perfused with essence and the disease will be cured in three days, for the patient in middle age in five days, and for the patient with less essence in seven days. The greenish and yellowish sputum coughed up is as thick as pus and as big as a

bolus which is expectorated from mouth or nose as otherwise it will damage lung, indicating approaching death.

Emperor: Some patients with kidney wind have swollen face and periorbital puffiness, which hinders speech, and can acupuncture be done in such cases?
Qibo: The deficiency syndrome shouldn't be treated with acupuncture, as otherwise the needling will trigger the arrival of reversal Qi.

Emperor: What is the outcome when reversal Qi arrives?
Qibo: When reversal Qi arrives, there will be less Qi, sometimes fever that starts from the chest and moves up to the head, hand heat after sweating, dry mouth and bitter thirst, yellow urine, puffiness below eyes, abdominal rumbling, heavy body with walking difficulty, pause of menstruation, vexation and failure to eat, failure to sleep flat, and cough when sleeping flat, which is termed wind water and discussed in *On Acupuncture Manipulation*.

Emperor: I'd like to know the mechanism.
Qibo: Where evils attack, there will be deficiency. The case with Yin deficiency must be attacked by Yang evil, so there will be less Qi, sometimes fever with sweating, yellow urine, and heat in the lower abdomen. Failure to sleep flat is due to disharmony in the stomach. Cough when sleeping flat is due to oppression upon lung. For any kind of water Qi diseases, slight edema is first seen below eyes.

Emperor: What is the reason?
Qibo: Water pertains to Yin and so does the region below eye while the abdomen is the place where the extreme Yin resides. Where there is water in the abdomen, there will be swelling

below eyes. The critical Qi ascending upwards leads to bitter mouth, dry tongue, failure to sleep flat, and coughing up clear water when sleeping flat. For any kind of water diseases, the patient cannot sleep and is frightened when sleeping, leading to more cough. Abdominal rumbling originates from the stomach. Oppression on spleen leads to vexation and failure to eat. Difficulty in swallowing food is due to obstruction of stomach and diaphragm. The body is too heavy to walk because stomach meridian is on the leg. The pause of menstruation is due to blockage of uterine vessels. Uterine vessels are attributed to heart and connected with womb. Now, reversal Qi ascends to oppress lung upwards and heart Qi fails to communicate downwards, so the menstruation pauses.

Emperor: Good.

Chapter 34

Disharmony of Diseases

Yellow Emperor: Some have unusual body temperature and abnormal fever with vexation and distention, why?
Qibo: There is less Yin Qi and Yang Qi dominance, so the patient has fever with vexation and distention.

Emperor: Though not wearing thin clothes and not attacked by cold, the patient still feels cold from inside the body, why?
Qibo: This is mostly due to impediment Qi with more Yin and less Yang, thus feeling body cold like being out of water.

Emperor: Some have fever over four limbs, feeling hot like being burned on fire when attacked by wind and cold, why?
Qibo: It is because the patient has deficient Yin Qi and exuberant Yang Qi. The four limbs correspond to Yang. When two Yangs meet while Yin Qi is deficient and less water fails to put out exuberant fire, that sole Yang will dominate. The governing of sole Yang cannot grow while the dominance of sole Yang will deprive body of vitality. With wind attacking, the four limbs feel hot like being burned on fire and the patient's muscles become emaciated.

Emperor: The patient has a cold feeling which cannot be relieved by hot water or fire or putting on more clothes, but he doesn't shiver with cold; what disease is it?
Qibo: The patient has innate dominance of kidney Qi and goes in for the job with water so that his Taiyang Qi declines, kidney lipid is withered without production, and then the sole water cannot dominate two fires. Since kidney is associated with water and governs bone growth, kidney lipid cannot be produced and the marrow cannot be filled fully, causing cold sensation deep in the bones. The patient doesn't shiver with cold in that liver corresponds to the first Yang and heart to the second Yang. Kidney is a sole viscus and solar water cannot dominate double fires, so that the patient doesn't shiver with cold, termed bone impediment and the patient must have spasm of joints.

Emperor: The patient with muscular numbness and heaviness still feels the same feeling though touching clothes or quilts, what disease is it?
Qibo: It is due to deficient nutrition Qi and excess defense Qi. Deficient nutritional Qi leads to numbness and deficient defensive Qi leads to failure of movement. The deficiency of both nutrition and defense leads to numbness and limb disability, but the muscles seem unchanged in appearance. The body doesn't cooperate with the mind, which indicates approaching death.

Emperor: With Qi reversal, some patients fail to sleep and breathe with adventitious sound, some fail to sleep and breathe without adventitious sounds, some can live a regular life and breathe with adventitious sound, some can sleep but walk with panting, some fail to sleep and walk with panting, and some fail to sleep and sleep with panting. What are the solid viscera involved, respectively? I'd like to know the reasons.

Qibo: Failing to sleep and breathing with adventitious sound is due to Qi reversal of Yangming meridian. Since three Yang meridians of foot run downwards, there will be breathing with adventitious sounds due to Qi ascending reversely now. Yangming is the stomach meridian, and stomach is the sea of six hollow viscera, whose Qi also runs downwards. If Yangming meridian has Qi reversal and cannot follow its normal course, it will induce failure of sleeping. It was said in *The Lower Set of Classics* that disharmony in stomach results in restless sleeping, which is the elucidation concerned. As to living a regular life and breathing with adventitious sound, it is concerned with disharmony in lung's collaterals, and Qi of collaterals fails to run through the course along with the meridians, and then lingers within the meridians. The conditions with morbid collaterals are moderate, so there will be regular life and breathing with adventitious sound. Failing to sleep and panting when sleeping are due to invasion of water Qi. Water is flowing with fluid and liquid, and kidney is the viscus of water, which governs fluid and liquid and is associated with sleeping and panting.

Emperor: Good.

Chapter 35

On Malaria

Yellow Emperor: Any lingering malaria is generally caused by evil wind, and the intermission and paroxysm have periodicity, why?
Qibo: A malarial paroxysm starts from the skin hair, is followed by yawning and stretching, shivering chill and teeth chattering, and then waist and spinal pain. After chill subsides, fever rises within the body, accompanied by split headache and extreme thirst with preference to cold drink.

Emperor: What kind of Qi causes this disease? I'd like to know the mechanism.
Qibo: Yang Qi and Yin Qi are wrestling up and down with alternating excess and deficiency and transferring to each other. When Yang is combined with Yin, Yin becomes excessive and Yang becomes deficient. Deficiency of Yangming causes chill and teeth chattering. Deficiency of Taiyang causes pain of the waist, back and nape. Deficiency of all three Yang meridians causes dominance of Yin. Dominance of Yin causes cold and bone pain. Then cold rises from the internal body, leading to cold of both internal and external body. Yang exuberance causes extreme heat, while Yin deficiency causes

internal heat. With both fevers, there will be panting with thirst and preference for cold water. The disease is generally affected by damage of summer heat. Heat Qi is exuberant and hidden in the skin but outside the stomach and intestine, where the nutrition Qi is housed. This change makes sweat pores loose and interstitial striae open. The condition is triggered by autumn Qi and the patient is attacked by wind when sweating or later when bathing. Water Qi lingers in the skin and resides with defense Qi. The so-called defense Qi runs along the Yang meridians during the daytime and the Yin meridians during the night, which obtains Yang to expose out and obtains Yin to stir internally; the Qi wrestling between the internal and external causes daily paroxysm.

Emperor: Why do some malarial paroxysms occur every other day?
Qibo: The evil Qi is lingering in deep focus and oppressing Yin, so that Yang Qi is dispersing solely. Yin evil is stagnated, and Yin and Yang are wrestling, which cannot be exposed outward, leading to paroxysm every other day.

Emperor: Good. Some paroxysm occurs late and some early, what kind of Qi makes it?
Qibo: The evil Qi invades the wind house and runs along the spine downwards. The defense Qi meets at the wind house every day and night while the evil Qi descends down the spine by one section a day, so the malaria paroxysm occurs later. It invades the back and spine. Whenever evil Qi arrives in the wind house, interstitial striae are open, which allows evil Qi to enter, leading to later occurrence of paroxysm. The evil Qi starts from the wind house and descends by one section a day; on the twenty-fifth day, it reaches the sacrum; on the

twenty-sixth day, it goes into spine again and hides in the thoroughfare channel; the evil ascends and on the ninth day comes out of the supraclavicular fossae. The evil ascends higher day by day, and its paroxysm occurs earlier day by day. Its paroxysm occurring every other day is due to evil internal oppression on five solid viscera and violating primordial membrane. Its spreading path is long, its Qi invading is deep and its expression is late; the evil Qi cannot run along with defensive Qi or go outside, so it leads to the paroxysm occurring every other day.

Emperor: You have said that when defense Qi arrives at the wind house, the interstitial striae are open and then the evil Qi takes the opportunity to invade and trigger the paroxysm. Now the defensive Qi descends down by one section a day and its evil Qi paroxysm doesn't occur at the wind house but occurs every other day, why?
Qibo: The evil Qi invades the head and nape and descends along the spine, which can attack the different foci due to alternative excess or deficiency in the body, so that it doesn't occur at wind house. Thus if evil attacks at the vertex, the defense Qi arrival triggers the disease of the vertex; at the back, it triggers the disease of the back; at waist and spine, it triggers the disease of the waist and spine; at the hands and feet, it triggers the disease of the hands and feet. Wherever the defense Qi approaches, it will be combined with evil to trigger the disease. Therefore, the so-called wind has no fixed house. If the defense Qi approaches, the interstitial striae must be open. The place where the defense Qi is combined with evil is just its house.

Emperor: Good! Wind and malaria are of the same category, but wind is always solely stirring while malaria is attacking on and off, why?

Qibo: Wind Qi lingers in a certain place, so it always exists there. Malaria Qi is running along with meridians and collaterals and invades deep, leading to oppression internally, so that the defensive Qi can react with it to cause paroxysm.

Emperor: The case with malaria first has chill and later fever, why?

Qibo: After the patient was damaged by great heat in summer, there will be profuse sweating and open interstitial striae in the summer. Then, the patient is exposed to the icy coldness of water in summer, the cold evil is hidden in interstitial striae of the skin, and the effect of wind in autumn will cause the malaria. The cold pertains to Yin Qi while the wind pertains to Yang Qi. During the first sign of affect by cold and later by wind, the patient will have chill and later fever with periodic paroxysms, which is termed cold malaria.

Emperor: There appears fever first and chill later, why?

Qibo: It is first affected by wind and later by cold, so the patient will first have fever and later chill, also with periodic paroxysm, which is termed warm malaria. If there is only fever without chill, Yin Qi is first exhausted and then Yang Qi is exposed solely, the patient will have short of breath, vexation, febrile hands and feet, and vomiting, which is termed as hot malaria.

Emperor: It is said in the classics that the excess should be purged while the deficiency be supplemented. Now the fever pertains to excess and chill to deficiency. The cold feeling in malaria cannot be improved by hot water and fire roasting and the fever is also not cooled down by ice, all of which pertains to excess or deficiency. At that time, the good doctor can do nothing to stop the condition, which could be needled when

the severity is reduced spontaneously, what is the reason? I'd like to know the mechanism.
Qibo: It is said in the classics to avoid needling for high fever, for the disturbed pulses and for profuse sweating because these conditions are the reversal disorders which must not be treated immediately. When the malaria starts to attack, Yang Qi is combined with Yin and Yang deficiency and Yin exuberance develop without external Yang Qi, leading to chill first and shivering later. If Yin Qi is extremely reversed, it will be exposed, overlapping Yang. If Yang is combined with Yin to be exposed outside, Yin is deficient and Yang is excessive, leading to fever first and thirst later. If malaria Qi is combined with Yang, Yang Qi will dominate, and if with Yin, Yin Qi will dominate; Yin dominance causes chill and Yang dominance causes fever. In malaria, wind and cold evil Qi are changing abnormally and the extreme condition will turn into attack. When the disease is attacking, the condition is hot, like fire, or like violent wind and rain that is out of control. So, it is said in the classics that purging treatment at the peak of severity will ruin the health Qi, and purging treatment during the subsiding of disease must be effective. This is the mechanism. When malaria hasn't attacked, Yin isn't combined with Yang and Yang isn't combined with Yin; it is the proper time to give regulation to calm the genuine Qi and make evil Qi die. So, the doctor cannot treat the paroxysm of diseases because of its incurable reversal Qi.

Emperor: Good. How about purging treatment then? How about the early and later timing for the treatment?
Qibo: The paroxysm of malaria is in fact the transference of Yin and Yang, which starts from four extremities. When Yang is damaged and Yin is involved, the focus should be confined prior to paroxysm of malaria, in order to make evil Qi not go

in and Yin Qi not go out. After observing the exuberant and firm conditions of collaterals with stagnated blood, all of them should be needled, which is a therapy directing genuine Qi that hasn't be combined with evil Qi.

Emperor: When malaria is in remittance, what is the response?
Qibo: Malaria Qi must alternate in dominance or deficiency along with the evil; if the evil arrives in the Yang, it causes fever and stirs pulse, and if in the Yin, it causes chill and quiet pulse; in the peak, Yin and Yang are both deficient and defensive Qi is divorced from evil Qi, so that the disease is in remittance; when the defensive Qi is gathering, the disease is in paroxysm.

Emperor: Malaria sometimes occurs every other day or every few days with or without thirst, what is the reason for this?
Qibo: The paroxysm occurring every other day is due to the evil Qi and the defensive Qi invading the six hollow viscera at different times; when sometimes they are divorced and not combined, remittance will be observed for several days followed by the next attack. In malaria, Yin and Yang alternate severely or moderately as well as with or without thirst.

Emperor: It is said in the classics that damage by heat in summer must cause malaria in autumn, but now the pathogenesis of malaria does not correspond to this rule; why?
Qibo: As a rule, malaria corresponds to four seasons, and the heterogenic malaria is opposite to four reasons. Notably, malaria in autumn causes severe chill, in winter causes moderate chill, in spring causes fearing wind and in summer causes profuse sweating.

Emperor: How do evils of warm malaria and cold malaria invade? In which solid viscera do they linger?
Qibo: Warm malaria is contracted by wind in winter and then cold evil is hidden in bone and marrow. When Yang Qi in spring revives, the evil Qi cannot be exposed by itself. Due to great heat in summer, the brain and marrow are depleted, muscle is emaciated, and interstitial striae are opened to discharge evil, or the evil goes out together with sweat, especially during great physical labor. Since the disease is hidden in kidney originally, the evil Qi first goes from the internal to external. In this way, deficient Yin causes exuberant Yang that causes fever. When the body condition declines, evil Qi enters repeatedly, after which Yang is deficient, leading to chills. So, the patient has fever first and later chill, which is termed as warm malaria.

Emperor: How about hot malaria?
Qibo: For the patient with hot malaria, there is heat in lung innately, and lung Qi is exuberant and surging reversely, but the middle Qi is too solid to leak out. When in physical labor, the interstitial striae are open and wind and cold evil are lingering and spreading between skin and intermuscles, by which Yang Qi is exuberant with no declining to cause the disease. The evil Qi doesn't have an effect on Yin, so the case has only fever with no chill; Qi is internally hidden in heart but externally invading intermuscle, resulting in depletion and emaciation, which is termed hot malaria.

Emperor: Good.

Chapter 36

Theory on Acupuncture for Malaria

The malaria involving foot-Taiyang meridian makes the patient suffer from lumbago, heavy head, chill arising from the back followed by fever with hot feeling like fire; if the fever subsides after sweating, it is still difficult for the patient to be cured; for treatment, acupoint Xizhong (BL40)* can be needled.

The malaria involving foot-Shaoyang meridian makes patient suffer from lassitude, moderate chill, moderate fever, fear of meeting people and other forms of fright, prolonged fever and profuse sweating; for treatment, the acupoints on foot-Shaoyang can be needled.

The malaria involving foot-Yangming meridian makes the patient suffer from chill first with shivering feeling, fever after prolonged chill, fever subsiding after sweating, preferring sunlight and moonlight as well as heat from the fire for a comfortable feeling; for treatment, the acupoints above tarsus of foot-Yangming can be needled.

---

*The acupuncture points are referred to by their traditional names in *Huangdi Neijing*. The meridians and numbers are added by the translator.

The malaria involving foot-Taiyin meridian makes the patient suffer from unhappiness, frequent long sigh, no appetite for food, and frequent intermittence of chill and fever and sweating; there is frequent vomiting at the stage of attack, and its severity will be reduced after vomiting; for treatment, the acupoints on this meridian can be needled.

The malaria involving foot-Shaoyin makes patients suffer from severe vomiting, frequent chill and fever, fever more than chill, and a preference to stay in the room with the doors and windows closed, and this, malaria is difficult to be cured.

The malaria involving foot-Jueyin makes patient suffer from severe lumbago, lower abdominal pain, difficulty in urination (like dysuria without urinary retention but with frequent urination), horrible feeling, less Qi and abdominal stagnation; for treatment, the acupoints on foot-Jueyin can be needled.

Malaria involving lung makes patient suffer from heart cold, chill more than fever, frequent fright between fevers as if seeing something; for treatment, the acupoints on hand-Taiyin and hand-Yangming can be needled. Malaria involving heart makes the patient suffer from much vexation, feeling of chills after drinking clear water and slight fever; for the treatment, the acupoints on hand-Shaoyin can be needled. Malaria involving the liver makes the patient suffer from having a green complexion and giving long sighs, as if dying; for treatment, the acupoints on foot-Jueyin can be needled till bleeding. Malaria involving spleen makes the patient suffer from chill, abdominal pain, abdominal rumbling during fever and sweating after rumbling stops; for treatment, the acupoints on foot-Taiyin can be needled. Malaria involving kidney makes the patient suffer from continuous chill, waist and spinal pain with difficult turning over, difficult defecation, blurred vision and cold hands and feet; for treatment, the acupoints on foot-Taiyang and foot-Shaoyin can be needled. Malaria involving stomach makes the patient suffer from sickness, frequent hunger with no appetite, sticking fullness and bulging abdomen after eating. For treatment, the acupoints on foot-Yangming and foot-Taiyin can be needled till bleeding.

When the patient is going to have fever at the stage of attack, the acupoint over the artery above tarsus can be needled to open its orifice and enable bleeding, instantly cooling the febrile body; just at the start of chill, the acupoints on Yangming and Taiyin of hand and foot can be needled.

If malaria pulse is full, large and swift, the back transporting acupoints can be needled and Wuqu acupoints in parallel with back transport (Shu) acupoints can be needled with medium-sized needles, each one time; according to the fat or thin body type, the bleeding should be controlled. If malaria pulse is small, solid and swift, the acupoints on foot-Shaoyin on tibia can be moxibusted on shank and the well acupoints can be needled. If malaria pulse is full, large and swift, the Wuqu acupoints as back acupoints can be needled, each one time till they are properly bleeding. If malaria pulse is slow, large and deficient, then medication is better than applying acupuncture. Whenever treating malaria, the treatment should be applied one meal time prior to the onset, and missing this timing means a missed opportunity.

For any case with malaria with no pulse felt, the inter-digital acupoints should be needled till bleeding, after which the disease must be cured; if rashes resembling small red beans are seen, all of them can be needled. Since the twelve kinds of malaria have different onset times, their manifestations should be observed in order to identify which meridian is involved in the disease. If needling treatment is applied one meal time prior to the onset, the first needling can reduce the severity, the second can result in obvious improvement and the third can cure the disease; if not cured, the acupoints on two sublingual vessels should be needled till bleeding; if still not cured, acupoint Xizhong (BL40) should be needled till bleeding; and again acupoints below the nape and beside both sides of the spine should be needled and the disease must be cured. The two sublingual vessels mentioned above are in fact Lianquan (RN23).

Before needling is applied for malaria, the focus of onset should be identified, which should be first needled. If headache and heavy head appear first, the acupoints on the head, above the temples, and between the eyebrows should be needled till bleeding. If backache is first seen, the acupoints on the neck and back should be first needled. If waist and spinal pain occur first, acupoint Xizhong (BL40) should be first needled till bleeding. If arm pain is the first sign, the ten interdigital acupoints on hand-Shaoyin and hand-Yangming meridians should be first needled. If shank and foot pain are seen first, the ten interdigital acupoints on foot-Yangming meridian should be first needled. In the case of wind malaria, sweating and fear of wind are seen at the stage of the attack; for this, the back acupoints on Taiyang meridian should be needled till bleeding. If there appears impalpable severe pain on shank, termed tarsus marrow disease, the acupoint Juegu (GB23) can be needled with arrowhead needle till bleeding, and the condition is cured immediately. For light pain in the body, acupoint Zhiyin (BL67) should be needled. For any well acupoint, bleeding is not allowed and it should be needled once every other day. If the patient with malaria has no thirst but paroxysm every other day, the acupoints on foot-Taiyang can be needled; if the patient has thirst and paroxysm every other day, the acupoint of foot-Shaoyang can be needled; in case of warm malaria with no sweating, Fifty-nine-needling therapy can be applied.

Chapter 37

Qi Reversal

Yellow Emperor: How is the transference of cold or heat among five solid viscera and six hollow viscera?

Qibo: Cold is transferred from kidney to liver, leading to carbuncles, swelling and shortness of breath. Cold is transferred from spleen to liver, leading to carbuncles, swelling and sinew spasm. Cold is transferred from liver to heart, leading to mania and obstruction in the diaphragm. Cold is transferred from heart to lung, leading to consumptive thirst disease of lung, with much urine — almost two times the amount of drink that is consumed — which is an incurable disease. Cold is transferred from lung to kidney, leading to ascites accompanied by soft abdomen. When pressing due to water Qi, cold invades the large intestine and there is a splashing sound like that made by a bag filled with fluid when walking rapidly, which is a watery disease.

Heat is transferred from spleen to liver, leading to sudden nose bleeding. Heat is transferred from liver to heart, leading to death. Heat is transferred from heart to lung, leading to consumptive thirst disease of diaphragm. Heat is transferred from lung to kidney, leading to body rigidity. Heat is transferred from kidney to spleen, leading to deficiency and dysentery, which is incurable. Heat is transferred from womb to bladder, leading to urinary retention and urinary bleeding. Heat is transferred from bladder to small intestine, leading to intestine stagnation and constipation and oral erosion due to heat Qi ascending. Heat is transferred from small intestine to large intestine, leading to hidden lump and hemorrhoids. Heat is transferred from large intestine to stomach, leading to eating excessively but still being thin, which is termed polyphgia. Heat is transferred from stomach to gallbladder, also leading to polyphagia. Heat is transferred from gallbladder to brain, leading to sour nose and chronic nasosinusitis, which is characterized by turbid nasal discharge continuously and progresses to nose bleeding and blindness. All these diseases above are caused by transference of Qi reversal.

Chapter 38

Cough

Yellow Emperor: The change of lung can make the patient cough; why?
Qibo: The changes of five solid viscera can all make the patient cough, not only changes in the lung.

Emperor: I'd like to know their mechanism.
Qibo: The skin and hair are the corresponding partner of lung; when the skin and hair are firstly affected by evil Qi, it then invades its partner correspondingly. Cold evil can also invade stomach with cold food, and through lung meridian it reaches the lung by moving upward, leading to lung cold, which can then invade the body by a combination of internal and external evil, leading to lung-cough. Five solid viscera can be affected by cough diseases in their due time, but not during the due time of lung, and lung-cough can be caused by evil transferred from other solid viscera. Since human body corresponds with the heavens and the earth, five solid viscera can be affected by cold evil in due time, in which the moderate case has cough and the more severe case has diarrhea and pain. Correspondingly, lung is first affected by evil in autumn, in spring liver is first affected, in summer heart is first

affected, in later summer spleen is first affected, and in winter kidney is first affected.

Emperor: How to differentiate the different conditions?
Qibo: Lung-cough manifests as panting with adventitious breathing sound, and even hemoptysis. Heart-cough manifests with heart pain, a sense of blockade, like a stick in the throat and even swollen pharynx and throat impediment. Liver-cough manifests in hypochondriac pain and even the inability to turn round; there will be distention below two armpits while turning round. Spleen-cough manifests in right hypochondriac pain and referred dull pain to shoulders and back, and even presents with failure to move and severe cough while moving. Kidney-cough manifests in dragging pain between waist and back, even spitting and drooling.

Emperor: How about the cough due to changes of six hollow viscera? How do these conditions develop?
Qibo: The chronic cough due to five solid viscera will be transferred to six hollow viscera. Spleen-cough, if incurable, can be transferred to stomach; stomach cough manifests in coughing with vomiting, and even vomiting out long worms. Liver-cough, if incurable, can be transferred to gallbladder; gallbladder cough manifests in coughing with vomiting bile. Lung-cough, if incurable, can be transferred to large intestine; large intestine cough manifests in coughing with fecal incontinence. Heart-cough, if incurable, can be transferred to small intestine; small intestine cough manifests in cough with flatus or simultaneous coughing and flatus. Kidney-cough, if incurable, can be transferred to bladder; bladder-cough manifests in cough with enuresis. Chronic cough, if incurable, can be

transferred to triple Jiao; triple Jiao cough manifests as coughing with the full abdomen and lack of a desire for food; all these changes converge in the stomach and are terminated in lung, which makes the patient have more snivel and sputum, facial swelling and cough due to Qi reversal.

Emperor: How to treat them?
Qibo: For the cough associated with solid viscera, the stream acupoints can be needled, for the cough due to hollow viscera, the estuary acupoints needled, and for the cough with edema, the river acupoints concerned are needled.

Emperor: Good.

Chapter 39

Listing and Analyzing Pain-Disease

Yellow Emperor: I'm told that those doctors good at the analysis of natural law should observe it in human affairs, those doctors good at history should relate it with the present society, and those doctors good at human affairs should restrain themselves. Thus, one won't be puzzled and master the principle, which is called enlightenment. Now I'd like to consult with you on the details about knowing by inquiry, observing by inspection and finding by palpation, thus helping me implement them without puzzles; shall I know them?
Qibo bowed and kowtowed twice, and said: What principles do you want to know?

Emperor: I'd like to know about the sudden pain with five solid viscera, and what kind of Qi causes pain?
Qibo: Qi and blood are flowing along meridians and vessels ceaselessly and cycling endlessly. Cold Qi invading into the meridians externally will stagnate and slow down the flow, and even cause damping and stopping; invasion into vessel externally will reduce blood, and invasion into intra-vessel will obstruct Qi, leading to sudden pain.

Emperor: The pain can stop suddenly, or become more severe and ceaseless, or become too severe to be pressed, or stop under pressure, or not be alleviated after pressing, or throb referring to hands, or drag between heart and the back, or drag between hypochondria and lower abdomen, or there could be abdominal pain dragging inner thigh, or it could linger into accumulation, or be so sharp that the patient loses consciousness and then comes round after a while, or it could cause vomiting, or diarrhea after abdominal pain, or even constipation. All of these pains are different — how to differentiate them?

Qibo: Cold Qi invades meridians externally, leading to meridian cold that causes constriction that causes meridian spasm that draws minute collaterals exteriorly which finally causes sudden pain, which can be stopped by warming; if affected by cold again, the pains will linger for long. If cold Qi invades meridians internally and wrestles with heat Qi, it will cause fullness of meridians and the pain that cannot be pressed. If cold Qi lingers interiorly, hot Qi will ascend, meridian will be full and blood Qi will be disturbed, so that the pain cannot be pressed. If cold Qi invades between intestines and stomach and below primordial membrane, blood cannot be distributed and small collaterals convulses leading to pain; blood and Qi can be dispersed after pressing, leading to pain relief. If cold Qi invades the meridian along both sides of spine, the pain is too deep to be pressed, so pressing is not helpful in providing relief. If cold Qi invades thoroughfare meridian, which starts from Guanyuann (CV04) acupoint and ascends straight along the abdomen, it will cause obstruction of meridians, which causes Qi to breakthrough, leading to throbbing pain involving hands. If cold Qi invades the meridians of back acupionts, it will cause meridian damping that causes blood deficiency that results in pain, and these acupionts are in communication with heart, so that there will appear referred pain between the back and heart. When pressed, heat Qi arrives and can stop the pain. If cold Qi invades the Jueyin meridian, which runs around the genitals and is connected with liver, it will invade the meridians internally and cause blood damping and meridian spasm, leading to referred pain between hypochondriac ribs and lower abdomen. If reverse cold Qi invades the inner thigh, the cold Qi will ascend into the lower abdomen and cause blood damping downward, leading to abdominal pain drawing into the inner thigh. If cold Qi invades the small intestine and primordial membranes and interior collateral blood, it will cause blood damping; blood fails to flow into the large meridians and blood Qi lingers without flowing, leading to chronic pain turning into accumulation. If cold Qi invades five solid viscera, Qi will ascend astray reversely, and Yin Qi will be exhausted and Yang Qi fails to enter, leading to sudden sharp pain with unconsciousness; if Yang Qi is restored, the patient can be resuscitated. If cold Qi invades intestine and stomach, reversal Qi will ascend to go out, leading to pain and vomiting. If cold Qi invades small intestine, small intestine fails to gather content, leading to diarrhea and abdominal pain. If heat Qi lingers in small intestine, intestinal pain, hot fever with burning thirst as well as firm and dry stool with constipation will develop, leading to pain and obstruction of defecation.

Emperor: There exists the so-called knowing something by inquiry. So, how about seeing something by inspection?
Qibo: Five solid viscera and six hollow viscera all have their corresponding parts on the face so that five complexions can

be seen. On inspection of complexion, the yellow and red indicate heat, the white indicates cold, and the blue and black indicate pain, and this is called seeing something by inspection.

Emperor: What about feeling something by palpation?
Qibo: The doctor should examine the pulse conditions that dominate the disease, in which the firm, full and sunken pulses due to abnormal blood-Qi can be all examined by palpation.

Emperor: Good. I have understood that hundreds of diseases are caused by Qi disorder. Rage causes Qi to ascend reversely, overjoy causes Qi to flow slowly, sorrow causes Qi to disperse, horror causes Qi to descend, cold causes Qi to constrict, hot evil causes Qi leakage, fright causes Qi disturbance, overstrain causes Qi consumption and contemplation causes Qi binding. These nine kinds of abdominal Qi are different; how will they cause the respective diseases?
Qibo: Rage causes Qi reversal and even vomiting of blood and diarrhea after indigestion, which is called Qi ascending. Overjoy causes Qi harmony and smooth Qi, which is called Qi moderation. Sorrow causes constriction of the heart system and lung distension and bloating, so that obstruction of upper Jiao will develop, and there will be accumulation of nutritive and defensive Qi and heat Qi will linger in the middle, which is called Qi consumption. Horror causes essence declination, which causes closure of upper Jiao that causes Qi regurgitation, which causes distention of lower Jiao, which is called failure of Qi flowing. Cold evil causes closure of interstitial striae and Qi stoppage, which is called Qi shrinkage. Hot evil causes opening of interstitial striae, unblocking of nutritive and defensive and profuse sweating, which is called Qi

leakage. Fright makes the heart have nothing to depend on, spirit no house to return to and mind no place to concentrate on, which is called Qi disturbance. Overstrain causes panting with perspiration and Qi floating astray, which is called Qi consumption. Contemplation causes deep thinking and concentrated spirit, which makes healthy Qi fail to flow. It is called Qi binding.

Chapter 40

Abdominal Disorders

Yellow Emperor: The patient with heart and abdominal diseases can have breakfast in the morning but no appetite in the evening; what is this disease?
Qibo: It is termed tympanites.

Emperor: How about the treatment?
Qibo: Chicken Poop Wine can be given to treat it, one dose of which can improve the conditions and the second dose can cure the disease.

Emperor: However, the disease sometimes relapses — why?
Qibo: It is the improper diet that sometimes results in the relapse. When the disease is being cured, it is influenced by improper diet that makes evil Qi accumulate in the abdomen.

Emperor: The patient with sticking distention in the chest and hypochondia has difficulty in eating, and there a fetor smell first appears, followed by thin nasal discharge, hemoptysis and then four cold extremities, blurred vision, and often urine or stool bleeding. What disease is this? What is the cause?
Qibo: It's termed blood exhaustion. It is a disease that was contracted during childhood when there was massive bleeding.

If the person has intercourse after getting drunk, there will be Qi exhaustion and liver damage, leading to scanty, or even paused, menstruation.

Emperor: How to treat it? What is the therapy to improve it?
Qibo: Four parts of cuttlebone and one part of Rubia are mixed with sparrow egg to make pills like small beans. Five pills are taken in with abalone juice after meals in order to smooth the intestine and relieve the liver damage.

Emperor: There is a patient with firm fullness in the lower abdomen which has root up and down or on right and left sides; what is the disease? Can it be cured?
Qibo: It is termed Fuliang.

Emperor: How to contract Fuliang?
Qibo: There is massive amount of pus and blood outside of stomach and intestine, which is incurable; in treatment, the patient would be dead because of heavy pressing.

Emperor: What is the reason?
Qibo: In the lower regions, it will oppress the anus and genitals, causing pus and blood to discharge out, and in the upper region it will oppress stomach and epigastrium and cause obstruction and carbuncles there, which is a chronic disease that is hard to cure. If it is above the navel it is a reversal syndrome, and when it is below the navel it is a complying syndrome, for which palpation is not allowed lest the lower part is destroyed. The discussion is recorded in *On Acupuncture Manipulation*.

Emperor: The patient has the swelling in the trunk, hip, thigh and shank accompanied by the pain around the navel, what is the disease?

Qibo: It is also termed Fuliang, which is caused by wind evil. The wind evil is spreading over the large intestine and stagnated in the mesentery that originates from below the navel, so there is pain around the navel. The condition cannot be stirred, as stirring will cause urinary difficulty.

Emperor: You the Master have mentioned several times heat in the middle and middle consumptive thirst disease; these cases cannot be given greasy food, aromatic herbs, or mineral drugs, because the mineral drugs will result in epilepsy while aromatic herbs will result in mania. Since the disease of heat in the middle and middle consumptive thirst disease are most common in rich people, now that greasy food is prohibited, it doesn't meet their preference and the prohibition of aromatic herbs also cannot cure their disease either. I'd like to know the reason.
Qibo: The aromatics are characterized by flying action and the mineral by drastic action, both of which are urgent and drastic but not moderate and harmonizing, so the two kinds of drugs cannot be medicated.

Emperor: The two drugs cannot be medicated — what's the reason for this?
Qibo answered: Because internal heat Qi is violent, and so is the Qi of the drugs; thus, when two heats meet together, they will damage the spleen. Since spleen corresponds to earth, the patient fears wood. After medication with the two kinds of drugs, the disease will be more severe on the first–second day.

Emperor: Good. The patient has swollen chest, painful nape, bloating chest and abdominal distention — what is the disease? And how to contract it?
Qibo: It is termed critical Qi reversal.

Emperor: How to treat it?
Qibo: Moxibustion leads to dysphonia and stone acupuncture leads to mania; when Yin Qi and Yang Qi are combined together, the treatment can be applied.

Emperor: What's the reason?
Qibo: Yang Qi tends to be in the upper and it is excessive also in the upper; if moxibustion is given, it will drive Yang Qi into Yin, which will result in dysphonia; stone acupuncture will cause deficiency of Yang Qi, leading to mania. When Yin Qi and Yang Qi meet together, the disease can be cured.

Emperor: Good. How to know that a woman is bearing a child and is in labor?
Qibo: The woman seems as if she is ill but without morbid pulse.

Emperor: The febrile case has pain and why?
Qibo: The febrile disease is associated with Yang meridian. Because the three Yang meridians are stirred, Renyin pulse one grade more than Cunkou reflects the disease in Shaoyang and two grades in Taiyang and three grades in Yangming. The so-called "into Yin" means three Yang into three Yin, which reflects the diseases in head and abdomen, leading to epigastric distention and headache.

Chapter 41

Treatment of Lumbago with Acupuncture

The disorder of foot-Taiyang meridian leads to lumbago involving the nape, back, spine and buttock, as if carrying heavy objects, for which Xizhong, the estuary acupoint on Taiyang meridian proper, should be needled till bleeding; however, in spring, bloodletting should be avoided.

The disorder of Shaoyang meridian makes patients have lumbago as if the skin being needled, and the lumbago gradually leads to slowing down of action so that the patients fail to even be able to bend forward and backward or turn their head to the right and left; for its treatment, the lateral tibia condyle (Yanglingquan, GB34)*, on Shaoyang meridian, the lateral prominence to the knee, can be needled till bleeding, but in summer bloodletting should be avoided.

The disorder of Yangming meridian leads to lumbago, which makes patients unable to turn their head or causes them to have visual hallucination if they turn their head and frequently feel sad. For this, Zusanli (ST36) acupoint on front

*The acupuncture points are referred to by their traditional names in *Huangdi Neijing*. The meridians and numbers are added by the translator.

shank should be needled three times combined with needling both Shangjuxu (ST37) and Xiajuxu (ST39) acupoints till bleeding, but in autumn bloodletting should be avoided.

The disorder of foot-Shaoyin meridian leads to lumbago involving the inner spine, for which Fuliu (KI07) acupoint above the medial malleolus should be needled twice, but in spring bloodletting should be avoided; if there is excessive bleeding, it is difficult to restore.

The disorder of Jueyin meridian leads to lumbago, with the patient feeling like a drawn bowstring, for which the region between the calf and the heel, which feels like something has been clustered, should be needled; if the patients tend to be over-talkative or silent, it can be needled three times.

The disorder of Jie collateral (the branch of foot-Taiyang meridian) leads to lumbago, which involves shoulders and causes blurred vision and frequent urinary incontinence, for which the transverse vessel at the inter-space lateral to the sinew muscle in Jie collateral on posterior knees should be needled till bleeding, and the needling should not be stopped until the dark blood turns red in color.

The disorder of Jie meridian makes patients have lumbago, which feels like being dragged by a band, and even as if waist being broken, and it is also characterized by frequent fright, for which, on Jie meridian, the interspace with stagnated collateral like millet can be needled till the dark blood shoots out and turns red.

The disorder of Tongyin collateral (divergent branch of foot-Shangyang) makes patients have lumbago, as if a small hammer being inside with sudden swelling, for which, on Tongyin meridian, Juegu (GB38) acupoint at the external ankle can be needled three times.

The disorder of Yangwei extra meridian makes patients have lumbago with sudden swelling, for which, on Yangwei meridian, the acupoint below the calf between Yangwei and Taiyang and one chi from the ground can be needled.

The disorder of Hengluo collateral makes patients have lumbago with inability to bend forward and backward, and they also easily fall down when bending backward, which is caused by lifting heavy things leading to obstruction of Hengluo collateral and congestion of bad blood; for the treatment, Xiyang (Weiyang, BL39) and the collateral Yinmen (BL37) acupoints between sinews several cun above Xizhong (BL40) can be needled two times till bleeding.

The disorder of Huiyin meridian (middle foot-Taiyang meridian) makes patients have lumbago with streaming of sweat, feeling thirst after sweating and upset after drinking, for which, on Zhiyang meridian, the transverse vessel above Yangqiao meridian and five cun below Xixia (Chengjin, BL56) acupoint (popliteal space) can be needled three times till bleeding from the full vessel.

The disorder of Feiyang collateral (divergent branch of foot-Taiyang) makes patients have lumbago with sudden swelling and even with sorrow and fear, for which, on Feiyang meridian, the acupoint five cun above the internal ankle, anterior to Shaoyin meridian and at the convergence with Yinwei meridian can be needled.

The disorder of Changyang collateral (divergent branch of foot-Shaoyin) makes patients have lumbago referring to the chest with blurred vision, and even the waist arches backward; there is also inability to speak due to a curled tongue, for which, Fuliu (KI07) acupoint, anterior to the major muscle and two cun above internal ankle behind Taiyin, can be needled two times.

The disorder of San collateral (divergent branch of foot-Taiyin) makes patients have lumbago with fever and even vexation due to fever, with feeling like transverse wood in the waist and urinary incontinence, for which, on San meridian, the acupoint at inter-space connecting the lateral of collateral can be needled.

The disorder of Rouli collateral (divergent branch of foot-Shaoyang) makes patients have lumbago with fear of cough and leads to sudden sinew spasm, for which, on Rouli meridian, the acupoint exterior to Taiyang and posterior to Juegu (GB38) on Shaoyang meridian can be needled twice.

For lumbago radiating to the spine and the head with nape and back stiffness, blurred vision and tendency to fall down, Xizhong (BL40) can be needled till bleeding; for lumbago with fearing cold in the upper, foot-Taiyang and foot-Yangming meridians can be needled; for lumbago with heat in the upper, foot-Jueyin meridian can be needled; for lumbago with inability to bend forward and backward, foot-Shaoyang meridian can be needled; for lumbago with the heat in the middle and panting, acupoint Xizhong on foot-Shaoyang meridian can be needled till bleeding.

For lumbago with cold sensation in the upper and inability to turn head, foot-Yangming meridian can be needled; for lumbago with the heat in the upper, foot-Jueyin meridian can be needled; for lumbago with the heat and panting, foot-Shaoyin meridian can be needled. For lumbago with difficulty in defecation, foot-Shaoyin meridian can be needled. For lumbago with abdominal fullness, foot-Jueyin meridian can be needled. For lumbago as if being broken as well as inability to bend forward or backward and inability to lift, foot-Taiyang meridian can be needled. For lumbago referring to the inner spine, foot-Shaoyin meridian can be needled. For lumbago referring to the lower abdomen and hypochodria with inability to face up, Xialiao (BL34) acupoint between the waist and buttock and above the muscles of two thighs spine can be needled, and its needling times depend on the moon's waxing and waning; the lumbago can be cured immediately after needle withdrawal. The right can be needled for pain on the left side, while the left be for the pain on the right.

Chapter 42

Wind Evil

Yellow Emperor: If wind evil attacks the body, it will give rise to chill-fever, heat in the middle, cold in the middle, leprosy, hemeplagia or wind syndrome. Different diseases with different terms develop, which are associated with five solid viscera and six hollow viscera; I do not know the mechanism and I'd like to know the explanation.

Qibo: The attacking wind tends to linger in the skin so that the meridian Qi fails to be communicated internally and the defense Qi fails to diffuse externally. Wind tends to be mobile and change rapidly. With the interstitial striae being open, the patient will feel continuously chilly; with the interstitial striae closed, the patient will feel feverish and stuffy. The cold can reduce appetite while the heat can consume the muscles, which makes the patient shiver and fail to take in food, termed chill-fever.

Wind evil enters stomach through Yangming meridian and then ascends to the inner canthus. If the patient is fat, wind evil cannot escape, causing the heat in the middle with yellowish eyes. If the patient is thin, Yang Qi can leak externally with chill and cause the cold in the middle with lacrimation.

Wind evil enters the body through Taiyang meridian and then runs to all the acupoints of meridians, spreading to inter-muscles and wrestling against defensive Qi. If its passage is obstructed, muscular swelling with ulceration will develop. If its Qi is congealed with stagnation, muscular numbness will develop. With leprosy, nutrition Qi is rotten due to the heat. Its unclean Qi destroys the bridge of the nose, deforms the facial complexion and ulcerates the skin, because wind-cold invades meridians and lingers there, which is termed as leprosy or chill-fever.

Affected by wind in spring and on the First or the Second day, the disease is termed liver-wind; affected by wind in summer and on the Third or Fourth day is termed heart-wind; affected by wind in late summer and on the Fifth or Sixth, the disease is termed spleen-wind; affected by wind in autumn and on the Seventh or Eighth day, the disease is termed lung-wind; affected by wind in winter and on the Ninth or Tenth day, the disease is termed kidney-wind.

If wind evil attacks body through acupoints of five solid viscera or six hollow viscera, it is also known as visceral wind; if wind evil enters body through respective acupoint as door, it will cause hemilateral wind. If wind evil ascends through Fengfu (GV16)* acupoint, it will cause brain-wind. If wind evil enters head tract, it will cause eye-wind, with a fear of cold. If wind evil attacks during drinking, it will cause leaking wind. If wind evil attacks during intercourse with sweating, it will cause internal wind. If wind evil attacks after hair-washing, it will cause head-wind. If affected by wind evil lingering internally, it will cause diarrhea after indigestion. If wind evil

---

*The acupuncture points are referred to by their traditional names in *Huangdi Neijing*. The meridians and numbers are added by the translator.

lingers in interstitial striae exteriorly, it will cause discharging wind. So, wind is the chief cause of all diseases. As to its alteration leading to other diseases, there is no constant rule, but the cause of all the diseases is wind evil.

Emperor: What are the differences of wind syndromes among five solid viscera? I'd like to know their diagnoses and manifestations.

Qibo: Lung-wind is characterized by profuse sweating, fearing cold, pale complexion, frequent cough and shortness of breath, which is alleviated in daytime and worsened at night. Its diagnostic examination should focus on the part above eyebrows with white color as feature. Heart-wind is characterized by profuse sweating, fearing wind, dry lips and tongue, frequent anger and fright, reddish complexion and slowing of speech if severe. Its diagnostic examination should focus on the mouth with red color as feature. Liver-wind is characterized by profuse sweating, fearing wind, frequent sorrow, slightly greenish complexion, dry throat, frequent anger and occasionally disliking females. Its diagnostic examination should focus on the part under eyes with green color as feature. Spleen-wind is characterized by profuse sweating, fearing wind, lassitude, unwillingness to move limbs, slightly yellow complexion and no appetite. Its diagnostic examination should focus on the nose with yellow color as feature. Kidney-wind is characterized by profuse sweating, fearing wind, puffy face with edema, spinal pain with inability to stand straight, sooty complexion, and difficulty in urination and defecation. Its diagnostic examination should focus on the cheeks with black color as feature.

Stomach-wind is characterized by profuse sweating on the neck, fearing wind, lack of appetite, blockage of the diaphragm, frequent abdominal fullness, gastric distension if wearing less clothes, and diarrhea after eating cold food. Its diagnostic examination should focus on a thin physique and bulging abdomen. Head-wind is characterized by profuse sweating on the head and face and fearing wind. It will be obvious one day prior to wind day, making the patient afraid to go out, but the disease will be slightly relieved when wind is blowing. Leaking wind syndrome is characterized by profuse sweating (usually the patient is unable to wear thin clothes), sweating right after eating, general sweating if severe, panting, fearing wind, clothes that become wet with sweat, dry mouth, frequent thirst and incapability to work hard. Discharging wind is characterized by profuse sweating, clothes being wet after sweating, dry mouth, soaking in the upper body, inability to work and general pain with chill.

Emperor: Good.

Chapter 43

Impediment Syndrome

Yellow Emperor: How is the impediment developed?
Qibo: The combination of wind, cold and damp Qi can cause impediment syndrome. Impediment disease caused by the dominant wind is termed migratory one; when caused by the cold, painful one; and when caused by the dominant damp, fixed one.

Emperor: There are five types of impediment diseases; what are they?
Qibo: Impediment syndrome occurring in winter is termed bone impediment; in spring, sinew impediment; in summer, vessel impediment; in late summer, muscle impediment; and in autumn, skin impediment.

Emperor: Impediment evil stays internally in five solid viscera and six hollow viscera, and what Qi makes it so?
Qibo: Five solid viscera all have the correspondent exteriors respectively, and the disease evil that lingers long and isn't removed will internally stay in the correspondent solid viscera. So, if not cured or complicated by evil Qi, bone impediment will linger in kidney; if not cured and complicated by evil Qi,

sinew impediment will linger in liver; if not cured and complicated by evil Qi, vessel impediment will linger in heart; if not cured and complicated by evil Qi, muscle impediment will linger in spleen; if not cured and complicated by evil Qi, skin impediment will linger in lung. The so-called impediment disease means that in the corresponding season the solid viscera are repeatedly affected by the Qi of the wind, cold and damp.

As a rule, impediment evil invades five solid viscera differently to cause respective impediment syndrome. Lung impediment is characterized by vexation, fullness, panting and vomiting. The cases with heart-impediment have vessel obstruction, followed by vexation with palpitating, Qi suddenly surging up with panting, dry throat, frequent belching and horror due to critical Qi ascending reversely. Liver-impediment is characterized by night fright, excessive drinking, frequent urination and bulging upper abdomen, just like in pregnancy. The cases with kidney-impediment frequently have distention, and when walking, the buttocks touches the ground instead of feet while the spine is higher than the head. The cases with spleen impediment have limb flaccidity, cough, vomiting of clear water and excess stagnation of the upper abdomen. The cases with intestine impediment drink frequently with passing of little urine, and even at times suffer from diarrhea after indigestion due to middle Qi struggling with evil Qi. The cases with bladder impediment have internal pain due to pressure on the lower abdomen akin to being filled with hot water, dripping urination and clear snivel.

As to Yin Qi of five solid viscera, if being calm, it will be kept internally, while if agitated and restless, it will be exhausted. With excessive diet, intestines and stomach will be injured.

Excessive Qi leading to panting indicates the accumulation of impediment evil in lung; excessive Qi leading to anxiety indicates the accumulation of impediment evil in heart; excessive Qi leading to enuresis indicates the accumulation of impediment evil in kidney; excessive Qi leading to exhaustion indicates the accumulation of impediment evil in liver; excessive Qi leading to emaciation indicates the accumulation of impediment evil in spleen. When not being cured, any type of impediment diseases will progress deeper to the interior. With wind domination, the patient can be easily cured.

Emperor: Impediment disease can sometimes lead to death, sometimes to lingering pain, and sometimes to easy cure; what is the reason?

Qibo: The impediment evil invading solid viscera leads to death, lingering between sinews and bones leads to chronic pain and staying in the skin leads to easy cure.

Emperor: What are factors that make impediment evil invade six hollow viscera? And why?

Qibo: It is also concerned with improper diet and living environment, which are origins of the disease. The six hollow viscera also have transport (Shu) acupoints respectively. If the wind, cold and damp hit the transport (Shu) acupoints involved, further complicated by improper diet, the evil can invade inside along the transport (Shu) acupoints and stay in the hollow viscera respectively.

Emperor: How to treat it with acupuncture?

Qibo: Five solid viscera have Shu acupoints, while six hollow viscera have estuary acupoints. According to the different meridians involved, the impediment syndromes have the respective expression, while according to the different focus, the disease will be cured after acupuncture treatment.

Emperor: Do nutrition Qi and defense Qi also make the patient get impediment syndrome?
Qibo: Nutrition Qi is the essence Qi from water and grain, which is peacefully distributed in five solid viscera and spread into six hollow viscera, and then can flow into vessels. Hence, both Qi can flow along the vessels up and down, link five solid viscera and connect six hollow viscera. Defense Qi is the valiant Qi from water and grain, which is swift and smooth in movement. It cannot enter vessels but can flow in the skin and inter-muscle, diffuse in mesentery membrane, and distribute in the chest and abdomen. Reversing the Qi leads to diseases and complying with the Qi leads to cure. If not combined with the Qi of wind, cold or damp, they won't cause impediment syndrome.

Emperor: Good. Impediment disease can lead to pain, no pain or no numbness as well as to cold, heat, dry or damp; what is the cause?
Qibo: As to the pain, it is due to the excessive cold, and while there is cold, pain will be manifested. Among the cases with numbness or with no pain, the disease lasts for long with deeper progression, and both nutrition Qi and defense Qi cannot flow smoothly, so that the meridians and collaterals are loose and stagnated, and the skin loses nutrition, leading to numbness. For the cold case, it is due to less Yang Qi and more Yin Qi, in which Yin Qi and the disease Qi interact, leading to cold impediment. For the heat case, it is due to more Yang Qi and less Yin Qi, in which the dominant disease Qi overcomes Yin Qi, leading to heat impediment. For the

case with profuse sweating and wet skin, it is due to excessive damp, and moreover there is less Yang Qi and excessive Yin Qi with the interaction of Yin Qi and the damp Qi, leading to sweating and wetness.

Emperor: Among the impediment diseases, some cause no pain, why is this so?
Qibo: The impediment in the bones leads to heaviness; in the vessels, to congealing and loss of blood flow; in the sinews, to contracture and inflexibility; in the muscles, to numbness; and in the skin, to cold. So, having any of these five impediments will not manifest any pain. For any impediment syndrome, it will cause spasm when meeting the cold while there will be flaccidity when meeting the heat.

Emperor: Good.

Chapter 44

Flaccidity Syndrome

Yellow Emperor: The changes of five solid viscera make the patient suffer from flaccidity, why?

Qibo: Lung governs the skin and hair of the body, heart governs the blood and vessels of the body, liver governs the sinews and membrane of the body, spleen governs the muscles of the body, and kidney governs the bones and marrow of the body, so lung Qi heat with withering lobes makes the skin and hair weak and thin rapidly, and stagnated heat will cause flaccidity of four limbs. Heart Qi heat makes the Qi of lower vessels ascend reversely, and then the lower vessels are deficient, thus leading to flaccidity of all vessels. There appears joint stiffness, shank flaccidity and failing to step on the ground. Liver Qi heat makes the patient suffer from gallbladder leakage and bitter mouth, dry sinew and membrane, and then spasm and contracture of the sinews, leading to sinew flaccidity. Spleen Qi heat makes the patient suffer from dry stomach, thirst and muscular numbness, leading to muscular flaccidity. Kidney Qi heat makes the patient fail to straighten the lower back due to withered bones and reduced marrow, leading to bone flaccidity.

Emperor: How to contract these diseases?

Qibo: Lung is the chief among solid viscera and the covering for heart. When lung is experiencing loss or frustration and seeking something in vain, it will be characterized by wheezing that causes lung heat and lobe withering. It's believed that five solid viscera will lose nutrition due to lung heat and withering lobes, leading to flaccidity of four limbs. It is dependent on the information concerned. If the patient is too grievous, the pericardium collaterals will be blocked, which stirs Yang Qi internally and causes collapse of heart blood downward and even bloody urine sometimes. As mentioned in *The Fundamentals of the Diseases*, the emptiness and deficiency of great meridians can progress into muscular flaccidity and be transmitted as vessel flaccidity. If longing for something endlessly but failing to get it, or if attracted by external temptation and indulgence in frequent intercourse, the patient will have flaccid feet and penis and develop sinew flaccidity with white oozing. As mentioned in *The Lower Set of Classics*, the sinew flaccidity originates from liver changes due to indulgence in sex. Some people are gradually affected by damp evil and engage in a job related with water. When damp lingers in the body during living in a wet environment, it will be stagnated in muscles with numbness, progressing into muscular flaccidity. As mentioned in *The Lower Set of Classics*, muscular flaccidity is associated with living in a wet field. When taking a long journey or suffering from physical fatigue, the patient will have thirst in hot weather, which damages internal Yang Qi and makes heat linger in kidney. Kidney is the organ of water, but now the water cannot dominate fire, so the bone will be withered, marrow reduced, and feet too weak to support the body, leading to bone flaccidity. As mentioned in *The Lower Set of Classics*, bone flaccidity is caused by great heat.

Emperor: How to differentiate them?
Qibo: Lung heat is associated with white complexion and withered hair, heart heat with red complexion and engorged veins, liver heat with green complexion and dry nails, spleen heat with sallow complexion and muscle tremor, and kidney heat with black complexion and toth decay.

Emperor: As you the Master have mentioned, treatment is feasible. Why is only Yangming meridian selected to treat the flaccidity syndromes according to some medical descriptions?
Qibo: Yangming is the sea of five solid visera and six hollow viscera and governs the moistening of all sinews that are in charge of controlling bones and smoothing joints. Thoroughfare meridian is the sea of the meridians, which governs irrigating intermuscular septa and is combined with Yangming in convergent sinews. All Yin and Yang meridians meet in convergent sinews locating at Qi street. Yangming is the chief of meridians, belonging to girdle meridian and connecting governing meridian. Therefore, if Yangming meridian is deficient, the penis and testicles will be flaccid and girdle meridian cannot guide it, leading to feet flaccidity and even disability of the feet.

Emperor: How about their treatment?
Qibo: The respective creek acupoints are supplemented, the Shu acupoints on meridians are dredged, deficiency and excess are regulated, and reversal and compliance are harmonized. If the sinews, vessels, bones and muscles are treated at the respective dominant time, the diseases can be cured.

Emperor: Good.

Chapter 45

Reversal Syndrome

Yellow Emperor: Why does reversal disease have the reversal cold or the reversal heat?
Qibo: Decline of Yang Qi in the lower leads to cold reversal, while decline of Yin Qi in the upper to heat reversal.

Emperor: Heat reversal leads to hot feeling starting from the sole center, why?
Qibo: Yang Qi starts from the exterior of five toes, gathers at the sole and converges at the sole center, so the domination of Yang Qi leads to sole heat.

Emperor: Cold reversal leads to cold feeling also from the five toes and goes up to below the knees, why?
Qibo: Yin Qi starts from the interior of five toes, gathers below the knees and converges above the knees, so the domination of Yin Qi leads to cold from five toes to above the knees, which isn't caused by external cold and instead by internal deficiency.

Emperor: What is depleted to cause the cold reversal?
Qibo: The external genital area is the region where all sinews converge, and where Taiyin and Yangming meet. In spring and summer, there is more Yang Qi and less Yin Qi, while in

autumn and winter Yin Qi is exuberant and Yang Qi is deficient. The patient with cold reversal is self-assured of his strong constitution, but Qi is depleted in autumn and winter by indulgence and overstrain, which makes lower Qi rob essence Qi in the upper for recovery in vain, and then essence Qi is drained downwards, leading to internal evil Qi ascending reversely. Evil Qi is stagnated in the middle, which makes Yang Qi decline and fail to distribute and nourish the meridians and collaterals; Yang Qi is damaged day by day and Yin Qi dominates alone so that hands and feet turn cold.

Emperor: How is the heat reversal caused?
Qibo: When wine is taken into stomach, the collaterals are full and the meridians are empty instead. Spleen is in charge of transporting the fluid for the stomach, and if Yin Qi is deficient, Yang Qi will enter; if Yang Qi enters, stomach is disharmonized; if stomach is disharmonized, the essence Qi is exhausted; if the essence Qi is exhausted, and it will fail to nourish four limbs. The patient with heat reversal must often have intercourse after getting drunk or a full meal, and after that Qi is accumulated in spleen without being dispersed, and wine Qi is struggling with grain Qi, turning into heat in the middle; as a result, heat is spread all over the body and internal heat causes dark urine. Wine Qi is exuberant and drastic, so kidney Qi is damaged and Yang Qi is dominant alone, leading to hands and feet heat.

Emperor: Qi reversal makes patient have abdominal fullness or become suddenly unconscious, and the patient will recover consciousness in half a day and even a day. Why is this so?
Qibo: Yin Qi is exuberant in the upper and so the lower will be deficient, and this lower deficiency will lead to abdominal

distention and fullness. Yang Qi is exuberant in the upper and then the lower evil Qi will ascend additionally and the evil Qi is reversed, which leads to Yang Qi disturbance and finally to unconsciousness.

Emperor: Good. I'd like to know the manifestations of critical reversal concerned with six meridians.

Qibo: The critical reversal of Taiyang manifests in swollen and heavy head and failing to walk on foot, leading to fainting spells due to vertigo. The critical reversal of Yangming manifests in mania with running and shouting, failing to sleep flat due to abdominal fullness, reddish and hot face, hallucination and incoherent speech. The reversal of Shaoyang manifests in sudden deafness, swollen and hot cheek, hypochondriac pain and failing to move the lower leg. The reversal of Taiyin manifests in abdominal fullness, epigastric distention, difficulty in defecation, lack of appetite, vomiting after eating, and failing to sleep flat. The reversal of Shaoyin manifests in dry mouth, dark urine, abdominal fullness and heart pain. The reversal of Jueyin manifests in swelling and pain in the lower abdomen, abdominal distention, difficulty in defecation and urination, sleeping with knees bent, shrinkage and swelling of genitals, and internal shank heat. For the exuberance, purgation therapy is applied; while for the deficiency, supplementing therapy is applied, and for non-exuberance and non-deficiency, the acupoints on the meridian involved are selected.

The critical reversal of foot-Taiyin manifests as shank cramp and heart pain referring to abdomen; the acupoints on the meridian involved are treated. The critical reversal of foot-Shaoyin manifests as deficient fullness, vomiting, and watery diarrhea, and the acupoints on the meridian involved are treated. The critical reversal of foot-Jueyin manifests as spasm and lumbago, deficient fullness, dysuria and delirious speech; the acupoints on the meridian involved are treated. If there is critical reversal involving all three Yin meridians, which manifests as difficulty in urination and defecation, and cold hands and feet, and the patient will die in three days. The critical reversal of foot-Taiyang manifests in sudden syncope, vomiting blood and frequent nosebleed, and the acupoints on the meridian involved are treated. The critical reversal of foot-Shaoyang manifests in rigid joints, which makes the waist fail to rotate and the nape fail to turn, and intestinal carbuncles, which is incurable, and so the patient will die when in fright. The critical reversal of foot-Yangming manifests as panting, cough, feverish body, frequent fright, nosebleed and vomiting blood.

The critical reversal of hand-Taiyin manifests as deficient fullness with cough, frequent vomiting and spitting, and the acupoints on the meridian involved are treated. The critical reversal of hand-Jueyin and hand-Shaoyin manifest as heart pain referring to throat, and feverish body, which is a fatal disease and incurable. The critical reversal of hand-Taiyang manifests as deafness, lacrimation, the nape failing to turn and the waist failing to bend and stretch; the acupoints on the meridian involved are treated. The critical reversal of both hand-Yangming and hand-Shaoyang manifest as throat obstruction, swollen pharynx and stiffness of the neck, and the acupoints on the meridian involved are treated.

Chapter 46

Manifestations of Seven Diseases

Yellow Emperor: When a patient suffers from stomach abscess, how to make the diagnosis?

Qibo: To diagnose this kind of disease, stomach pulse should be taken, which should be sunken and thin. This pulse indicates Qi reversal, which will make Renying pulse beat forcefully so as to cause fever. Renying pulse belongs to stomach pulse, and if it is in reversal and exuberant, the heat will accumulate in the stomach and not be dispersed, thus leading to stomach abscess.

Emperor: Good. What is the reason for those who cannot sleep calmly?

Qibo: It is because the solid viscera are damaged in some way and the essential Qi is deviated, so the patient cannot sleep calmly, and thus the patient cannot get rid of their disease.

Emperor: What is the reason for those who are unable to lie on the back?

Qibo: Since lung is the canopy of solid viscera, the exuberance of lung Qi will make the meridian dilate, and then the patient cannot lie on his back, which is discussed in *Extraordinary & Ordinary Diseases with Their Yin & Yang*.

Emperor: For the patient with critical reversal, the right pulse is sunken and tight while the left is floating and slow in pulse examination. I don't know what the primary disease is in these conditions.
Qibo: In winter, the right pulse should be sunken and tight, which complies with the season; the left pulse is floating and slow, which reverses with the season; the left pulse indicates the primary disease is in kidney, which is similar to lung pulse, leading to lumbago.

Emperor: Why is it so?
Qibo: The Shaoyin meridian runs through the kidney and connects lung, and now the patient has lung pulse but contracts the disease in kidney, leading to kidney disease with lumbago.

Emperor: Good. The patient with neck abscess can be treated with either stone needles or acupuncture, which can be both helpful in the cure, what is the real reason for this?
Qibo: It is because they share the same name with different properties. So, the neck abscess due to Qi stagnation should be opened and removed with the treatment of acupuncture, while the neck abscess due to Qi exuberance and blood accumulation should be purged with the treatment of stone needles, which is so called treating the same disease with different therapies.

Emperor: Some patients have rage and mania; how does this develop?
Qibo: It is originated from Yang.

Emperor: How can Yang make the patient have mania?
Qibo: If Yang Qi is suddenly disturbed and hard to control, it will cause frequent rage, termed Yang reversal.

Emperor: How to know it?
Qibo: Normally Yangming constantly pulsates while Taiyang and Shaoyang do not. Now the latter two, which shouldn't have pulsated forcefully, indeed cause major disease, and this is the sign of Yang reversal.

Emperor: How to treat it?
Qibo: It can be cured by reducing the intake of food. Since the food is digested into Yin to grow Yang Qi, the patient can be cured after the intake of food is reduced. The patient can be given some decoction with iron fillings because iron fillings can calm down Yang Qi.

Emperor: Good. There is a disease with general fever, lassitude, sweating like bathing, fearing wind and breathlessness; what is the disease?
Qibo: It is called wine wind.

Emperor: How to treat it?
Qibo: It can be treated with ten fen of Zexie, ten fen of Baizhu and five fen of Mixian, which are ground into a powder, and three pinches of this is taken before meal. The so-called deep and thin pulse means that it feels like a thin needle under fingers, and it should be felt and pressed carefully. Qi accumulation leads to the firm pulse, and the pulse drumming under the fingers means large pulse. *The Upper Set of Classics* discusses the communication of Qi with nature. *The Lower Set of Classics* describes the changes of diseases. *The Golden Chest* introduces diagnosis and prognosis about life and death. *The Measurement and Judgement* states palpation and their analysis. *The Extraordinary and Ordinary Diseases* focuses on uncommon diseases. The so-called extraordinary means that

the deadly diseases are not consistent with the changes of four seasons. The so-called ordinary means that the deadly diseases are consistent with the changes of the four seasons. The so-called measurement means that the diagnosis of the disease is based on the pulse-taking and its mechanism analysis. The so-called judgment means to find the focus and judge the severity of the confirmed diseases assisted by the changes of the four seasons.

Chapter 47

Uncommon Diseases

Yellow Emperor: Some women bearing a child suffer from aphonia in the third trimester; what is the cause of this?
Qibo: It is because the uterine collaterals are oppressed.

Emperor: Why do you say so?
Qibo: The uterine collaterals communicate with kidney. As kidney meridian of Shaoyin runs from kidney to the root of tongue, they cannot speak then.

Emperor: How to treat it?
Qibo: It needs no treatment, the patient will recover after the ten-month pregnancy. It is said in the *On Acupuncture Manipulation* that the insufficiency shouldn't be reduced and the excess shouldn't be nourished, which otherwise will lead to disorders, which would then necessitate treatment actually. The so-called "to avoid reducing the insufficiency" means that the emaciated patient cannot be treated with stone needles. The so-called "to avoid nourishing the excess" means that if the woman bearing a child is given purging therapy, it will disperse essence and let the evil retain solely, and then the heat disease is formed.

Emperor: There is fullness below hypochondria and Qi reversal, which lasts for two or three years without being cured; what is the disease?
Qibo: The disease is termed hypochondriac Qi accumulation, which doesn't affect ingestion and can't be treated with moxibustion and acupuncture. This accumulation can be treated with both Daoyin and medication, and only drug therapy has no effect.

Emperor: Some patients suffer from the swelling of the hip, thigh and shank as well as pain around the navel. What is the disease?
Qibo: It is termed Fuliang, and it originates from lingering wind evil. The wind Qi overflows over the large intestine and stagnates at Huang membrane (mesentery), which is below the navel, and then the pain around the navel develops. It shouldn't be treated with pressing manipulation, otherwise it will lead to dysuria.

Emperor: Some patients have more rapid Chi pulse and obvious spasm of sinews and vessels, and what is this disease?
Qibo: It is called Zhenjin, in which there must be a cramp in the area of abdomen. If there appears white and black on skin, it indicates worsening disease.

Emperor: Some patients suffer from headache for years without relief; how does the disease occur, and what is the disease?
Qibo: If the great cold evil invades into bone marrow deeply, which belongs to brain, there appears Qi reversal of brain, leading to headache and also toothache, which is termed critical reversal.

Emperor: Good.

Emperor: Some patients have sweet taste in the mouth; what is the disease and how does the disease occur?

Qibo: It is caused by reversal overflow of essential Qi from five flavors, termed spleen heat syndrome. Five flavors are ingested into the mouth and stored in stomach. Spleen transports the essential Qi, while fluid and liquid encumber spleen, hence leading to the sweet taste in the mouth. The disease is usually caused by addiction to sweet and fatty food. These people often binge on sweet and fatty food and become obese. Obesity makes heat linger inside the body, while sweetness causes the middle distension, so the spleen loses the normal function and its Qi overflows upward, leading to consumptive thirst. It can be treated with boat orchids to clear and drain stagnated heat Qi.

Emperor: Some patients have a bitter taste in the mouth, which can be treated by needling acupoint Yanglingquan (GB34)*. What is the disease of this bitter taste in mouth? How does it occur?
Qibo: It is termed gallbladder heat syndrome. Liver, serving as general, is governed by the gallbladder, which is responsible for decision-making, and the throat is its external indicator. These patients tend to contemplate with irresolution, leading to gallbladder deficiency and the ascent of reversal Qi and bitter taste in the mouth. It can be treated with needling Curtain (Mu) and transport (Shu) acupoints of gallbladder, which is recorded in *Mutual Synergy of Yin–Yang Twelve Organs*.

Emperor: Some people suffer from enuresis with dozens of urination a day which is regarded as Qi deficiency. There is body heat like charcoal burning, the obstruction between the throat and chest, restless surging Renying pulse, and panting and Qi reversal, which is regarded as five kinds of Qi excess.

---

*The acupuncture points are referred to by their traditional names in *Huangdi Neijing*. The meridians and numbers are added by the translator.

Taiyin pulse is thin like hair due to Qi deficiency. Where is the disease focus? And what is the disease?
Qibo: The disease originates from Taiyin; the excessive evil exists in stomach, but its manifestation appears in lung, whose disease is termed critical Qi reversal, indicating incurable disease and death. These are the so-called five kinds of excess and two kinds of deficiency.

Emperor: What are five kinds of excess and two kinds of deficiency?
Qibo: The so-called five kinds of excess mean the excessive Qi due to five kinds of diseases. Two kinds of deficiency mean the deficient Qi due to diseases concerned. Now there are five kinds of excess outside and two kinds of deficiency inside, which embodies non-exterior and non-interior syndromes, indicating doomed death.

Emperor: Someone was born with epilepsy, and what is the disease? How does it occur?
Qibo: It is called fetal disease. The baby acquired it during the mother's pregnancy when the mother was frightened, Qi ascended adversely and failed to descend, and then the essence and Qi were combined together, which made her child suffer from epilepsy before birth.

Emperor: Some diseases manifest with swollen face and eyes like water, the pulse is large and tense, and there is no general body pain, no emaciation and less ingestion of food; what is the disease?
Qibo: The disease originates from kidney, termed kidney wind. Kidney wind is characterized by failure to eat and frequent fright. If there is heart Qi flaccidity after fright, the patient will die.

Emperor: Good!

Chapter 48

Extraordinary Diseases

The fullness conditions of liver meridian, kidney meridian and lung meridian all have excess pulse, indicating edema. The congestion of lung causes panting and hypochondriac fullness bilaterally. The congestion of liver causes fullness of bilateral hypochondria, fright when sleeping and difficulty in urination. The congestion of kidney causes the fullness from hypochondrium to the lower abdomen, varying degrees of roundness of bilateral shanks, swelling of thighs and shanks with lameness as well as susceptibility to paralysis.

The full and large heart-pulse is associated with epilepsy, convulsion and sinew spasm, and the small and rapid liver-pulse is also associated with epilepsy, convulsion and sinew spasm. If the rapid and irregular liver-pulse is associated with fright, and if it cannot be felt or if there is sudden loss of voice, the disease could be spontaneously cured without any treatment. If kidney-pulse, liver-pulse and heart-pulse are all small and rapid without overt drumming sense, they are associated with abdominal lump.

If kidney-pulse and liver-pulse are both sunken, it indicates stone-water; if both are floating, it indicates wind-water; if both are insufficient, it indicates the death; and if both are small and stringy, it indicates the approaching convulsion. If kidney-pulse and liver-pulse are both large, rapid and sunken, they indicate hernia. If heart-pulse beats in a slippery manner and rapidly, it indicates heart-hernia. If lung-pulse beats deep, it indicates lung-hernia. The rapid pulse of third Yang (gallbladder meridian of foot-Taiyang and small intestine meridian of hand-Taiyang) indicates abdominal lump, of third Yin (spleen meridian of foot-Taiyin and lung meridian of hand-Taiyin) indicates hernia, of second Yin (kidney meridian of foot-Shaoyin and heart meridian of hand-Shaoyin) indicates epileptic reversal, and of second Yang (stomach meridian of foot-Yangming and large intestine meridian of hand-Yangming) indicates convulsion.

The drumming and sunken spleen-pulse indicates dysentery, and it would heal by itself after a long time. The small and slow liver-pulse indicates dysentery, which is easy to treat. The small, forceful and sunken kidney-pulse indicates dysentery with bloody stool, and if there develops heat in blood and general fever, it indicates death. If the dysentery with bloody stool is associated with heart and liver disorders, the two solid viscera sharing the same disease could be treated, but if the dysentery has the small, sunken and unsmooth pulse with general fever, it indicates death, in which the patient tends to die after seven successive days of fever.

If stomach-pulse is sunken, unsmooth, outward drumming and large and heart-pulse is small, firm and rapid, they are all associated with hemiplegia; in male the disease occurs on the left and in female on the right, and they can speak normally and the tongue is flexible. In this case, the disease could be treated in thirty days; if the male or female has the condition in the opposite way with aphonia, the disease can be treated in three years; if the patient is under twenty, he will die in three years. The pulse, coming forcefully with bleeding and general fever, indicates death. The pulse that comes like a suspending hook indicates the normal condition. The pulse that is rapid and surging is called as sudden reversal, and this person fails to speak with others. The pulse that comes rapidly causes sudden fright, and the patient would be cured spontaneously in three or four days.

The pulse that comes like waves rolling on so rapidly, over ten times in one breath, indicates the insufficiency of meridian Qi; this patient would die in about ninety days. The pulse that is like hay burning indicates exhaustion of heart essence, so the patient would die when grass becomes dry. The pulse coming like leaves falling indicates deficiency of liver Qi, and the patient would die when leaves of trees have fallen down. The pulse that is like a visitor going and coming, which is obstructive and drumming, indicates the insufficiency of kidney Qi, and the patient would die when jujube flowers are in blossom and then fall. The pulse that is like a muddy ball indicates insufficiency of stomach essence, and the patient would die when elm seeds fall. The pulse that comes like a transverse wood pole indicates insufficiency of gallbladder Qi, and the patient would die when the grains are ripe. The pulse that is like a tense string indicates insufficiency of uterine-essence; if the patient speaks repeatedly, he would die when frost falls; if he fails to speak, the disease could be treated. The pulse, coming like sticky lacquer that lingers left and right indicates the patient would die in about thirty days from the onset. The pulse that comes like a surging spring and floats in the muscles indicates insufficiency of Taiyang meridian Qi and shortness of breath, and the patient would die when fresh Chinese chives are tasted. The pulse that is like rotten soil that cannot be felt indicates insufficiency of muscle Qi; if the complexion first appears black among the five colors, the patient would die when white kudzu vine is in blossom. The pulse that comes like uvula that can be felt larger under lighter pressure indicates essential insufficiency of twelve visceral acupoints, and the patient would die when water is frozen. The pulse that comes like a knife-edge that can be felt floating and small even under light pressure, and firm, large and rapid under heavy pressure, indicates the depressive heat of five solid viscera; the cold and the heat are constrained in kidney in this case, and the patient with this condition would die at the beginning of spring. The pulse that is like a slippery pill that cannot be felt by fingers indicates essential insufficiency of large intestine, and the patient would die when jujube trees grow leaves. If the pulse comes like flowers, the patient tends to be frightened, would find it difficult to sit and sleep and would be sensitive to sound when walking and standing, which indicates insufficiency of small intestine, and the patient would die at the end of autumn.

Chapter 49

Explanations of Twelve Meridians

In Taiyang meridian, there will appear the disease so-called swelling and pain of the waist and buttocks, because the first lunar month corresponds to Taiyang, which just starts from the 3rd Earthly Branch. In the first lunar month, Yang Qi begins to emerge in the upper while Yin Qi is exuberant but Yang hasn't been in the peak, leading to swelling and pain of the waist and buttocks. There will appear the disease due to partial deficiency so-called lameness, because in the first lunar month Yang Qi melts the frozen earth and earthly Qi emerges, leading to the partial deficiency. In winter Yang Qi is rather deficient, so the deficiency occurs partially leading to lameness. There will appear the disease so-called neck stiffness dragging the back, because Yang Qi surges greatly and tenses up, leading to neck stiffness. There will appear the disease so-called tinnitus, because Yang Qi of everything is exuberant and leaping, leading to tinnitus. There will appear the disease so-called mania and vertex disease, because Yang Qi is constrained in the upper while Yin Qi is constrained in the lower, with deficiency in the upper and excess in the lower, leading to mania and vertex diseases. There will appear the disease so-called deafness with floating Qi, which is rooted in Qi dysfunction. There will appear the disease so-called aphonia due to evil attacking the internal, because Yang Qi has declined after its peak, leading to aphonia. The critical reversal caused by excessive sexual activities will result in dysphonia and flaccid limbs, because kidney Qi is deficient but Shaoyin Qi fails to arrive, leading to the critical reversal.

In Shaoyang, there will appear the disease so-called pain of heart and hypochondria, because Shaoyang just starts from the 11th Earthly Branch which is the branch of heart meridian. In the ninth lunar month Yang Qi is exhausted and Yin Qi is exuberant, leading to pain of heart and hypochondria. There will appear the disease so-called inability to turn over, because Yin Qi can store everything which is in the still status, leading to inability to turn over. There will appear the disease so-called jerk, because in the ninth lunar month everything is declining, and grass and woods are withering and falling, in which Qi leaves the Yang aspect and enters the Yin aspect, so that Yin Qi is exuberant while Yang Qi descends to the lower, leading to jerk.

In Yangming, there will appear the disease so-called chill and shivering with cold, and Yangming just starts from the 7th Earthly Brach, because Yin goes into exuberant Yang in the fifth lunar month and Yang exuberance is overlapped by Yin Qi, leading to chill and shivering with cold. There will appear the disease so-called shank edema and thigh flaccidity, because the Yin goes into the exuberant Yang in the fifth lunar month. Yang is declining after its peak in fifth lunar month while Yin Qi (Jueyin) is ascending to wrestle with Yang, leading to shank edema and thigh flaccidity. There will appear the disease so-called Qi surging due to water evil, because Yin Qi goes from the lower to the upper and the evil invades the viscera in the upper, leading to water evil. There will appear the disease so-called chest pain and shortness of breath, because the water Qi is lingering in the viscera; the water is of Yin Qi and Yin Qi is in the middle, leading to chest pain and shortness of breath. There will appear the severe disease so-called critical reversal characterized by fearing to see people and fire, timidity and fright when hearing wood-sound, because Yang Qi and Yin Qi wrestle mutually, and the water and the fire dislike each other, leading to timidity and fright. There will appear the disease as preferring staying alone in the room with doors and windows closed, because Yin and Yang wrestle with each other while Yang is exhausted and Yin is exuberant, leading to preferring staying alone in the room with doors and windows closed. There will appear the disease as climbing high to sing and throwing away clothes to run, because Yin and Yang wrestle continuously which is constrained in Yang meridians, leading to throwing away clothes to run. There will appear the disease so-called headache, nasal obstruction and abdominal distension after invasion into minute collaterals, because evil Qi of Yangming is constrained in the upper which invades its own minute collaterals or Taiyin meridian, leading to headache, nasal obstruction and abdominal distension respectively.

In Taiyin meridian, there will appear the disease so-called distention because Taiyin just starts from the 1st Earthly Branch, while everything is in the status of storage in the eleventh lunar month, which is termed distension. There will appear the disease so-called belching after Yin Qi ascending to heart, because exuberant Yin goes up to Yangming whose collaterals correspond to heart, leading to belching after Yin Qi ascending to heart. There will appear the disease so-called vomiting after meal, because receiving too much will cause overflow, leading to vomiting. There will appear the disease as feeling relieved and comfortable after defecation or breaking wind, because in the eleventh lunar month Yin Qi begins to decline while Yang Qi to emerge, leading to feeling relieved and comfortable after defecation or breaking wind.

In Shaoyin meridian, there will appear the disease so-called lumbago, because Shaoyin just starts from the 9th Earthly Branch and the Yang Qi of everything is damaged in seventh lunar month, leading to lumbago. There will appear the disease so-called vomiting, cough and Qi surging, because Yin Qi is in the lower, Yang Qi is in the upper and all the Yang Qi is floating and has nothing to depend on, leading to vomiting, cough and Qi surging. There will appear the diseases as inability to stand and sit for long or vertigo and temporary blindness when rising after long-sitting, because Yin-Yang collision of everything is uncertain and has no domination. When autumn Qi is coming, a light frost falls to conquer everything and Yin-Yang is damaged internally, leading to vertigo and temporary blindness. There will appear the disease so-called shortness of breath and frequent anger, because Yang Qi fails to administer which makes itself not discharge outward while liver Qi should have been treated, leading to frequent anger. The frequent anger is termed scotching reversal. There will appear the disease as fright as if being arrested, because in autumn everything hasn't been exhausted, its Yin Qi has been thin while Yang Qi intrudes, and Yin and Yang wrestle mutually, leading to fright. There will appear the disease as disliking food smell, because stomach Qi is insufficient, leading to disliking food smell. There will appear the disease as blackish complexion like soil, because autumn Qi is exhausted internally, leading to the change of complexion. There will appear the disease as hemoptysis, because the Yang meridians are damaged and its

Qi fails to infuse fully in the upper, but the vessels are filled with blood, leading to cough, and nosebleed is also seen.

In Jueyin meridian, there will appear the disease so-called swollen scrotum in male and swollen lower abdomen in female, because Jueyin just starts from the 5th Earthly Branch, and in the third lunar month Yin Qi in Yang is accumulated in the middle as evil, leading to swollen scrotum in male and swollen lower abdomen in female. There will appear the disease so-called difficulty in bending forward and backward, because in the third lunar month, Yang Qi begins to emerge and awaken the living things but everything hasn't fully grown due to remaining Yin, leading to bending forward with no bending backward. There will appear the disease so-called swollen scrotum and testes with dysuria and skin distention, because Yin is exuberant and distension meridians are obstructed, which is termed swollen scrotum and testes with dysuria. There will appear the severe case with dry pharynx and internal heat, because Yin and Yang wrestle mutually producing internal heat, leading to dry pharynx.

Chapter 50
Keys of Needling

Yellow Emperor: I'd like to know the keys of needling.
Qibo: Diseases can be external or internal, and needling can be shallow or deep accordingly, both of which should be controlled in a reasonable way without exceeding the threshold. Too deep needling will cause internal injuries, while too shallow needling will cause external congestion of Qi that can give an opportunity for evil to invade. Thus, improper shallow or deep depth reversely causes catastrophic harm, which will internally disturb five solid viscera, and later give rise to serious diseases. It's believed that there are different diseases occurring in the body hair and interstitial striae, in the skin, in the muscles, in the vessels, in the sinews, in the bones or in the marrow. Hence, when needling the body hair and interstitial striae, the skin shouldn't be injured as otherwise it will internally stir lung, which makes the patient suffer from warm malaria in autumn with continuous chill and shivering cold. When needling the skin, the muscles mustn't be injured as otherwise it will stir spleen, which makes patient suffer from disease with abdominal distension, full vexation and anorexia in the last seventy-two days in four seasons. When needling the muscles, the vessels shouldn't be injured as otherwise it

will stir heart, which makes the patient suffer from heart pain in summer. When needling the vessels, the sinews shouldn't be injured as otherwise it will disturb liver, which makes the patient suffer from heat disease with sinew flaccidity. When needling the sinews, the bones shouldn't be injured as otherwise it will disturb kidney, which makes the patient suffer from abdominal distension and lumbago in winter. When needling the bones, the marrow shouldn't be injured as otherwise it will cause emaciation, shank sourness, and lingering lassitude of body.

Chapter 51

Restrictions of Needling

Yellow Emperor: I'd like to know the difference between deep needling and shallow needling.
Qibo: With deep needling, the acupuncturist should avoid injuring sinews while needling bones, avoid injuring muscles while needling sinews, avoid injuring vessels while needling muscles, and avoid injuring skin while needling vessels; with shallow needling, the acupuncturist should avoid injuring muscles while needling skin, avoid injuring sinews while needling muscles, and avoid injuring bones while needling sinews.

Emperor: I still haven't understood the reasons concerned; so I'd like to know the explanations.
Qibo: The so-called avoiding of injury to sinews while needling bones means that the needle shouldn't be withdrawn till it reaches the sinews without touching bones. Avoiding injury to muscles while needling sinews means that the needle shouldn't be withdrawn till it reaches muscles without touching sinews. Avoiding injury to vessels while needling muscles means that the needle shouldn't be withdrawn till reaching vessels without touching muscles. Avoiding injury to skin while needling vessels means that the needle shouldn't be

withdrawn till it reaches skin without touching vessels. Avoiding injury to muscles while needling skin means that, if the disease is in the skin, the needle should be inserted into the skin without injuring muscles. Avoiding injury to sinews while needling muscles means that penetrating muscles will cause injury to sinews. Avoiding injury to bones while needling sinews means that penetrating sinews will cause injury to bones. The above-mentioned outline incorrect manipulations.

Chapter 52

Contraindications of Acupuncture

Yellow Emperor: I'd like to know the contraindications of acupuncture.

Qibo: The solid viscera have their respective critical parts that cannot be observed; liver Qi emerges on the left, lung Qi is stored on the right, heart regulates the exterior, kidney administers the interior, spleen serves as envoy and stomach serves as a market. Above the diaphragm there is parental heart and lung in the chest and pericardia beside the seventh thoracic vertebra, for which the compliance means safety and the reversal means the danger.

Accidental puncturing of heart will result in death within a day, with warning sign of belching. Accidental puncturing of liver will result in death in five days, with warning sign of delirium. Accidental puncturing of kidney will result in death in six days, with warning sign of sneeze. Accidental puncturing of lung will result in death in three days, with warning sign of cough. Accidental puncturing of spleen will result in death in ten days, with warning sign of frequent swallowing. Accidental puncturing of gallbladder will result in death in one day and a half, with warning sign of vomiting.

Accidental puncturing of the large vessel on the back of the foot (Chongyang, ST34)* will cause endless bleeding and even death. Accidental puncturing of the Liu meridian on face will cause endless bleeding till blindness. Accidental puncturing of Naohu (GV17) acupoint in the head will cause death immediately after needling into the brain. Needling the Lianquan (CV23) acupoint under the tongue too deep will cause endless bleeding with aphonia. Accidental puncturing of the small vessels network on sole of foot cannot cause bleeding internally with local swelling. Accidental puncturing of the large vessel at Xizhong (BL40) acupoint will make the patient have sudden syncope and pale complexion. Accidental puncturing of the vessel at Qijie (ST30) acupoint will cause internal bleeding with inguinal swelling. Accidental puncturing of the marrow at intervertebral space will make the patient have stoop. Accidental puncturing of the breast at Ruzhong (ST17) acupoint will cause breast swelling with internal erosion. Accidental puncturing of the subclavicular fossa deeply will cause air leakage and make the patient suffer from panting, cough and Qi reversal. Needling Yuji (LU10) acupoint deeply will cause local swelling.

The acupuncturist should avoid needling the patient who is drunk, as otherwise it will make the patient have Qi disorder. The acupuncturist should avoid needling the patient who is in anger, as otherwise it will cause Qi reversal. The acupuncturist should avoid needling the patient who is overstraining, overeating, overthirsty and overfrightful.

Accidental puncturing of the large vessel on the inner thigh (SP11) will cause endless bleeding and even death. Accidental

---

*The acupuncture points are referred to by their traditional names in *Huangdi Neijing*. The meridians and numbers are added by the translator.

puncturing of the vessel deeply at Kezhuren (GB03) acupoint will cause suppuration in the ear and even deafness. Accidental puncturing of the kneecap will cause leakage of synovial fluid, and even lameness. Needling hand-Taiyin meridian (LU03) accidentally will cause immediate death if there appears massive bleeding. Needling foot-Shaoyin meridian accidentally will cause severe deficiency of kidney Qi with bleeding and even difficulty in speech due to tongue inflexibility. Needling the lung in the chest cavity deeply will cause panting, Qi reversal and breathing while facing up. Needling the elbow deeply (LU05, PC37) will cause Qi gathering and make the elbow fail to extend and flex. Needling the part three cun below the thigh on the internal side deeply will cause urine incontinence. Needling the part between the armpit and hypochondria deeply will make the patient cough. Accidental puncturing of bladder while needling the lower abdomen will cause urine leakage and make the patient have fullness in the lower abdomen. Needling the calf of the lower leg deeply (BL56) will cause local swelling. Accidental puncturing of the vessel while needling at the ocular orbit deeply (TE23) into the bone will cause tear leakage and even blindness. Accidental puncturing of the joint deeply will cause fluid leakage and inability of flexion and extension.

Chapter 53

Notes of Needling

Yellow Emperor: I'd like to know the keys concerned with deficiency and excess.
Qibo: Qi sufficiency with physique sufficiency and Qi deficiency with physique deficiency are normal conditions, and their contrary conditions are diseases. Sufficient intake of grain causes Qi sufficiency, while insufficient intake of grain causes Qi deficiency. These are normal conditions; their contrary conditions are diseases. Sufficient meridians with blood sufficiency and insufficient meridians with blood deficiency are normal conditions; their contrary conditions are diseases.

Emperor: What is the contrary condition?
Qibo: Qi deficiency with body heat is called abnormality. Sufficient intake of grain with Qi insufficiency is called abnormality. No intake of grain with Qi sufficiency is called abnormality. Exuberant pulse with insufficient blood is called abnormality. Small pulse with sufficient blood is called abnormality. Qi exuberance with cold body is caused by cold damage. Qi deficiency with body fever is caused by summer heat. Sufficient intake of grain with insufficient Qi is caused by blood loss or retention of damp in the lower body. Insufficient

intake of grain with sufficient Qi is caused by invasion of evil into stomach and lung. Small pulse with sufficient blood is caused by heat in the middle due to excessive drinking. Large pulse with insufficient blood is caused by invasion of wind Qi and no intake of water and fluid, which is the abnormality concerned. The excess syndrome is associated with evil Qi entry. The deficiency syndrome is associated with healthy Qi exit. Qi excess causes the heat. Qi deficiency causes the cold. When treating excessive syndrome with acupuncture, the pinhole on acupoints should be opened with no pressing of the left hand. When treating deficient syndrome with acupuncture, the pinhole on acupoints should be closed by pressing of the left hand.

Chapter 54

Explanations of Needling

Yellow Emperor: I'd like to know the introduction for the nine needles and the principle of deficiency and excess.
Qibo: To treat the deficiency with needling, the supplementing method should be adopted, and there will be heat sensation under the needle just due to Qi being supplemented there. To treat the excess, the purging method should be applied, and there will be cold sensation under the needle just due to evil Qi being purged there. To treat the stagnated blood, the elimination method should be applied to remove the evil blood. To treat the evil domination, the purging method should be applied, avoiding pressing when withdrawing the needle. The so-called "slowly and quickly" refers to the supplementing method, in which the needle is withdrawn slowly and the acupoint is pressed quickly. The so-called "quickly and slowly" refers to a purging method, in which the needle is withdrawn quickly and the acupoint is pressed slowly. The differentiation for excess and deficiency depends on the degree of cold and warm sense as well as Qi fullness. There may appear a vague sense of coldness or warmness because the rapid transient variation is hard to detect. If the priority of arrival sense can be detected, the early or late occurrence of the diseases can be

identified. Also, the principle of excess–deficiency shouldn't be ignored by the doctors. An uncertain sense of arrival Qi may also be seen, indicating that the principle hasn't been observed. The key of deficiency and excess is mostly associated with application of nine needles, which should be used on their own merits. The timing for applying the supplementing or purging method should conform to the opening and closing of Qi movement. The nine needles have different names and different shapes, and their best manipulation can be done according to the application of supplementing or reducing.

To treat the excess, the purging method should be applied and the needle should be retained till Yin Qi is in exuberance, when the needles can be withdrawn. To treat the deficiency, the supplementing method should be applied, and then the exuberant Yang Qi will appear, and needle cannot be withdrawn until a warm sense is felt under the needle. When meridian Qi is arriving, one should wait and then keep it carefully, while avoiding changing the manipulation during that time. To decide on whether to use deep or shallow depth of needling by sense, one should analyze whether the disease is internal or external. The far and near Qi arrival share one property, which means that both shallow and deep needling have the same method to wait for Qi arrival. As if being on the brink of an abyss means one shouldn't perform needling with careless attitude. Hand holds the needle firmly as if grasping the tiger's tail. All this means that, without being influenced by anything or anyone, one should attentively observe the patient without glancing to either the left or right. Avoiding inserting needle obliquely means one should keep the needle straight when needling. Tranquilizing one's mind means one should observe the patient and calm down his spirit by eye contact, making his meridian Qi smooth. The so-called Zusanli (ST36)* is located at the acupoint three cun below the knee. The so-called Chongyang (ST42) on acrotarsium can be easily found when lifting the knee. Juxu (ST39) acupoint is located at the acupoint with the depression only on the shank when raising the foot. Xialian (LI08) is also located below the depression.

Emperor: I have heard of nine needles that correspond to the earth and the heavens, the four seasons as well as Yin and Yang. I'd like to know the theory which can be passed down from generation to generation as a conventional method.
Qibo: There are nine natural factors in order from the first to the ninth, with the heavens as one, the earth as two, the human as three, the seasons as four, the scales as five, the pitches as six, the stars as seven, the kinds of wind as eight and divisions of the field as nine; the parts of the human body correspond to each of these, respectively, and the various kinds of needles can have nine shapes based on the similar correspondence, which are called nine kinds of needles. In the human body, the skin corresponds to the heavens (one); the muscles to the earth (two); the meridians to the human beings (three); the sinews to the seasons (four); the voice to the scales (five); the combination of Yin and Yang to the pitches (six); the teeth, face and eyes to the stars (seven); inhalation and exhalation to the wind (eight); and the nine orifices (nine) and the 365 collaterals to the divisions of field. Thus, the first type of needle (the arrowhead) can be used for needling the skin, the second (ovoid-tip) for the muscles, the third (the spoon) for meridians, the fourth (the ensiform) for sinews, the fifth (the stiletto) for bones, the

---

*The acupuncture points are referred to by their traditional names in *Huangdi Neijing*. The meridians and numbers are added by the translator.

sixth (the round-sharp-tip) for regulating Yin–Yang, the seventh for (the filiform) nourishing essence, the eighth (the long) for expelling wind and the ninth (the large) for communicating with the nine orifices, which can all expel evil Qi in the 365 acupoints, and each of the nine types of needles has its own dominant role. Similarly, the human mind corresponds to eight (wind); the human Qi to the heavens; the human hair, teeth, ears and eyes to the five scales and six pitches; the human's Yin–Yang, meridians and blood to the earth; and human liver and eyes to the number nine.

Chapter 55

Extension of Needling Manipulation

Listening to the complaint of the patient prior to examination, the acupuncturist can perform needling. If there is disease on the head with severe headache, one can perform the needling deeply to the bone and the disease can be cured. However, one should avoid injuring the bone, muscles and the skin, especially because the skin is the only passage for the needling.

The so-called technique of Yang needling is to insert the needle in the center with four needlings around. To treat the cold-heat disease, if the evil intrudes deeply, one should needle collection acupoints of five solid viscera, and if the evil is approaching solid viscera, one should needle the back transport (Shu) acupoint where solid viscera Qi converge, till the cold or heat in the abdomen is dispelled. The key for this needling is to needle shallowly till slight bleeding.

To treat carbuncle, one should needle the affected part, and the depth of the needling varies with the sizes of carbuncles. For the large carbuncle, one should let out more blood, and for the small, one should needle deeply with the needle being held vertically into the interior till the cure is achieved. For the disease in the lower abdomen with evil accumulation, one should needle the acupoints from sub-umbilical part to the lower abdomen and then needle the acupoints on both sides of the fourth vertebrae as well as the acupoints on two iliac crests (Juliao, GB29) and lower rib cage, so as to guide the heat Qi in the abdomen to move downward till the cure is achieved.

If there is disease in the lower abdomen characterized by pain and difficulty in defection and urination, it is termed hernia due to the cold. One should needle the acupoints between the lower abdomen and thighs as well as the waist and hip, appears sensation of heat is felt, indicating cure with multiple manipulations.

If there is disease in sinews characterized by spasm, joint pain and inability to walk, it is termed sinew impediment. One should needle the acupoint above sinews, in which the needle is inserted through inter-muscle to avoid injuring the bone. The cure has been achieved and the needling can be stopped if there appears a sensation of heat in the sinews.

If there is the disease in the muscles and skin with general pain, it is termed muscle impediment due to the cold and damp. One should needle multiple acupoints at large and small muscles deeply till there appears the heat sensation locally. One should avoid injuring the sinews and bones. If the sinews and bones are injured, it will give rise to carbuncles and other changes. If cure is indicated, the needling can be stopped when a sensation of heat is felt in inter-muscle.

If there is the disease in the bone with heaviness and inability to lift objects as well as sour pain of the bone marrow, due to the cold Qi arrival, it is termed bone impediment. One should needle deeply without injuring the vessels and muscles. Also, the needles are inserted through the large and small muscles till a sensation of heat is felt around the bone, indicting cure, and then needling can be stopped.

If there is the disease in all the Yang meridians with alternative chill and fever, and especially with alternative cold and heat in inter-muscle, it is termed mania. One should needle the deficient meridians. It indicates cure, and needling can be stopped if a sensation of heat is felt in all the inter-muscle.

The initial disease may recur once a year. If not treated, it may recur once a month; if not treated further, it may recur four or five times a month, which is termed epileptic disease. One should needle inter-muscle and related meridians. If there is no cold sensation, Qi-blood can be regulated with acupuncture and the disease can be cured.

If there develops disease due to wind attacking with alternating episodes of chill-fever and sweating, with several paroxysms a day, one should needle muscles, interstitial striae and collaterals; if there is still sweating with alternating chill or fever, the patient should be subjected to one acupuncture treatment every three days, and the disease can be cured after a course of 100 days.

If there is disease due to violent wind with heaviness of bones and joints as well as loss of beards and eyebrows, it is termed Big Wind (leprosy). One should needle muscles to induce sweating for 100 days, and then needle the bone marrow to induce sweating for another 100. After a total of 200 days of therapy, the beards and eyebrows will grow again, and the needling course can be finished.

Chapter 56

Skin Regions

Yellow Emperor: I have heard that the skin has divisional parts, the meridians have vertical and horizontal ones, sinews have knots and collaterals, and bones have various measurements, so that their diseases are different accordingly. The divisional parts of the skin should be distinguished so as to define if the disease is on the left or right, in the upper or lower, with Yin or Yang, and also to assess its cause and outcome. I'd like to know the theory behind this.

Qibo: To know about the skin parts, one should use meridians as principle lines, which is the same case with all the meridians.

The Yang collateral of Yangming meridians is called Haifei (gate). The upper and the lower (foot-Yangming) share the same method. Any floating collaterals seen in the skin part are the ones of Yangming meridians. If green is mostly seen on the collaterals, it indicates pain, black indicates impediment, yellow and red indicate heat, and white indicates cold. If all the five colors are seen, it indicates intermingled chill and heat. If evil Qi in the collaterals is exuberant, it will invade meridians, in which collaterals dominating the external are Yang while meridians dominating the internal are Yin.

The Yang collateral of Shaoyang meridians is called Shuchi (axis). The upper (hand-Shaoyang) and the lower (foot-Shaoyang) share the same method. Any floating collaterals seen in the skin part are ones of Shaoyin meridians. If evil Qi in the collaterals is exuberant, it will invade meridians, in which the evil in Yang is transmitted into internal meridians while the evil in Yin is transmitted out of the meridians and into the viscera, which is the case with all the meridians.

The Yang collateral of Taiyang meridians is called Guanshu (pivot). The upper (hand-Shaoyang) and the lower (foot-Shaoyang) meridians share the same method. Any floating collaterals seen in the skin part are ones of Taiyang meridians. If evil Qi in the collaterals is exuberant, it will invade meridians.

The Yin collateral in Shaoyin is called Shuru (switch), and the upper (hand-Shaoyin) and the lower (foot-Shaoyin) meridians share the same rule. Any floating collaterals seen in the skin part are of Shaoyin meridians. If evil Qi in the collaterals is exuberant, it will invade meridians. When invading the meridians, the evil is transmitted from Yang collaterals into the meridians. When leaving the meridians, the evil is transmitted from Yin aspect into the bones.

The Yin collateral in Jueyin is called Haijian (carrier), and the upper (hand-Jueyin) and the lower (foot-Jueyin) meridians share the same rule. Any floating collaterals seen in the skin part are the ones of the pericardium meridians. If evil Qi in the collaterals is exuberant, it will invade meridians.

The Yin collateral in Taiyin is called Guanzhe (concealer). The upper (hand-Taiyin) and the lower (foot-Taiyin) meridians share the same method. Any floating collaterals seen in the skin part are the ones of Taiyin meridians. If evil Qi in the collaterals is exuberant, it will invade meridians. All the collaterals of the twelve meridians have divisional parts of the skin.

Hence, the onset of all the diseases necessarily starts from the skin and hair, after which the interstitial stiare are open and the evil can go through and invade the collaterals; if lingering in the collaterals, the evil is transmitted into meridians; if lingering in the meridians, the evil is transmitted into the hollow viscera and constrained in stomach and intestines. When the evil first invades the skin, it will cause chill, with hair standing up and interstitial striae opening; after it invades the collaterals, they will be filled with evil and their colors will change. When invading the meridians, the meridian Qi is deficient and then the evil intrudes deeply. When lingering between the sinews and bones, it will cause sinews spasm and bone pain due to more cold, and it will cause flaccid sinews, bone loss, emaciation, and dry and brittle hair due to more heat.

Emperor: You have mentioned the twelve parts of the skin, but how do they contract diseases in general?
Qibo: The skin is the part where the collaterals innervate. When the evil invades the skin, the interstitial striae will open and then the evil will intrude the collaterals. If the collaterals are filled with evil, it will flow into the meridians. If the meridians are filled with evil, it will intrude and linger in the solid and hollow viscera. Thus, the skin is divided into the twelve parts, and if the skin isn't given preventive therapy, the body is doomed to suffer from drastic disease.

Emperor: Good.

Chapter 57

Meridians and Collaterals

Yellow Emperor: The collaterals can become visible, and their five colors are different, varying in shade from green, yellow, red and white to black; what is the mechanism behind this?
Qibo: The meridians have a constant color while the collaterals have no constant colors, that is, they are changeable colors.

Emperor: What are the constant colors of each of the meridians respectively?
Qibo: Heart corresponds to the color red, lung to white, liver to green, spleen to yellow and kidney to black, all of which correspond to the constant colors of the related meridians.

Emperor: Do the Yin and Yang of the collaterals also correspond to the dominant color of meridians?
Qibo: The colors of Yin collaterals correspond to the meridians, but the colors of Yang collaterals are changeable but follow the changes of four seasons. Excessive cold will cause congealing and damping that is expressed as green and black colors; excessive heat will cause moist distention of Qi-blood that is expressed as yellow and red colors. These are all the constant colors and indicate no diseases. If the five colors all appear, it indicates disorder of cold-heat.

Emperor: Good.

Chapter 58

Qi-Acupoint

Yellow Emperor asked: I have heard that there are 365 acupoints, which correspond to the days of a year, but I don't know their positions; so, I would like to know further details.
Qibo kowtowed and bowed to answer: What a profound question you have asked! Who can explore such a profound theory unless he is the saint emperor? So, please allow me to explain all the locations carefully.

Emperor, cupping one hand in the other, said with humility: You the Master have enlightened me about the theory; though not seeing the locations nor hearing the numbers of the acupoints, I can see clearly and hear keenly about them.
Qibo answered: This is exemplified by the so-called 'It is easy for the sage to understand and for good horses to be driven.'

Emperor said: I'm far from a sage to understand readily, but it is said that the actual number of Qi acupoints can really broaden one's mind. I have asked this question just to enlighten my darkness and solve my puzzle, so it's not such a profound theory. However, I hope you, the Master, can explain all the locations in detail and help me fully understand them. I will store them in the golden chest and not be ready to show them off.

Qibo bowed again and said: Please allow me to talk about it. The back and heart drag each other and cause the pain, and the treatment is to needle Tiantu (CV22)* acupoint, the tenth thoracic vertebra (Zhongshu, GV07) and Shangji (CV12). Shangji (CV12) is the Weiwan acupoint (Zhongwan, CV12), and Xiaji (CV04) the Guanyuan (CV04) acupoint. Meridians between the back and the chest are related with Yin and Yang as well as left and right by evils, so that their disease is characterized by the referred pain of back and heart; with the chest and hypochondriac pain, the patient has difficulty in breathing and sleeping, reversal ascending Qi, shortness of breath and lateral pain. The full evil in the meridian overflows obliquely to the buttock meridian, and connects the chest and hypochondria; its branch reaches heart and penetrates through the diaphragm, and then ascends to Tiantu (CV22), crosses over the shoulders and meets beneath the tenth thoracic vertebra.

There are fifty acupoints for solid viscera, seventy-two for hollow viscera, fifty-nine for treating febrile diseases, and fifty-seven for treating water diseases. There are five lines on the head, with five in each line, accounting for a total of twenty-five. There are also five along the vertebral column on each side, leading to a total of ten. There is one (Dazhu, BL11) above Dazhui (GV14) at each side, one Tongziliao (GB01) and one Fubai (GB10), one (Huantiao, GB30) in each acetabulum, two Dubi (ST35), two Duosuowen (Tinggong, ST19), two Meiben (Zanzhu, BL02), two Wangu (GB12), one (Fengfu, GV16) in the center of the nape, two Zhengu (Qiaoyin, GB11),

---

*The acupuncture points are referred to by their traditional names in *Huangdi Neijing*. The meridians and numbers are added by the translator.

two Shangguan (GB03), two Daying (ST05), two Xiaguan (ST07), two Tianzhu (BL10), two pairs of Shangjuxu (ST37) and Xiajuxue (ST39), two Quya (Jiache, ST06), one Tiantu (CV22), two Tianfu (LU03), two Tianyou (TE16), two Futu (LI18), two Tianchuang (SI16), two Jianjie (GB21), one Guanyuan (CV04) acupoint, two Weiyang (BL39), two Jianzhen (SI09), one Yinmen (GV15), one Navel (Shenque, CV08), twelve transport (Shu) acupoints on the chest, two transport (Shu) acupoints on the back (Geshu, BL17), twelve acupoints on anterior chest (Yingshu), two Fenrou (Yangfu, GB38), two pairs of Fuyang (KI06) and Jiaoxin (KI08) at horizontal striae above ankle and four Yinqiao (Zhaohai, KI06) and Yangqiao (Shenmai, BL62) acupoints. The acupoints for treating water diseases are located in the inter-muscle, while the acupoints for treating febrile diseases are located in the place where meridian Qi converges. The two acupoints (Yangguan, GB33) for treating chill-fever diseases are in the lateral depressions of the knees, and the twenty-five forbidden acupoints are five cun below Tianfu (LU03) acupoints. All these 365 acupoints are the ones where the needles can be inserted.

Emperor said: I have known clearly that the locations of Qi acupoints are places for acupuncture, and I'd like to know whether the minute collaterals and inter-muscular space also correspond to a year.

Qibo answered: There are 365 acupoints connecting minute collaterals, which also correspond to the days of a year, for expelling extraordinary evil and communicating with nourishment Qi and defensive Qi. If evil lingers in minute collaterals, scattering of defense Qi and overflow of nourishment Qi will occur, leading to subsequent Qi exhaustion and blood stagnation, which are indicated by external heat and internal Qi insufficiency. So, the patient should be given purgation by acupuncture immediately so as to enable communication between nourishment Qi and defensive Qi, and any stagnation should be purged whether it is a convergence acupoint or not.

Emperor said: Good. I'd like to know the convergence of inter-muscular interspace.
Qibo answered: The convergence of larger muscles is called the valley, and the convergence of smaller muscles is called the creek. Nourishment Qi and defensive Qi travel through to communicate with the great Qi between the muscle boundaries and in the convergence of inter-muscular space. If there is evil exuberance and Qi stagnation, heat will develop in meridians, muscles will decay, and nourishment Qi and defensive Qi will be blocked. The evil will necessarily result in suppuration and internal consumption of bone marrow, external erosion of large muscles, and linger in the joints and interstitial striae, which must result in deterioration. If cold evil accumulates and lingers there, the nourishment Qi and defensive Qi cannot function normally, leading to cramp of muscles, contracture of sinews and inability to extend the elbows and rib cage. Also, internal bone impediment and external numbness will develop, which indicates insufficiency due to great cold lingering in inter-muscular space. The convergence of 365 acupoints of inter-musclar space also corresponds to the days in a year. For the minor impediment with evil spreading and going along meridians, the small needles can be used with the same manipulation as that of the minute collaterals.

Emperor sent away the other companions and rose up, bowed again and said: Today you have resolved my puzzles through enlightenment, and I will keep it in the golden chest, never to show it off.

So, the emperor stored it in the gold-fragrance treasure room and gave it the plaque of Location of Qi Acupoints.

Qibo said: The minute collaterals are the branches of meridians, and if there is exuberance of blood, it should be purged, whose manipulations are the same as that of the 365 meridians. Evil lingering here long will pour into the collaterals and then to the 12 large collaterals and not only be limited within the 14 collaterals (affecting all the collaterals). For internal invasion, the ten meridians (five solid viscera) concerned can be purged.

Chapter 59

Qi-House

There are 78 acupoints for communication of Qi from foot-Taiyang meridian Qi: there is one (Cuanzhu, BL02)* at each interior side of the brows. There are five lines from the hairline to the nape, three and a half cun in length and three cun in width off the middle line. Its Qi is floating in the scalp, and there are five lines with five acupoints on each line with a total of 25 acupoints. There is one (Tianzhu, BL10) at each side of the big sinews on the nape and one (Fengchi, GB20) at each side beside the Fengfu (GV16) acupoint. There are 21 vertebrae along the back till the tailbone, among which any of the 15 intervertebral spaces has one on each side. There are five transport (Shu) acupoints of five solid viscera at each side and six transport (Shu) acupoints of six hollow viscera at each side. There are six acupoints at each side from Weizhong (BL40) acupoint to the little toe.

There are 62 acupoints for communication of Qi from foot-Shaoyang meridian: two at each frontal angle (Qubin, GB07; Tianchong, GB09), five on each line directly from the eyes into the hairline (Toulinqi, GB15; Muchuang, GB16;

* Editor's note: The names, meridians and numbers in brackets are added by the translator.

Zhengyins, GB17; Chegling, GB18; Naokong, GB19), one on each side of the anterosuperior ear, one on each side of the anteroinferior ear (Hanyan, GB04), one on each side of temple hair (Heliao, TE22), one Kezhuren (Shangguan, GB03) on each side, one at each depression behind ear (Yifeng, TE17), one Xiaguan (ST07) at each side in front of the ear, one at each side below the ear and behind the dental bed at the mandibular angle (Jiache, ST06), one at each supraclavicular fossa (Quepen, ST12), one at each side three cun from the armpit (Yuanye, GB22; Zhejin, GB23; Tianchi, PC1), one at each intercostal space from the armpit to the hypochondrium (Riyue, GB24; Jingmen, GB25; Daimai, GB26; Wushu, GB27; Weidao, GB28; Juliao, GB29), one at each acetabulum (Huangtiao, GB30), and six (Yanglingquan, GB34; Yangfu, GB38; Qiuxu, GB40; Zulinqi, GB41; Jiaxi, GB43; Zuqiaoyin, GB44) on each side from below the knee to between the fourth toe and little toe.

There are 68 acupoints for communication of Qi emitting from foot-Yangming meridian: three on each side beside the hairline in the head (Xuanlu, GB05; Yangbai, GB14; Touwei, ST08), one on each side in the cheekbone foramen (Sibai, ST02), one at each side in the foramen of Daying ST5 acupoint, one at Renying (ST09) acupoint on each side, one at each side in the infraclavicular foramen (Tianliao, SJ15), one at each side in the intercostal space of the chest (Qihu, ST13; Kufang, ST14; Wuyi, ST15; Yingchuang, ST16; Ruzhong, ST17; Rugen, ST18), five on each side beside the epigastric region three cun below breast and stomach (Burong, ST19; Chengman, ST20; Liangmen, ST21; Guanmen, ST22; Taiyi, ST23), three at each side three cun beside the navel (Huaroumen, ST24; Tianshu, ST25; Wailing, ST26), two at each side two cun below the navel (Daju, ST27; Shuidao, ST28; Guilai, ST29), one at each side of Qijie (Qichong, ST30) acupoint with pulsation, one above each Futu (ST32) acupoint (Biguan, ST31), and eight on each line from Zusanli (ST36) to the middle toe; all these acupoints have their own foramen of bone (Zusanli, ST36; Shangjuxu, ST37; Xiajuxu, ST39; Jiexi, ST41; Chongyang, ST42; Xiangu, ST43; Neiting, ST44; Lidui, ST45).

There are 36 acupoints for communication of Qi coming from hand-Taiyang meridian: one at each inner canthus (Jingming, BL01), one at each outer canthus (Tongziliao, GB01), one below each cheekbone (Quanliao, SI18), one above each auricle (Jiaosun, SJ20), one at each ear (Tinggong, SI19), one at each Jugu acupoint, one above each acromion (Naoshu, SI10), one above each clavicle (Jianjing GB21), one four cun above each Tianchuang (SI16) acupoint (Touqiaoyin GB11), one at each Jianjie (Bingfeng SI12), one three cun below each Jianjie (Tianzong SI11), and six from the elbow to the little finger at each side (Shaoze, SI01; Qiangu, SI02; Houxi, SI03; Wangu, SI04; Yanggu, SI05; Xiaohai, SI08).

There are 22 acupoints for communication of Qi coming from hand-Yangming meridian: two on each side between the outside nostril (Yingxiang, LI20) and above the nape (Futu, LI18), one in the foramen of Daying (ST05) at each side, one at the convergence of clavicle on each side (Tianding, LI17), one at the convergence of humeral head on each side, and six from the elbow to the thumb and index finger on each side (Shangyang, LI01; Erjian, LI02; Sanjian, LI03; Hegu, LI04; Yangxi, LI05; Shousanli, LI10).

There are 32 acupoints for communication of Qi emerging from hand-Shaoyang meridian: one at each side below cheekbone (Quanliao, SI18), one at each tip of the eyebrow (Sizhukong, SJ23), one above the frontal angle at each side (Hanyan, GB04), one behind the temporal mastoid process at each side (Tianyou, SJ16), one before foot-Taiyang meridian in the nape at each side (Fengchi, GB20), one beside Futu (LI18) acupoint at each side (Tianchuang, SI16), one Jianzhen (SI09) acupoint at each side, one at each side three cun below each Jianzhen(SI09) and in the inter-muscle (Xiaoluo, SJ12; Naohui, SJ13; Jianliao, SJ14), six from the elbow to the fourth finger and the little finger at each side (Guanchong, SJ01; Yemen, SJ02; Zhongzhu, SJ03; Yangchi, SJ04; Zhigou, SJ06; Tianjing, SJ10).

There are 28 acupoints for communication of Qi that come from Du meridian: two in the center of the nape (Yamen, DU15; Fengfu, DU16); eight from frontal to the back hairline (Naohu, DU17; Qiangjian, DU18; Houdins, DU19; Baihui, DU20; Q1anding, DU21; Xinhui, DU22; Shangxing, DU23; Shenting, DU24), three in the center of the face (Suliao, DU25; Shuigou, DU26; DuiDuan, DU27), and 15 along the line from Dazhui acupoint to the sacrococcyx (Changgqian, DU01; Yaoshu, DU02; Yaoyangguan, DU03; Mingmen, DU04; Xuanshu, DU05; Jizhong, DU06; Zhongshu, DU07; Jinsuo, DU08; Zhiyang, DU09; Lingtai, DU10; Shendao, DU11; Shenzhu, DU12; Taodao, DU13; DaiZhui, DU14), and one (Huiyang, BL35) beside the sacrococcyx. There are 21 vertebrae, which are the vertebral landmarks for locating the acupoints.

There are 28 acupoints for communication of Qi emitting from Ren meridian: there are two at the center of the throat (Tiantu, RN22; Lianquan, RN23), six along the breastbone in the chest on each side (zhongting, RN16; Danzhong, RN17; Yutang, RN18; Zigong, RN19; Huagai, RN20; Xuanji, RN21), three acupionts which are three cun below xiphoid process (Shangwan, RN13; Juque, RN14; Jiuwei, RN15), five acupoints which are five cun above the stomach (Shenque, RN08; Shuifen, RN09; Xiawan, RN10; Jianli, RN11; Zhongwan, RN12), and six acupoints from stomach to the pubis running the length of six and a half cun (Qugu, RN02; Zhongji, RN03; Guanyuan, RN04;Shimen, RN05;Qihai, RN06;Yinjiao, RN07). These are the abdominal landmarks for locating acupoints. There is one acupoint between the anus and genital region (Huiyin, RN01), one below each eye on each side (Chengqi, ST01), one below the lip and one on the upper gums (Chengjiang, RN24) and Yinjiao (DU28).

There 22 acupoints for communication of Qi emerging from Chong meridian: there are six on each side half a cun off the xiphoid process to the navel with one cun for one acupoint (Huangshu; KI16; Shangqu; KI17; Shiguan; KI18; Yindu; KI19; Futonggu; KI20; Youmen; KI21) and five on each side from five Fen off the navel to the pubis with one cun for one acupoint (Henggu; KI11; Dahe; KI12; Qixue; KI13; Siman; KI14; Zhonszhu; KI15), which is the abdominal landmark for locating acupoints.

There are two acupoints for communication of Qi from foot-Shaoyin meridian, one at each side in the pubic hair on foot-Jueyin meridian (Jimai, LR12), one at each side on hand-Shaoyin meridian (Yinxi, HT06), one at Yinqiao and one at Yangqiao meridians (Jiaoxin, KI08; Shenmai, BL62), and there are acupoints in the thenar eminence of hand and foot for Qi communication. Totally, 365 acupoints have been described.

Chapter 60

Bony Foramen

Yellow Emperor: I have heard that wind is the leading evil for various diseases; how to treat it with acupuncture?

Qibo: Wind evil invades from outside, which makes people suffer from chill, sweating, headache, heavy body and fearing cold, and it should be treated by needling Fengfu to balance Yin and Yang. When there is deficiency, supplementing therapy is used; when there is excess, purging therapy is used.

If big wind evil invasion causes the pain of neck and nape, it can be treated by needling Fengfu (GV16)*, which is located above the midpoint of the atlas. If high wind invasion causes sweating, it can be treated by moxibustion over acupoints Yixi (BL45), located below the sixth thoracic vertebra and three cun on both sides of the backbone; pressing the acupoints can make the patient utter sound "Yixi", which reflects pain beneath the finger.

If the patient fears wind anyhow, it can be treated by needling acupoints Cuanzhu (BL02) near the medial end of the eyebrows. Stiff neck with tension between upper shoulders can be treated by moxibustion over Jizhong (DU06), which is

---

*The acupuncture points are referred to by their traditional names in *Huangdi Neijing*. The meridians and numbers are added by the translator.

found by bending both elbows and locating the intersection between the horizontal line between the elbows and the vertebrae. The pain and distention of the lower abdomen referred from hypochondriac region can be treated by needling acupoints Yixi (BL45). If lumbago makes lifting heavy objects difficult and results in inability to turn around and if the muscular spasm draws testes, it should be treated by needling acupoints Baliao (BL31) and Pain-point; Baliao (BL31) is located in dorsal sacral foramina. Tuberculous fistula with chill-fever can be treated by deeply needling Hanfu (Xiyangguan) (GB33) located in the lateral seam beside the knee cap. The patient should take a posture of bowing to enable selection of the acupoint on lateral knee; the patient should take a posture of kneeling to enable selection of acupoint Yongquan (KI01) on the center of the sole.

Conception channel starts from Huiyin (RN01) below Zhongji (RN03), goes anteriorly to the pubic region and ascends along internal abdomen, through Guanyuan and into the throat; then it ascends across the cheeks and enters the eyes. Thoroughfare channel starts from Qijie together with Shaoyin meridian, ascends by both sides of the navel and then spreads into the chest. When there is pathologic change in Reception channel, the male will suffer from seven kinds of accumulative hernias internally while the female will suffer from leukorrhagia and abdominal lump and aggregation. When there is pathologic change in Thoroughfare channel, there will be Qi reversal and internal spasm and pain.

When there is pathologic change in Governor channel, there will be rigid spine and opisthotonus. Governor channel starts from the middle of the pubic symphysis below the lower abdomen; in females, it runs into the external orifice of the uterus and below the urinary opening; its collateral passes along the external genital and converges at the perineum and bypasses posterior perineum; it diverges and runs around the buttock to meet the collaterals of foot-Shaoyin meridian and to combine with foot-Taiyang, which ascends together with foot-Shaoyin along the posteromedial thigh, penetrates through the spine and connects kidney; the divergent branches also start together with foot-Taiyang meridian from inner canthus, ascend to the forehead, converge on the vertex, then go into the brain; the divergent also comes out of the brain, descends along nape, runs inside the shoulders, along the spine and to the waist, and connects kidney; in males, Governor channel descends along the penis to the perineum, which shares the same course with the female; it ascends straight along the lower abdomen, by the middle of the navel, through the heart, and into the throat; it ascends along the cheeks, goes around the lips and connects the middle acupoints below the eyes. When there is pathologic change in Governor channel, there will be heart pain due to Qi surging into heart from the lower abdomen as well as difficulty in defecation and urination, which is termed thoroughfare hernia. Females will suffer from infertility, or there will be urinary retention, hemorrhoids, enuresis and dry throat. For the disease of Governor channel, it should be generally treated by targeting Governor channel by needling Qugu (RN02) at the midpoint above the pubic bone, and the severe case of disease should be treated by needling acupoint Yinjiao below the navel.

For the patient with reversal Qi with wheezing, treatment should be done by needling acupoint Tiantu (RN22) at the throat center and between supraclavicular fossae. For the patient with Qi surging to the throat, treatment should be by needling acupoint Jian, i.e. Daying (ST05) at anterior cheek. For the patient with lameness and inflexibility of the knee, treatment is by needling the thigh where Biguan (ST31) is located. For the patient with knee pain when sitting, needling the hip where Huantiao (GB30) is located is the treatment strategy. For the patient with internal heat of the knee when standing, treatment is by needling the knee where Xiyangguan (GB33) is located. For the patient with knee pain involving hallux, the popliteal fossa where Weizhong (GB40) is located should be needled for treatment. For the patient with knee pain that feels like something is hiding inside it when sitting, needling of thigh joint where Chengfu (BL36) is located is the form of treatment. For the patient unable to flex and extend due to knee pain, needling the acupoints on the back is recommended. When the pain involves the shank with fracture-like feeling, it should be treated by needling acupoint (ST36) over sacrum on Yangming. Or it should be treated by needling creek (Xing)acupoint on foot-Taiyang and foot-Shaoyin meridians. For the patient with sore shank and pain due to long-term soaking in water and failing to stand long, it should be treated by needling acupoint Guangming (GB37) on collateral from foot-Shaoyang meridian, five cun above the lateral angle. Above the assistant bone and below the pubic bone is the femur bone; beside the hip is the acetabulofemoral joints; the junction of the knee is the knee joint; inside the knee is the patella; below the patella is the assistant bone; above the assistant bone is the popliteal fossa; above the popliteal fossa is the knee joint; horizontally behind the head and above the neck is occipital bone.

There are 57 acupoints for treating water-disease: there are five rows with five acupoints each above the sacrum and coccyx; there are two rows with five acupoints each above Futu (ST32); there is one row, respectively, with five acupoints each on both sides; there are six acupoints each in each row above the malleolus. There are three foramina in occiput three fen under the sharp bone of the skull marginal, one under the sutural bone of the skull, one under the middle of cervical vertebrae, and one above Fengfu (ST32) on the cervical spine. The lower spinal foramina are located in the sacrococcyx. There are several marrow foramina in the facial region and beside both sides of the nasal bones, and also at the bottom of the oral bone, being flush with the level of the two shoulders. The bony foramina of the two shoulders are on the lateral scapula. Arm bony foramina are on lateral arm, four cun away from epicondyle and between two bones. Upper femoral foramina are on lateral femurs, four cun above the knee. Shank bone foramina are on the upper end of assistant bones. The bony foramnia between femurs are under the pubic artery region. Sacrococcyx foramina are behind and four cun away from the femurs. Flat bones have striae to infiltrate, having no marrow foramina for exchange.

For treating cold-heat disease with moxibustion, firstly Dazhui (GV14) on the nape should be moxibusted and the number of moxa-cone is equivalent to the patient's age; secondly Changqiang (Weilue GV01) on coccyx be moxibusted, and here also the number of moxa-cone is equivalent to the patient's age; moxibustion should be given after inspecting the depression on the back transport (Shu) acupoints, for the depression of the shoulders when the arms are raised, for Jingmen (GB25) between the hypochondria, for Juegu (GB38) above the lateral malleolus, for Xiaxi (GB43) acupoint between the little and fourth toes, for depression below the shank, for

Kunlun (BL60) behind lateral malleolus, for a painful region as hard as sinew above the supraclavicular fossa, for Tiantu (CV22) the depression in the chest, for Daling (PC07) below the wrist, Guanyuan (RN04) three cun below the navel, Qichong (ST30) over the artery in the pubic artery region, Zusanli (ST36) three cun below the knee, Chongyang (ST42) on foot Yangming above tarsus, and Baihui (DU20) on the vertex. The wound area arising due to being bitten by a dog should be given moxibustion with three cones. Totally, 29 regions for moxibustion have been mentioned above. Maldigestion can be also treated with moxibustion, and if not cured, according to the meridians concerned with hyperactive Yang, the acupoints can be needled repeatedly together before administering medication to the patient.

Chapter 61

The Acupoints for Water-Disease and Heat-Disease

Yellow Emperor: Why can Shaoyin govern kidney? And why can kidney govern the water?
Qibo: Kidney is the extreme Yin that is responsible for regulating water; since lung is associated with Taiyin and Shaoyin with winter pulse, the root is in kidney and the branch is in lung, both of which can cause accumulation of water.

Emperor: How can kidney accumulate water and cause diseases?
Qibo: Kidney is the gate of stomach, and if kidney fails to close normally, it will accumulate water and show its water property. The water overflows up and down the skin, leading to edema. Edema is the disorder caused by accumulation of water.

Emperor: Do all types of water retention originate from kidney?
Qibo: Kidney is a Yin-organ, and all earthly Qi from the lower ascends to kidney to generate fluid, which is then termed the extreme Yin. Sweating will be one manifestation that

originates from kidney because of overstraining with boldness; if kidney-sweat encounters the wind, the evil cannot enter the viscera internally and go away from the skin externally, but can only invade the sweat pores and overflow beneath the skin to cause edema; it is originated from kidney and termed wind-water. The so-called black-house refers to sweat pores.

Emperor: There are 57 acupoints related with water disease; which viscera govern these acupoints?
Qibo: There are 57 acupoints related with kidney where Yin is accumulated and water comes in and goes out. There are five lines of acupoints with five acupoints at each line above the sacrum, which are acupoints related with kidney. So, water diseases are characterized with edema, bulging abdomen in the lower, panting in the upper and inability to sleep, indicative of disease involving both root and branch; so the water evil in lung causes panting and the evil in kidney causes edema; additionally, the evil in lung causes Qi reversal and inability to sleep, and then the water disease in both kidney and lung show different manifestations that affect mutually, whose original cause is water retention. Above Futu (ST32) acupoints there are two lines of acupoints, with five in each line, which are the Qi passage of kidney. Three Yin meridians converge in the feet. There is one line of acupoints with six acupoints above the medial malleolus, and it is the descending branches of kidney meridian, termed Taichong (LR03). All the 57 acupoints are located deeply in Yin collaterals, where water evil tends to invade.

Emperor: The collaterals and inter-muscle are selected in spring, why?
Qibo: In spring, the wood Qi begins to administer and liver Qi begins to emerge; liver Qi is irritable and its wind is urgent;

however the meridian tends to run in deep with less Qi, and therefore only collaterals and inter-muscle are selected.

Emperor: The inter-muscle and interstitial striae of exuberant meridian are selected in summer; why is this so?
Qibo: In summer, the fire Qi begins to administer and heart Qi begins to grow; then the vessels are thin and Qi is weak because the meridians are full of Yang Qi and heat overflows inter-muscle and interstitial striae to diffuses in the meridians; therefore the exuberant meridians as well as inter-muscle and interstitial striae are selected; the disease can be cured just by penetrating the skin with needling because evil Qi is only in the shallow region. The so-called exuberant meridian refers to the Yang meridians.

Emperor: In autumn, river (Jing) acupoints and stream acupoints (Shu) are selected; why?
Qibo: In autumn, the metal Qi begins to administer and lung is going to constrict and conquer; metal Qi is about to dominate the fire Qi and Yang Qi returns to estuary acupoints (He); since Yin Qi begins to dominate and the damp Qi is invading the body, Yin Qi isn't exuberant and the evil cannot intrude deeply, so that river (Shu) acupoints are selected to purge Yin evil and estuary acupoints (He) are selected to purge the Yang evil; since Yang Qi begins to decline, estuary acupoints (He) are selected.

Emperor: In winter well points (Jing) and creek points (Ying) are selected, and why?
Qibo: In winter the water Qi begins to administer and kidney Qi begins to close; Yang Qi is declined while Yin Qi is firmed and exuberant; Qi in Taiyang meridian sinks and hides itself and Yang meridian is fading out, so that well acupoints (Jing)

is selected to purge Yin evil and creek acupoints (Ying) is selected to supplement Yang Qi. It's believed that in winter well acupoints (Jing) and creek acupoints (Ying) can be selected so as to prevent running nose and epistaxis. It's the information concerned.

Emperor: After you the Master have mentioned the 59 acupoints for treating heat diseases, I can understand their action but still don't know their locations; I'd like to know their locations and their action in detail.
Qibo: There are five lines with five acupoints in each on the head, which are responsible for purging reversal heat of all Yang meridians. There are a total of eight acupoints including Dazhu (BL11)*, Yingshu (Zhongfu LU01), Quepen (ST12) and Beishu (Fengmen BL12) on both sides, which can be used to purge the heat in chest. There are a total of eight acupoints including Qijie (Qichong ST30), Sanli (ST36), Shangjuxu (ST37) and Xiajuxu (ST39) on both sides, which can be used to purge the heat in the stomach. There are a total of eight acupoints including Yunmen (LU2), Yugu (Jianyu LI15), Weizhong (BL40) and Suikong (Yaoshu GV02) on both sides, which can be used to purge the heat of the four limbs. Beside the back-transport acupoints of five solid viscera, there are totally ten acupoints on both sides which can be used to purge heat in the five solid viscera. All the 59 acupoints are the ones on the right or left to treat fever.

Emperor: One is affected by the cold that can turn into heat, and why?
Qibo: Because excessive cold Qi will give rise to fever.

---

*The acupuncture points are referred to by their traditional names in *Huangdi Neijing*. The meridians and numbers are added by the translator.

Chapter 62

Regulation of Meridians

Yellow Emperor: I've learnt a quotation from *On Acupuncture Manipulation* that the excess should be purged while the insufficiency supplemented; what is the excess and what is the insufficiency?
Qibo: There are five types of excess and also five types of insufficiency, so which one would you like to know?

Emperor: I'd like to know both.
Qibo: The spirit has excess or insufficiency, and so does Qi, blood, physique and mind. There are totally ten conditions, and they present different levels of Qi.

Emperor: The body is composed of essence, Qi, fluid, liquid, four limbs, nine orifices, five solid viscera, sixteen meridians and 365 acupoints, all of which can contract hundreds of diseases. These diseases can be divided into excess and deficiency. Now you the Master state that there are five types of excess and five types of insufficiency — how do they come about?
Qibo: They all originate from the five solid viscera. Among them, heart stores spirit, lung stores Qi, liver stores blood,

spleen stores muscular essence and kidney stores mind, all of which compose the physique. Only when the mind is communicative and connected with bone and marrow can it integrate a human body with physique and five solid viscera. The paths of five solid viscera originate from meridians, in which the Qi and blood can circulate, and if there is disharmony between Qi and blood, it will give rise to changes and further to hundreds of diseases; hence, the meridians should be kept intact.

Emperor: What are manifestations if spirit is excessive or insufficient?
Qibo: Excessive spirit manifests in laughing endlessly, and insufficient spirit with sorrow. If evil isn't combined with blood-Qi, five solid viscera will be peaceful; if evil only invades the physique, chill will be from the skin-hair but not into meridians, which is termed slight spiritual disease.

Emperor: How to do the purging or supplementing techniques when needling?
Qibo: For excessive spirit, the small collaterals should be purged with shallow needling till bleeding and the large meridians should be avoided, so that the spirit can be calmed down. For deficient spirit, deficient collaterals should be observed, the acupoints can be located by palpating and then acupoints can be needled to soothe Qi and blood, during which bleeding and Qi leakage should be avoided, so that the meridians can be communicated to calm down spirit.

Emperor: How to do the needling for slight evil?
Qibo: With massaging for longer time and avoiding needling too deep, the Qi can be moved to the location with insufficient Qi and then spiritual Qi can be calmed down.

Emperor: Good. What are the manifestations of Qi excess or Qi deficiency?
Qibo: Excessive Qi causes panting and cough due to surging Qi, and insufficient Qi causes labored respiration and less Qi. If the evil isn't combined with blood-Qi, five solid viscera are peaceful and only slight skin disease develops, which is termed slight leakage of white Qi.

Emperor: How to do supplementing or purging manipulation when needling?
Qibo: For Qi excess, one should purge the divergent collaterals of meridians purged without injuring great meridians, bleeding and leakage of Qi. For Qi deficiency, the divergent collaterals of meridians should be supplemented avoiding leaking Qi leakage.

Emperor: How to do the needling for slight evil?
Qibo: The acupoint should be massaged for a longer time; then the doctor can take out the needle and show it to the patient, saying: 'I'd like to insert the needle deep into your body'. However, the needle should be actually inserted to the proper depth of the body, during which the patient can concentrate the spirit by himself, evil Qi can be dispersed and driven away through interstitial striae, and finally the genuine Qi can be restored.

Emperor: Good. What are the manifestations of excessive or deficient blood?
Qibo: Excessive blood causes anger and deficient blood causes fright. If the evil isn't combined with Qi and blood, five solid viscera are peaceful; the evil can only attack and overflow the minute collaterals to cause blood stasis there.

Emperor: How to do supplementing or purging manipulation when needling?

Qibo: For excessive blood, the exuberant meridians should be purged till bleeding. For deficient blood, the deficient meridians should be identified and needled internally on the meridian; the needle should be retained for observation; when the meridians become dilated, the needle should be withdrawn quickly without bleeding.

Emperor: How about the needling for blood stasis?
Qibo: The collaterals with blood stasis should be identified and then be needled till bleeding, avoiding driving bad blood into meridians to cause the diseases accordingly.

Emperor: Good. What are the manifestations of excessive or deficient physique?
Qibo: Excessive physique causes abdominal distention and difficulty in urination and defecation, and insufficient physique causes disability of four limbs. If the evil isn't combined with Qi and blood, five solid viscera are peaceful and the evil only attacks the muscle, leading to muscle twitch, which is termed the slight wind.

Emperor: How to do supplementing or purging techniques when needling?
Qibo: For excessive physique, foot-Yangming meridian should be purged, and for deficient physique, the Yangming collaterals should be supplemented.

Emperor: How to do the needling for slight evil?
Qibo: Inter-muscle should be needled with avoiding meridians and injuring collaterals, so that defensive Qi can be restored and evil can be eliminated.

Emperor: Good. What are the manifestations of excessive or deficient mind?

Qibo: Excessive mind causes abdominal distention and diarrhea after indigestion, while deficient mind causes cold limbs. When the evil isn't combined with Qi-blood, five solid viscera are peaceful and the evil Qi only attacks the bone, leading to joint tremor.

Emperor: How to do supplementing and purging manipulations when needling?
Qibo: For excessive mind, acupoint Rangu (KI02)* should be needled for purging the blood of sinews; for deficient mind, Fuliu (KI07) should be needled for supplementing Qi.

Emperor: When evil isn't combined with Qi-blood, how to do the needling?
Qibo: The joint with tremor should be needled, avoiding inserting the meridians; thus the evil can be driven away.

Emperor: Good. I have learnt the manifestations of excess and deficiency syndromes, but I don't know how they are caused.
Qibo: If evil is combined with Qi-blood, Yin and Yang will deviate mutually, Qi will be disturbed in the defense aspect, blood will flow reversely in the meridian, and blood will divorce Qi, leading to one deficiency and one excess. If blood is combined with Yin evil or Qi with Yang evil, it will cause mania. If blood is combined with Yang evil and Qi with Yin evil, it will cause the middle overheating. If blood is combined with evil in the upper and Qi is combined with evil in the lower, there will be heart vexation, depression and frequent anger. If blood is combined with evil in the lower and Qi is combined with evil in the upper, there will be derangement and amnesia.

---

*The acupuncture points are referred to by their traditional names in *Huangdi Neijing*. The meridians and numbers are added by the translator.

Emperor: When blood is combined with Yin evil and Qi with Yang evil, blood and Qi can be divorced; then which is the excess and which is the deficiency?
Qibo: Blood and Qi prefer warm and fear cold; cold can make Qi and blood fail to flow due to damping, and warm can disperse and eliminate their stagnation; thus the evil combined with Qi pertains to blood deficiency while the evil combined with blood to Qi deficiency.

Emperor: Blood and Qi are the important substances in the human body. As you the Mister have mentioned that double blood pertains deficiency and double Qi also to deficiency, could it be said that there is no excess?
Qibo: To gain means excess and to lose means deficiency; so the double Qi causes blood deficiency while the double blood causes Qi deficiency, which leads to blood and Qi divorcing, leading to deficiency. By contrast, collaterals and minute collaterals infuse Qi and blood into meridians, in which double blood is combined with double Qi, leading to excess. If blood and Qi are combined toward meridians, it will cause critical reversal that in turn causes sudden deaths; if Qi and blood flow can be restored, the patient can survive; otherwise he will die.

Emperor: Where does the excess come from? And where does the deficiency go to? I'd like to know the cause of excess and deficiency.
Qibo: Both Yin and Yang meridians have acupoints for infusion and convergences. If Yang Qi infuses Yin meridian and Yin meridian is full of Qi and blood, Yin and Yang can keep the balance to nourish the physique sufficiently, leading to the consistency of the nine positions of the human body, and such a person is termed the normal person. As to the origin of the evil, it might originate from either Yin or Yang. The

diseases with the Yang evil can be caused by wind, rain, cold and summer heat. The disease with Yin evil can be caused by improper diet and living styles as well as abnormal emotion.

Emperor: How do wind and rain attack the body?
Qibo: When the wind and rain attack the body, the evil firstly invades the skin and then it is transmitted to minute collaterals; if the minute collaterals are full, the evil is transmitted to the collaterals; if the collaterals are full, the evil is transmitted to the meridians. If evil is combined with Qi-blood, it will invade between muscles and interstitial striae, and the pulse must be firm and large, which is termed the excess. The excess syndrome is characterized by the firm and full surface that cannot be felt and the person feels pain under pressure.

Emperor: How do cold and damp attack the body?
Qibo: When cold and damp attack the body, the patient will have numb skin, firm and tense muscles, damping of nutrition Qi and blood, and exhaustion of defense Qi, which is termed deficiency. The deficiency is characterized by loose skin and insufficient Qi; after being pressed, the skin will become warm due to the sufficient Qi and the person will feel no pain.

Emperor: Good. What are the manifestations of excess syndrome in Yin-phase?
Qibo: The abnormal emotion can cause Yin Qi reversal that causes in deficiency in the lower that causes Yang Qi to move away, which is termed excess.

Emperor: What are the manifestations of deficiency syndrome in Yin-phase?

Qibo: Joy can make Qi descend and sorrow leads to Qi exhaust, which result in empty pulse. Under this condition, cold food will make cold Qi diffuse into the internal to cause blood stagnation and Qi exhaustion, which is termed deficiency.

Emperor: It is said in the classics that Yang deficiency can cause external cold while Yin deficiency internal heat, and Yang exuberance can cause external heat while Yin exuberance internal cold. I have learnt that but I don't know the mechanism.

Qibo: Yang aspect receives Qi in upper Jiao to warm the skin and inter-muscle; if cold Qi attacks the external and causes obstruction of upper Jiao, it can make cold Qi linger alone in the skin, resulting in trembling.

Emperor: How about Yin deficiency to cause the internal heat?

Qibo: Overstrain can cause Qi deficiency, grain Qi insufficiency, stagnation of upper Jiao and obstruction of stomach in the lower; the heat of stomach Qi fumigates the chest, which is termed internal heat.

Emperor: How about Yang exuberance; how does it cause the external heat?

Qibo: If upper-Jiao isn't smooth, the skin will have condensation, blockage of interstitial striae and obstruction of sweat pores, all of which prevent defensive Qi from diffusing, leading to external heat.

Emperor: How about Yin exuberance; how does it cause the internal cold?

Qibo: Critical Qi surges reversely and accumulates in the chest without being discharged, making warm Qi leave and cold Qi linger alone; it will result in blood congealing and obstructed meridians with full, large and unsmooth pulse, indicating internal cold.

Emperor: How to do the needling when the disease has been caused by abnormal combination of Yin and Yang as well as Qi and blood?
Qibo: To treat the disease with acupuncture, the divergent collaterals should be selected. The blood should be directed for the disease in nutritional aspect and the Qi should be directed for the disease in the defensive aspect. Considering the build of the body and climate of the four seasons, the number and location of the acupoints can be determined.

Emperor: When blood and Qi is combined with evil, the disease has formed, and Yin and Yang deviate from each other; how to do supplementing and purging therapy in treatment?
Qibo: For excess syndrome with Qi exuberance, the needle should be inserted together with Qi to open the door like freeing the inlet; the needle should be drawn together with Qi in order to avoid damaging the essence Qi and to purge evil Qi; the outlet shouldn't be closed so as to drive the evil out; the needle hole should be enlarged for freeing its way, which is termed large purgation; the needle should be drawn out after pressing the skin around and then the severe evil Qi can be dispersed.

Emperor: How to do supplementing manipulation for deficiency?
Qibo: The doctor shouldn't hesitate to insert the needle after holding the needle. He should relax the mind to wait for patient's expiration and then insert the needle after the exhalation. The needle hole should be tight to avoid essential Qi leakage and the needle should be quickly withdrawn after having a replete sense when inhaling; then the heat cannot be retained internally, the needle hole can be closed, the evil Qi can be dispersed, and the essence Qi can be preserved. The doctor should wait for the timing to draw the needle according to the sense of Qi arrival; in this way, the local Qi cannot be lost and

Qi in other regions can come here, which is termed pursuing supplementation.

Emperor: As you the Master have mentioned, there are ten types of excess and deficiency syndromes, all of which are caused by five solid visceral disorders. However, there are only five meridians related to five solid viscera. In fact, there are 12 meridians in the body and each meridian can cause diseases. Just now, you the Mister only discussed the five solid viscera. Furthermore, all the 12 meridians connect with the 365 joints, by which diseases can also involve the 12 meridians. The meridian diseases also include excess and deficiency syndromes. How to match up the excess and deficiency syndromes to those of five solid viscera?

Qibo: The five solid viscera are related with six hollow viscera in exterior–interior relationships. Both meridians and joints can cause diseases of excess and deficiency, and according to their focus the treatment should be regulated. Blood should be regulated for the diseases in meridians; collaterals, for the diseases in blood; defense aspect, for the diseases in Qi; intermuscle, for diseases in flesh; sinews, for diseases in sinews; and bone, for the diseases in bone. Diseases in sinews can be treated by heated needling at the region below the focus or the cramp region; diseases in bone can be treated by heated needling and medicated compress; diseases without feeling pain can be treated by needling both Yinqiao and Yangqiao meridians; diseases with pain but nine divisions with no manifestations can be treated by needling contralateral collaterals; for example, for pain on the left with abnormal pulse felt on the right, contralateral meridian needling should be applied. All in all, only when the pulse conditions in nine divisions are clear can the needling techniques be properly applied.

Chapter 63

Contralateral Needling

Yellow Emperor: I have heard about contralateral needling, but I know little about its profound meaning. What exactly is called contralateral needling?

Qibo: After invading the body, evil Qi lingers first in the skin and hair; if not dispelled, it will involve the minute collaterals; if still not dispelled, it will invade the collaterals; if lingering without being dispelled, it will invade the meridians connecting five solid viscera, be distributed among stomach and intestines, involve both Yin and Yang, and damage the five solid viscera; it is the order of evil invasion, starting from the skin and hair and moving finally into five solid viscera, so the disease can be treated by acupuncture on the meridians concerned. Now evil Qi invades the skin and hair, lingers in the minute collaterals without being dispelled but with blockage; it is unable to invade meridians, and thus gets scattered in the large collaterals, leading to uncommon diseases. After invading the large collaterals, evil Qi will shunt from the left to the right and vice versa. Flowing down and up or invading left or right, evil Qi will interfere with meridians and spread over the ends of four limbs; its flow is indefinite and it doesn't run through acupoints on meridians, so the therapy is termed contralateral needling.

Emperor: I'd like to know what contralateral needling is, and why using this treating of disease on the left can be done by needling on the right or vice versa. Also, how to distinguish it from opposite needling?
Qibo: Invading meridians, the luxuriance of evil Qi on the left will cause disease on the right or vice versa; there is also transference and interchange such as the presence of unrelieved pain on the left followed by corresponding disease on the right meridian, for which the opposite needling should be applied on only the meridians instead of collaterals affected. Because the pain of collateral disease doesn't affect the same part of the body as that of meridian disease, the therapy is termed contralateral needling.

Emperor: I'd like to know how to apply contralateral needling and what acupoints are selected?
Qibo: Invasion of evil into the collaterals of foot-Shaoyin causes sudden heart pain, sticking fullness of chest and the hypochondria; without accumulation, the acupoint Rangu (KI02)* is needled till bleeding, and the disease can be cured in the time of a meal; if not relieved, the disease on the left is treated on the right and vice versa; the new disease can be cured in this way in five days.

Invasion of evil into the collaterals of hand-Shaoyang causes throat obstruction, curled tongue, dry mouth, vexation, pain in the lateral border of the arm, and failure to put hands upon the head, which can be treated with needling acupoints Guanchong (TE01) lateral to little finger and on the ring finger by the width of one leaf of Chinese chive each once; the

*The acupuncture points are referred to by their traditional names in *Huangdi Neijing*. The meridians and numbers are added by the translator.

patient of middle age can be cured at once and the elderly patient can be cured after a while; the disease on the left should be treated on the right and vice versa; newly occurred disease can be cured in several days.

Invasion of evil into the collaterals of foot-Jueyin causes sudden hernia and pain. It can be treated with needling the acupoints Dadun (LR01) above nail of hallux toe near the muscle each once. The male patient can be cured at once and the female patient after a while. The disease on the left can be treated on the right side and vice versa.

Invasion of evil into the collaterals of foot-Taiyang causes pain of the head, the nape and shoulders, which can be treated with needling the acupoints Zhiyin (BL67) above the nail of the little toe near the muscle once, and the patient can be cured at once. If it is not cured, the acupoints Jinmen (BL63) below the lateral ankle can be needled three times, needling the right for the left and vice versa; then, the disease can be cured in a meal of time.

Invasion of evil into the collaterals of hand-Yangming causes chest bloating, panting, distention in the hypochondria and heat in the chest, which can be treated with needling acupoints Shangyang (LI01) lateral to the thumb, above the nails of index finger and away from the nails by width of one leaf of the Chinese chive once. The disease on the left can be treated on the right and vice versa, and be cured in a meal of time.

Invasion of evil into the collaterals of hand-Jueyin between the arm and the palm causes difficulty of joint flexion; it can be treated with needling the acupoints posterior to the wrist, indicated by pressing pain. The needling frequency varies with the waxing and waning of the moon; it is done once on the first day of the lunar calendar, twice on the second day, 15 times on the fifteenth day and 14 times on the sixteenth day, decreasing progressively.

Invasion of evil into the foot Yangqiao meridian causes eye pain starting from the inner canthus, which can be treated with needling the acupoints Shenmai (BL62) half a cun below the lateral ankle twice with the method of needling the right for disease on the left and vice versa, and the disease can be cured in a period of time equivalent to a 10-mile walk.

If there is internal blood stasis, abdominal fullness and distension, and difficulty in urination and defecation due to tripping or falling, purging drugs can be taken first; if the disease damages the Jueyin meridian in the upper and collaterals of Shaoyin in the lower, the acupoints below the internal ankle and before the navicular bone can be needled till bleeding, and the artery acupoint on the foot back be needled; if the disease is not cured, acupoints Dadun (LR01) over hallux hairs can be needled one time each, treating the left with needling the right and vice versa, and the disease can be cured right after bleeding; for frequent sorrow, fright and unhappiness, the needling method used is the same as the above.

Invasion of evil into the collaterals of hand-Yangming causes deafness or intermittent hearing loss, which can be treated with needling the acupoints Shangyang (LI01) lateral to thumb, above the nails of index finger and away from the nails by width of one leaf of the Chinese chive once, and the disease can be cured at once; if it is not cured, the needling can be performed on the acupoints Zhongchong (PC09) above the nail of the middle finger near the muscle, so it can be cured at once; for the complete hearing loss, acupuncture cannot be administered; for tinnitus, which sounds like wind in the ears, the same method mentioned above can be used for treatment, including needling the right for the left and vice versa.

The patient with migratory arthralgia can be treated with needling the pain acupoint of inter-muscle, and the needling frequency varies with the waxing and waning of the moon or with the excess or deficiency of Qi; if needling number surpasses the number of days, the healthy Qi will be damaged, and if it is the opposite, the evil Qi cannot be dispelled. Needling is done on the right is to treat the disease on the left and vice versa; if the disease is cured, the needling should be stopped, and if not cured, the same needling process can be repeated. The needling is performed once on the first day of the lunar calendar, twice on the second day; the number increases with the passing days till needling is done 15 times on the fifteenth day, followed by 14 times on the sixteenth day, with the number decreasing day by day.

Invasion of evil into the collaterals of foot-Yangming causes nasal obstruction and epistaxis as well as cold sense in the upper teeth, which can be treated with needling the acupoints Lidui (ST45) lateral to the middle toe and above the nails of the second toe near the muscle once, and needling is done on the right to treat the disease on the left and vice versa.

Invasion of evil into the collaterals of foot-Shaoyang causes breathing difficulty due to hypochondriac pain and cough followed by sweating. It can be treated with needling the acupoints Zuqiaoyin (GB44) lateral to little toe and above the nails of the fourth toe near the muscles once; the difficulty in breathing and sweating can be relieved at once; the patient with cough can be given warm clothes and food, and the cough can be stopped in a day, with needling the right to treat disease on the left and vice versa; the disease can be cured at once; if not, the same treatment can be applied again.

Invasion of evil into the collaterals of foot-Shaoyin causes sore throat, difficulty in swallowing, frequent anger without any causes and Qi surging up on the diaphragm, which can be treated with needling acupoints Yongquan (KI01) at the center of the sole three times; after needling six times, the disease can be cured at once, by using needling the right side to treat disease on the left and vice versa. If the patient with swollen pharynx has difficulty in swallowing saliva or spitting it out occasionally, it can be treated with contralateral needling the acupoints Ranggu (KI02) anterior to navicular bone and the disease can be cured at once after bleeding; here also, the right side is needled to treat disease on the left and vice versa.

Invasion of evil into the collaterals of foot-Taiyin causes lumbago referring to the lower abdomen and hypochondria, and difficulty in breathing while facing up, which can be treated with needling the acupoints in the lumbosacral foramen and muscles on the both sides of lumbar spine, termed Yaoshu acupoints (GV02); the needling frequency varies with the waxing and waning of the moon and the disease can be cured at once after withdrawing the needle, and in this case, the right side is treated for diseases on the left and vice versa.

Invasion of evil into the collaterals of foot-Taiyang causes spasm and pain of the back, radiating to the hypochondria. The acupoints are selected by pressing along both sides of the neck and the spine with thee hand to locate the painful area. The disease can be cured at once after three times of acupuncture.

Invasion of evil into the collaterals of foot-Shaoyang causes pain of Huantiao (GB30) and difficulty in lifting the thigh, which can be treated with needling Huantiao (GB30) using filiform needles, and the needle should be retained for a certain amount of time in case of cold evil. The needling frequency should be based on the waxing and waning of the moon, and the disease can be cured at once.

Any diseases involving meridians can be treated with acupuncture, and if no route of meridian is involved, contralateral needling can be indicated. Deafness can be treated with needling acupoints Shangyang (LI01) on hand Yangming meridian. If it is not cured, the preauricular acupoints Tinggong (SI19), where the meridian runs through, can be needled. Dental caries can be treated with needling acupoints Shangyang (LI01) on hand Yangming meridian; if not cured, the collateral entering the teeth can be needled and the disease can be cured at once.

Invasion of evil into five solid viscera causes the disease characterized by referred pain of the meridian on and off, which can be treated with contralateral needling the acupoints above nails of the fingers and toes according to the condition; the collaterals with stagnation are observed and needled till bleeding; the needling is performed once every other day; if not cured once and for all, the disease can be cured after five times of needling. When the evil Qi is cross-transmitted into the upper teeth leading to cold pain of the lips and teeth, it can be relieved with needling the vessel with blood stasis seen on the back of the hand till bleeding; by needling the acupoints above the nails of the middle toe on foot-Yangming meridian once and the acupoints Shangyang (LI01) lateral to the thumb and above nail of index finger each once, the disease can be cured at once, needling the right side treats disease on the left and vice versa.

Invasion of evil into the collaterals of hand-Shaoyin, foot-Shaoyin, hand-Taiyin, foot-Taiyin and foot-Yangming meridians all converge in the ear and connect the left forehead angle; if evil Qi invading the five collaterals exhausts all their healthy Qi, it will stir all the meridians, leading to loss of general sense of the body, resembling a corpse, termed sudden corpse-like syncope. For treatment, the acupoints Yinhai (SP01) above the nail of hallux toe by a width of a Chinese chive leaf can be needled first; then, the acupoints Yongquan (KI01) and Lidui (ST45) on the center of the sole and above the middle toe nail are needled once; next, the acupoints Shangyang (LI01) on the radial side of the thumb by the width of a Chinese chive leaf are needled; and finally the acupoints Zhongchong (PC09) on hand-Juryin meridian and acupoints Shenmien (HT07) of styloid process on hand-Shaoyin meridian are needled once; then the disease can be cured at once; if not cured, a small bamboo pipe can be used to blow into the ears, and one cun of hair over the left forehead angle is cut off, burnt into ash and taken in with a cup of wine, and the disease can be cured at once; if the patient fails to drink it, the ash can be poured with the wine and disease can be cured at once.

As for the method of acupuncture, the meridians should be first inspected and then palpated carefully in order to differentiate between deficiency and excess. If the meridians aren't harmonized, the meridians involved can be needled; if there is no pain occurring in the meridians, contralateral needling can be applied; any blood stasis in the collaterals should be located, and all must be needled till bleeding; that is the method of contralateral needling.

Chapter 64

Needling for Reversing or Complying with the Changes in Four Seasons

In Jueyin meridian, Qi excess can cause Yin impediment while Qi insufficiency can cause heat impediment, and the slippery pulse indicates inguinal hernia while the unsmooth pulse indicates Qi accumulation in the lower abdomen. In Shaoyin meridian, Qi excess causes skin impediment and urticaria while Qi insufficiency causes lung impediment; and the slippery pulse indicates lung-wind-hernia while the unsmooth pulse indicates abdominal mass and blood in urine. In Taiyin meridian, Qi excess causes muscles impediment and cold attacking the middle while Qi insufficiency causes spleen impediment; and the slippery pulse indicates spleen-wind-impediment while the unsmooth pulse indicates evil accumulation and occasional fullness of heart and abdomen. In Yangming meridian, Qi excess causes meridian impediment and frequent fever while Qi insufficiency causes heart impediment; and the slippery pulse indicates heart-wind-impediment while the unsmooth pulse indicates evil accumulation and frequent fright. In Taiyang meridian, Qi excess causes bone impediment and heavy body while Qi insufficiency causes kidney impediment; and the slippery pulse indicates kidney-wind-hernia while the unsmooth pulse indicates evil accumulation and frequent paroxysms of head disease. In Shaoyang meridian, Qi excess causes sinew impediment and hypochondriac fullness while insufficient Qi causes liver impediment; and the slippery pulse indicates liver-wind-hernia while the unsmooth pulse indicates evil accumulation, sinew spasm and eye pain. Thus, spring Qi is in meridians, summer Qi in minute collaterals, late summer Qi in muscles, autumn Qi in skin and winter Qi in the bone and marrow.

Emperor: I'd like to know the reason.
Qibo: In spring, heavenly Qi begins to spread, earthly Qi begins to emerge, the ground thaws and ice is melting, water is flowing and meridian Qi is circulating, so human Qi is in meridians. In summer, the meridians are full of Qi, the minute collaterals are receiving blood and the skin is replete. In late summer, meridians and collaterals are both exuberant and Qi and blood are diffused in the muscles. In autumn, heavenly Qi begins to astringe, interstitial striae are blocked and the skin is tightened. In winter, it is responsible for coverage and storage, Qi and blood are in the middle and stored inside the bone and marrow and internally connected with five solid viscera. Hence, evil Qi invades the body following the variation of Qi and blood in four seasons, but its variation is hard to measure; so the meridian Qi should be made compliant in order to expel the evil, and it is by this process that Qi disorder won't develop.

Emperor: If one performs acupuncture in the way of reversing the variation of four seasons, what are the outcomes?

Qibo: Needling collaterals in spring will cause external leakage of blood and Qi with less breath; needling muscles in spring will cause reverse circulation of blood and Qi with Qi surging up; needling sinews and bones in spring will cause internal stagnation of blood and Qi with abdominal distension. Needling meridians in summer will cause exhaustion of blood and Qi and lassitude; needling muscles in summer will cause internal blockage of blood and Qi with frequent fear; and needling sinews and bones in summer will cause blood and Qi to ascend in the reverse with frequent anger. Needling meridians in autumn will cause blood and Qi to ascend reversely with frequent amnesia; needling collaterals in autumn will cause failure of Qi spreading out, with sleepiness and lassitude; needling collaterals in autumn will cause internal scattering of blood and Qi with chill and shivering. Needling meridians in winter will cause depletion of blood and Qi with blurred vision; needling collaterals in winter will cause external leakage of internal Qi with great impediment as a sequela; needling muscles in winter will cause exhaustion of Yang Qi with amnesia. The needling methods mentioned above severely reverse variation in four seasons, leading to drastic diseases, so one cannot but comply with the rules; otherwise, Qi disorder will develop that disturbs function leading to diseases. Therefore, if not knowing the rules of variation in four seasons and the mechanism of diseases, one will take compliance for reversal, leading to internal disorder of healthy Qi and making evil Qi collide with essence Qi; the nine positions should be observed so that the healthy Qi cannot be disturbed and essence Qi cannot be deviated by evil.

Emperor: Good! Accidentally puncturing one of five viscera will give rise to disastrous outcomes; if heart is accidentally punctured, the patient will die in one day with warning sign of belching. If liver is accidentally punctured, the patient will die in five days with warning sign of incoherent speech. If lung is accidentally punctured, the patient will die in three days with warning sign of cough. If kidney is accidentally punctured, the patient will die in six days with warning sign of sneezing and yawning. If spleen is accidentally punctured, the patient will die in ten days with warning sign of swallowing. As a rule, if one of five solid viscera is injured by accidental puncturing, the patient is doomed to die with critical warning signs varying with the organ under consideration, and the death date can be anticipated after watching out for the respective warning signs.

Chapter 65

Branch–Root and Transmission of Diseases

Yellow Emperor: Any disease has two basic manifestations — branch or root; acupuncture has two basic methods — reversal and compliance. Why is this so?
Qibo: Generally, prior to needling, Yin and Yang should be distinguished, time-order must be considered, reversal or compliance therapies must be properly applied and the treatment should be regulated for branch and root. It's believed that for the disease with branch manifestation, the treatment can be directed at the branch; for the disease with the root cause, the treatment can be directed at root; for the disease with the root, the treatment can be also directed at branch, and for disease with the branch, the treatment can be also directed at root. So, the corresponding therapies are effective, respectively, in directing at the branch disease or at the root disease as well as with reversal method or with compliance method. So, if knowing the reversal or compliance methods, there will be no doubt with regard to the proper treatment; if knowing the branch and root, the therapies are always successful. If not knowing the branch and the root, the medical behavior is blind.

Yin–Yang, reversal–compliance and the branch–root are the principle; the principle seems minor, but it is great and can cover the harm caused by all the diseases under one principle; it seems less but is more, or seems narrow but is broad, and so hundreds of cases can be summed up based on this principle. It's possible to know the deep from the shallow and to observe the future from the present; however it is easier said than done when branch and root are concerned.

Treating the evil with purgation against meridian Qi is called reversal method, while with supplementation along meridian Qi is called compliance method. For the disease followed by reversal condition, treatment should be directed at the root; for the reversal condition followed by disease, treatment should be directed at the root. For chill followed by disease, treatment should be directed at the root; for the disease followed by chill, treatment should be directed at the root. For the fever followed by disease, treatment should be directed at the root; for the fever followed by full distention in the middle, treatment should be directed at the branch. For the disease followed by diarrhea, treatment should be directed at the root; for diarrhea followed by other diseases, treatment should be directed at the root; only when diarrhea is cured can other diseases be treated. The disease followed by full distention in the middle should be treated by directing at the branch; for the disease followed by dysphoria, treatment should be directed at the root. The human body can suffer from disease either due to external evil Qi or internal disharmonious Qi. Any disease manifested by difficulty in defecation or urination should be treated by directing at the branch; any disease manifested by smooth defecation or urination should be treated directing at the root. The disease starting with the excess should be treated from the root to the branch, i.e., treating the root first and the branch second. The disease starting with the deficiency should be treated from the branch to the root, i.e., treat the branch first and the root second. The condition of the disease, moderate or severe, should be regulated attentively; for the moderate one, it can be treated by directing the branch and the root simultaneously, while for the severe one, it can be treated by directing the root alone. If there is difficulty in urination and defecation followed by disease, treatment should be directed at the root.

In view of transmission of diseases, heart disease first manifests in heart pain, which is transmitted (to lung) as coughing on the first day; (to liver) as sticking hypochondriac pain in three days; and then (to spleen) as obstruction and heavy body in five more days; if not cured in three days, the patient will die at midnight in winter or at noon in summer.

Lung disease manifests in panting and cough, which is transmitted (to liver) as sticking distension and pain on hypochondria, and on the third day; (to spleen) as heavy body and general pain one day later; (to stomach) as distension in five days; if not cured in ten days, the patient will die at sunset in winter or at sunrise in summer.

Liver disease manifests as vertigo and blurred vision, which is transmitted (to spleen) as a feeling of a heavy body on the third day; (to stomach) as abdominal distention in five more days; as pain of waist, spine and lower abdomen and sour shank in three more days; if not cured in three more days, the patient will die at sunset in winter or at breakfast in summer.

Spleen disease manifests as general pain and heavy body, which is transmitted (to stomach) as distention on the first day; (to kidney) as pain of lower abdomen, waist and spine and sour shank in two more days; and (to bladder) as pain of the back, spine and sinews and dysuria in three more days; if not cured in ten more days, the patient will die after midnight in winter or at dusk in summer.

Kidney disease manifests in pain of lower abdomen, waist and spine and sour shank, which is transmitted (to bladder) as pain of the back, spine and sinews, and anuria on the third day; (to stomach) as abdominal distention in three more days; (to liver) as sticking pain on hypochondria in three more days; if not cured in three more days, the patient will die at dawn in winter or at dusk in summer.

Stomach disease manifests as distention and fullness, which is transmitted (to kidney) as lower abdominal pain, lumbago and sour shank; as pain of the back, spine and sinews, and anuria in three more days; and (to spleen) as heavy body in five more days; if not cured in six more days, the patient will die after midnight in winter or after noon in summer.

The bladder disease manifests with anuria, which is transmitted (to kidney) as abdominal distention, waist and spinal pain, and sour shank on the fifth day; (to stomach) as abdominal distention in one more day, and (to spleen) as general pain in one more day; if not cured in two more days, the patient will die after midnight in winter or after noon in summer.

If the different diseases are transmitted in the full order mentioned above with a certain death date, the patient cannot be needled. If transmitted to every other organ, the disease is difficult to be transmitted, and if it is transmitted to the third or fourth organ, the patient can be needled.

Chapter 66

Great Theory on Law of Primordial Qi in Nature

Yellow Emperor asked: In the universe, there are five elements that control five aspects, giving rise to cold, heat, dry, damp and wind; in the human body there are five solid viscera that are expressed as five kinds of emotional Qi, giving rise to joy, anger, contemplation, anxiety and fright. It is said in classics that five evolutionary phases succeed with their respective dominating time, and at the end of a year, it will go round and begin again, all of which I know. Now I'd like to know how the evolutionary phases are related with the expression of three Yin and three Yang as well as six seasonal Qi?

Guiyuqu kowtowed again and kneeled to say: How wonderful your question is! The revolving five phases and Yin–Yang are the law of the heavens and the earth, the principle of all creatures small and great, the parents of changes and alterations, the origin of life and death, and the house of spirit; how can't we be familiar with them? So, the origin of the matter is called transformation, the extreme of the matter is called alteration, the uncertainty of Yin and Yang is called spirit, and indefinite application of spirit is called the Saint. The alteration can be expressed variously, in the heavens as metaphysics, in human being as the law, and on the earth as transformation. The transformation is associated with five flavors, and the law with wisdom and metaphysics with the spirit. The spirit in the heavens is expressed as wind, while on the earth as wood; in the heavens as heat, while on the earth as fire; in the heavens as damp, while on the earth as soil; in the heavens as dry, while on the earth as metal; and in the heavens as cold, while on the earth as water. Therefore, those in the heavens are expressed as Qi and on the earth as form, in which Qi and shape influence each other leading to the being of all creatures great and small. The heavens and the earth are the upper and lower of all creatures in the world; the left and the right are the route of Yin and Yang; water and fire are representatives of Yin and Yang; metal and wood are the end and origin of growth and development. Qi has large and small quantity, the shape has exuberance and decline, the upper Qi and lower matter cooperate with each other, and the excess and deficiency can all be shown obviously.

Emperor asked: I'd like to know the dominating time of revolving five phases; what are they?
Guiyuqu answered: Five evolutionary phases can dominate one year, respectively, but not only for seasons.

Emperor said: Please tell me the rule about it.
Guiyuqu answered: I have checked the *Primeval Genesis Volume of the Universe*; it is said in the book that the universe is an endless space, the basis of creation, and the origin of all creatures. Five phases are evolving round and round in the universe to distribute the genuine Qi and to control all the creatures on the earth. Nine stars twinkle high in the sky, and seven luminaries are revolving around; so, there are Yin and Yang changes,

which have the property of being soft and solid. Both Yin and Yang have immergence or emergence in due position, cold and heat shifting according to the season, and life and growth in nature lasting forever with various forms. After ten generations of research, they are just the rules concerned in my family.

Emperor asked: Good. What does it mean that Qi has large and small quantity and the shape has exuberance and decline?
Guiyuqu answered: Yin and Yang have large and small quantity, so there are triple Yin and triple Yang. The shape has exuberance and decline, which is associated with dominating time of revolving five phases and there will be excess or deficiency. Therefore at the beginning, there is excess to come, followed by deficiency, while there is deficiency to come, followed by the excess. Knowing the leading and the following, the phasing Qi can be expected. The phasing Qi coinciding with heavenly Qi is called the heavenly correspondence, coinciding with the year of earthly branches called as the year suitability, and together coinciding with heavenly Qi and year of earthly branches called as triple harmony.

Emperor asked: How about the influence between the upper Qi and the lower forms?
Guiyuqu answered: The cold, heat, dry, damp, wind and fire are the Yin and Yang in the heavens, which are embodied as the triple Yin and triple Yang meridians in the upper. Wood, fire (monarch), earth, metal, water, and fire (minister) are the Yin and Yang on the earth, which are embodied as birth, growth, development, harvest and storage in the lower. So, Yang has Yin while Yin has Yang. The heavens take charge of Yang's growth and Yin's development, while the earth takes charge of Yang's killing and Yin's storage. The heavens have Yin and

Yang, so does the earth. Therefore, the changes of Yin and Yang between the heavens and the earth should be known along with the five phases corresponding to the heavenly solar terms that are dynamic forever and shifted towards the right every five years; six earthly Qi corresponding to the earthly branches are static at each position and finish a circle every six years. With the influence between the dynamic and the static, overlapping between the upper and lower as well as interleaving of Yin and Yang, changes of the phasing Qi occur.

Emperor asked: Is there any definite number for the circulation of the upper and the lower Qi?
Guiyuqu answered: The heavenly Qi takes six as the definite number, while the earthly Qi takes five. The heavenly Qi finishes one circle with six years as one Bei, while the earthly Qi finishes one circle with five years as one Zhou. The monarch-fire has a nominal position, while the ministerial fire has a position to implement. Five phasing Qi is combined with six heavenly Qi; there are 720 heavenly Qi as one Ji with 30 years each; 1440 heavenly Qi as one Zhou with 60 years each. All excess and deficiency can be covered at one glance.

Emperor said: The theory that you the Master have mentioned can cover the heavenly Qi in the upper and the earthly Qi in the lower, which are, as it were, quite detailed. I'd like to know and preserve it. Since it can resolve the suffering of people first and foremost and culture the human body secondly, it is helpful if people understand these principles, harmonize the relationship, and enjoy the benefits everywhere; thus it should be passed on to the future generations for endless time; can I learn more?
Guiyuqu said: The mechanism of the extreme theory sticks to the point with deep elucidation, which can be seen when

coming and be retraced when going. Anyone will be prosperous if complying with it or extinguished if violating it. The selfish behavior against natural law must deserve the disasters that befall. Please allow me to follow the natural law and tell you the genuine truth.

Emperor said: Those good at discussing the origin can foresee the future and those who are good at discussing the close can know the distant, so that anybody can master the extreme theory and avoid puzzles, meaning elucidation. I wish you the Master could make a further inference, proper and logical, simple and clear, permanent and ceaseless, and applicable and unforgettable, which can be used as the outlines and genuine key.

Guiyuqu said: How wonderful your question is! How bright your statement is! It is as if a stick were striking a drum with the sound echoing. I've known that the first and sixth year is dominated by the earth phase; the second and seventh year by metal phase, the third and eighth year by water phase, the fourth and ninth year by wood phase, and the fifth and tenth year by fire phase.

Emperor asked: How is six-Qi combined with triple Yin and triple Yang?

Guiyuqu answered: The first and seventh earthly year is coincided with the Shaoyin in the upper Qi, the second and eighth year with Taiyin, the third and ninth year with Shaoyang, the fourth and tenth year with Yangming, the fifth and eleventh with Taiyang, and the sixth and twelfth year with Jueyin. Shaoyin meridian is marked as the start, while Jueyin meridian marks the end. Jueyin in the upper governs wind, Shaoyin governs heat, Taiyin governs damp, Shaoyang governs fire, Yangming governs dry, and Taiyang governs cold. The so-called origin of triple Yin and Yang are six primordial origins.

Emperor said: How bright your statement is! How clear your discussion is! I will inscribe them in jade and store it in the golden chest, with the title of *Universal Genesis Record*.

Chapter 67

Great Theory on Movement of Five Phases

Sitting in the bright hall, the Yellow Emperor began to follow the discipline of heavens, observe the eight directions of the earth, and consider establishing the principle of five-phase Qi.

Yellow Emperor invited Master Qibo and asked him: It was recorded in previous medical literature that the dynamics and statics in the heavens and the earth had set the natural changes as their laws and the alternation of cold winter and hot summer as the manifestation in the ascending and descending of Yin and Yang. I've learned from you the law of five phases that explains the governing of one year by each phase Qi and the determination of year phase starting from the primary-1st year, and therefore I once discussed it with Master Guiyuqu. Guiyuqu responded: 'The earth phase governs the first and sixth heavenly years, metal governs the second and seventh heavenly years, water governs the third and eighth heavenly years, wood governs the fourth and ninth heavenly years, and fire governs the fifth and tenth heavenly years. In the 1st and the 7th earthly years, the Shaoyin governs the heavenly Qi; in the 2nd and the 8th earth years, the Taiyin governs the heavenly

Qi; in the 3rd and the 9th earth years, the Shaoyang governs the heavenly Qi; in the 4th and the 10th earth years, the Yangming governs the heavenly Qi; in the 5th and the 11th earth years, the Taiyang governs the heavenly Qi; and in the 6th and the 12th earth years, the Jueyin governs the heavenly Qi. These all don't correspond to Yin and Yang, and what is the rule for it?'
Qibo: He did explain the laws, and it all refers to the Yin and Yang in the heavens and the earth. The Yin and Yang in human body are countable and all the corresponding parts can be deduced accordingly. The general Yin and Yang can be deduced from tens to hundreds, from hundreds to thousands, and from thousands to millions in numbers. But the Yin and Yang in the heavens and the earth cannot be deduced by numbers but only determined by manifestation.

Emperor: I'd like to know its initiation.
Qibo: How brilliant the question is! I had read the record in the *Primeval Genesis Volume of the Universe* that the red heavenly Qi travels through the Altair and Vega as well as the fifth heavenly phase (in the northwest), the yellow heavenly Qi travels through the Heart and Tail constellations as well as the sixth heavenly phase (in the southeast), the blue heavenly Qi travels through the Rooftop and Encampment as well as Willow and Ghost constellations, the white heavenly Qi travels through the Neck and Root as well as Hairy Head and Net constellations, and the black heavenly Qi travels through the Extended Net and Wings as well as Bond and Stomach constellations. The so-called fifth and sixth heavenly phases refer to the constellations of Legs, Wall, Horn and Chariot, which are the gates of the heavens and the earth. These are the initiation of deducing climates and the generation of heavenly law, and you cannot keep uninformed with them.

Emperor: Good. It's said in last chapter "Great theory on law of heavens and nature" that the heavens and the earth are the space between the upper and lower for all creatures in the world; the right and the left are the path for triple Yin and triple Yang. I don't know what it means.
Qibo: The so-called upper heavens and lower earth mean the position where Yin and Yang locate according to the Qi of heaven-governing and earth-governing yearly. The so-called right and left are the left Shaoyang interval Qi and right Taiyang interval Qi which are seen under Jueyin as governing-heaven Qi; left Taiyin and right Jueyin, when seen under Shaoyin; left Shaoyang and right Shaoyin, when seen under Shaoyin; left Yangming and right Taiyin, when seen under Shaoyin; left Taiyang and right Shaoyang, when seen under Shaoyin; and left Jueyin and right Yangming, when seen under Shaoyin. The so-called determined positions when facing north are the governing-heaven Qi on the left and right.

Emperor: What's the meaning of lower earth (governing-earth Qi)?
Qibo: When Jueying is in the upper heavens, Shaoyang is in the lower earth with left Yangming internal Qi and right Taiyin internal Qi; when Shaoyin is in the upper, Yangming is in the lower with left Taiyang and right Shaoyang; when Taiyin is in the upper, Taiyang is in the lower with left Jueyin and right Yangming; when Shaoyang is in the upper, Jueying is in the lower with left Shaoyin and right Taiyang; when Yangming is in the upper, Shaoyin is in the lower with left Taiyin and right Jueyin; when Taiyang is in the upper, Taiyin is in the lower with left Shaoyang and right Shaoyin. The so-called determined positions when facing south is the Governing-earth Qi on the left and right. The upper and the lower communicate

mutually, and the cold and the summer heat follow one after another; when the host-Qi and guest-Qi coincide in the proper position, harmony will be found, otherwise diseases will develop.

Emperor: Sometimes the Host Qi and Guest Qi are in the proper positions, which also lead to diseases, and why?
Qibo: The lower Guest Qi processes position over the upper position wrongly.

Emperor: How about their dynamics and statics?
Qibo: The Qi in the upper moves right, while Qi in the lower moves left; the right and the left movements consist of one year after a great circle.

Emperor: I'm told by Guiyuqu that the response to the earth is quiet. Today, you mention the Qi in the lower moves left; I don't understand this; I'd like to know why the Qi is in movement?
Qibo: The dynamics and statistics of the heavens and the earth are associated with the shifting and rotating of the five elements; though he knows the movement of the heavens, Guiyuqu hasn't understood the movements on the right and the left. As to the function of the natural changes, the heavens takes on the star phenomena while the earth forms all creatures, with the seven bright stars encircling in the heavens while the five elements attaching to the earth. The earth is the place to embrace the formed things, while the sky is the space to display Qi of heavens. The movement of the formed things and star-Qi is just like the root and branches, and through observing the star phenomena, the situation in the universe can be known.

Emperor: Is the earth located in the lower?
Qibo: The earth is located below humans, yet in the middle of the sky.

Emperor: Has it any proof?
Qibo: It's the atmosphere that supports it. The dry Qi dries it, the summer-heat evaporates it, the wind moves it, the damp moistens it, the cold hardens it, and the fire warms it. So, the wind and cold are in the lower, the dry and heat in the upper, the damp Qi in the middle, the fire wanders among them, and the six-Qi moves between changes of cold-winter and hot-summer, causing the heavens and the earth to create and transform all things. Therefore, the domination of the dry leads to the dry earth, domination of summer-heat to heat earth, domination of wind to stirred earth, domination of damp to muddy earth, domination of cold to cracked earth, and domination of fire to hardened earth.

Emperor: How to observe the correspondence to the Qi of the heavens and the earth?
Qibo: The Qi of the heavens and the earth with their domination or retaliation cannot be expressed in the pulse. It's said in *Methods for Pulse-Taking* that the changes of the heavens and the earth cannot be observed by pulse-taking, which is just the reason for it.

Emperor: How about the interval Qi?
Qibo: According to the position of interval Qi in shifting, its correspondence can be observed on the left or the right.
Emperor: How to detect them?
Qibo: The compliance of the internal Qi indicates harmony, while reversal of the internal Qi indicates diseases; if the shift

is not in due position, it indicates diseases, if in an interchanged position indicates diseases, and losing the due position indicates the crisis; reversion of Chi and Cun pulses indicate death, and reversion of Yin and Yang pulses indicate death as well. After the Year Phase is recognized in order to know the interval Qi and the corresponding pulses on the left and right, the death and survival as well as the reversal and compliance can be predicted.

Emperor: There is six-Qi as cold, summer-heat, dryness, damp, wind and fire, and what correspond to them in the human body? How do they cause the creation and transformation of all things?
Qibo: The east generates the wind that generates the wood that generates the sour taste that generates liver that generates the sinews that generate heart. The Qi corresponds to mystery in the heavens, to law in humans, and to transformation in the earth; the transformation generates five flavors, the law generates wisdom, the mystery generates the spirit and the transformation generates Qi. Its spirit corresponds to the wind Qi in heavens, to the wood in the earth, to the sinews in body, to the softness in Qi, and to liver in solid viscera. The property is warm, the nature is in harmony, the function is movement, the color is dark green, the transformation is blossom, and corresponding insect is the hairy; its administration is distribution, the climatic action is breezing, the change is destruction, the disaster is falling, the flavor is sour and the emotion is anger. The anger damages liver, while the sorrow dominates the anger; the wind damages liver, while the dryness dominates the wind; the sour taste damages the sinews, while the pungent taste dominates the sour.

The south generates the heat that generates the fire that generates the bitter taste that generates heart that generates the blood that generates spleen. Its spirit corresponds to the heat in heavens, to the fire in earth, to the vessel in humans, to growth in air, and to heart in solid viscera. The property is summer-heat, the nature is exposure, the function is stirring, the color is red, the transformation is exuberance, and corresponding insect is the winged; its administration is bright, the climatic action is depressive steaming, the change is consumption due to heat; the disaster is burning, the flavor is bitter, and the emotion is joy. Over-joy damages heart, while horror dominates the joy; the heat consumes Qi, while cold dominates the heat; the bitter taste damages Qi, while salty taste dominates bitter.

The center generates the damp that generates the earth that generates the sweet taste that generates spleen that generates muscles that generate lung. Its spirit corresponds to the damp in the heavens, to the soil in the earth, to muscles in body, to fullness in Qi, and to spleen in solid viscera. The property is quiet and various, the nature is moistening, the function is transformation, the color is yellow, the transformation is fullness, and corresponding insect is the naked; its administration is silent, the climatic action is cloud and rain, the change is pouring rain, the disaster is muddy landslide, the flavor is sweet, and the emotion is contemplation. Contemplation damages spleen, while anger dominates contemplation; damp damages muscles, while wind dominates damp; the sweet taste damages the spleen, while the sour taste dominates the sweet.

The west generates the dryness that generates the metal that generates the pungent taste that generates lung that generates skin and hair that generate kidney. Its spirit corresponds to the dryness in the heavens, to the metal in the earth, to the skin and hair in body, to the mature in Qi, and to lung in solid viscera. The property is cool, the nature is purity, the function is hardening, the color is white, the transformation is astringency, and corresponding insect is the cyprid; its administration is vigorous, the climatic action is fog and dew, the change is constriction and conquering, the disaster is withering of the green, the flavor is pungent, and the emotion is anxiety. Anxiety damages lung, while joy dominates anxiety; the heat damages skin and hair, while the cold dominates the heat; the pungent taste damages the skin and hair, while the bitter taste dominates the pungent taste.

The north generates the cold that generates the water that generates the salty taste that generates kidney that generates marrow that generates liver. Its spirit corresponds to the cold in the heavens, to the water in the earth, to the bones in body, to firmness in Qi, and to kidney in solid viscera. The property is chilly, the nature is cold, the function is storage, the color is black, the transformation is constriction, and corresponding insect is the scaled; its administration is silent, the climatic action is sleet and snowflake, the change is congelation and chill, the disaster is hailstones; the flavor is salty, and the emotion is horror. Horror damages kidney, while contemplation dominates horror; the cold damages the blood, while the dryness dominates the cold; the salty taste damages the blood, while the sweet taste dominates the salty. The climatic five-Qi alternates in respective time-order; so the appearance in improper position will lead to abnormality, while when in due position it leads to normality.

Emperor: How about the changes of the disease caused?
Qibo: The identification of Qi leads to mild diseases, while non-identification of Qi leads to severe diseases.

Emperor asked: How about the Qi in the Dominating Year?
Qibo answered: If excessive, the Qi will overcome the dominated one and retro-strain the non-dominated one; if insufficient, the dominating Qi will restrain it while the dominated one will restrain it. Any retro-straining when in excess or insufficiency is affected by evil, which is not afraid of dominating Qi.

Emperor said: Good.

Chapter 68

Great Theory on Movement of Six-Qi

Yellow Emperor asked: Oh! How profound it is! To understand the law of nature is just like to look up at floating clouds or look down into a deep pool; nevertheless, it is possible to measure the deep pool but it is impossible to have ultimate knowledge of the clouds. You have mentioned several times that the law of nature should be observed carefully, which I've learnt and kept in my mind; however, I'm still puzzled about it and don't understand what it means. I hope that you can enthusiastically and explicitly explain it, so that it won't die out and will be eternally distinguishable. Can I learn the law of nature?
Qibo kowtowed, bowed again and answered: What a clever question! The law of natural climate varies with the order of the heavens and with time of the exuberance and decline.

Emperor: I'd like to know the system of six-sixty and what the exuberance and decline are?
Qibo: The Qi in the upper or in the lower has the throne, and the interval Qi on the left or the right has the rule of motion. Then to the right of Shaoyang is Yangming; to the right of Yangming is Taiyang; to the right of Taiyang is Jueyin; to the

right of Jueyin is Shaoyin; to the right of Shaoyin is Taiyin; and to the right of Taiyin is Shaoyin. This is the so-called branch of six-Qi, which is determined when facing south. It's believed that, based on the celestial motion and the time of exuberance and decline, the sun shadow can be measured and shifting position can be determined when standing and facing south. That is the information concerned.

When Shaoyang is in the upper, the fire Qi is governing and the intermediate is Jueyin; when Yangming is in the upper, the dry Qi is governing and the intermediate is Taiyin; when Taiyang is in the upper, the cold Qi is governing and the intermediate is Shaoyin; when Jueyin is in the upper, the wind Qi is governing and the intermediate is Shaoyang; when Shaoyin is in the upper, the heat Qi is governing and the intermediate is Taiyang; when Taiyin is in upper, the damp Qi is governing and the intermediate is Yangming. This is the so-called root, below the root is the intermediate, and below the intermediate is the branch of Qi. Due to the difference between branch and root, there are different correspondences of pulses and manifestations.

Emperor: There appear conditions that the climatic Qi arrives in due time, the Qi doesn't arrive in due time and the Qi arrives ahead of the due time excessively, and why?
Qibo: The climatic Qi arriving in due time indicates harmony; the Qi not arriving in due time indicates insufficiency; the Qi arriving ahead of the due time indicates the excess of arrival Qi.

Emperor: When the Qi does not arrive in due time or if the Qi arrives ahead of the due time, what are the outcomes?
Qibo: The compliance indicates smooth condition while the contrary indicates reversal condition that results in changes that leads to diseases.

Emperor: Good! Please explain the correspondence.
Qibo: On things, the growth is their correspondence; on Qi, the pulses are their correspondence.

Emperor: Good! I'd like to know what the correspondence between geographic locations and six-Qi is.
Qibo: To the right of grand position (the Spring Equinox) is monarch-fire; to the right of monarch-fire and with one backward step is the position where minister-fire governs; with another backward step is the position where earthly Qi governs; with another backward step is the position where metal Qi governs; with another backward step is the position where water Qi governs; with another backward step is the position where wood Qi governs; with another backward step is the position where monarch-fire governs. Minister-fire position is opposed below by water Qi; water position is opposed below by earthly Qi; earth position is opposed below by wind Qi; wind position is opposed below by metal Qi; metal position is opposed below by fire Qi; monarch-fire is held below by Yin essence.

Emperor: Why?
Qibo: Hyperactivity will cause harm, while the opposite can lead to harmony, so that they can ensure generation and transformation expressed in exuberance or decline; if hyperactivity actually turns into harm, there will be deterioration and disorder, causing severe disease.

Emperor: How about the exuberance and decline?
Qibo: The Qi in the improper position is the evil, while Qi in the proper position is healthy. The climate changes greatly with evil Qi, while the climate changes slightly with healthy Qi.

Emperor: What is the so-called proper position?
Qibo: In view of heavenly stem, wood phase encounters the fourth year, fire phase encounters the seventh year, earth phase encounters the fifth, eleventh, second or eighth year, metal phase encounters the tenth year and water phase encounters the first year, which are termed year-identification with peaceful Qi.

Emperor: What is the condition in the improper position?
Qibo: It is the year when yearly Qi isn't identified with the earthly branch.

Emperor: Earth phase encounters Taiyin as heaven-governing Qi; metal phase encounters Yangming as heaven-governing Qi; wood phase encounters Jueyin as heaven-governing Qi; water-phase encounters Taiyang as heaven-governing Qi; what does it mean?
Qibo: It is the year when the Yearly Phase corresponds to the heaven-governing in terms of five elements, so it is called Heavenly Identification in the book *The Origin of the Heavens*.

Emperor: How does the year pertain to both the Heavenly Identification and Yearly Identification?
Qibo: It is the year of the Triple Heavenly Identification.

Emperor: How about the role of nobility or humbleness?
Qibo: The year of heavenly identification is like a tipstaff, the year of yearly identification is like an executor, and the year of triple heavenly identification is like a nobleman.

Emperor: How is it different after evil attacks?
Qibo: When the tipstaff is attacked, the diseases occur rapidly and critically; when the executor is attacked, the diseases occur

gradually and persistently; and when the nobleman is attacked, the diseases occur suddenly and can be deadly.

Emperor: What is the condition when six-Qi shifts their positions?
Qibo: The monarch Qi falls on the position of minister Qi, which is the smooth condition, while the minister Qi usurps the position of monarch Qi, which is the reversal condition; with the reversal, the disease is acute and the outcome is severe; with the smoothness, the disease is chronic and outcome is mild. They are the so-called two fires.

Emperor: Good! I'd like to know about the step.
Qibo: The so-called step is composed of 60 days and remaining notches, and in terms of 24 steps, 100 notches accumulated makes a day.

Emperor: What are the changes when six-Qi corresponds to five elements?
Qibo: The six phases of Qi have different positions including primary and intermediate, in each year, in which heavenly Qi and earthly Qi are not the same either, and hence the calculation is also different.

Emperor: How to calculate them?
Qibo: Heavenly Qi starts from the first and earthly Qi from the first; when the first encounters the primary, it means the beginning of a year. If the time of Yearly Phase is observed closely, every yearly Qi can be calculated.

Emperor: I'd like to know the yearly Qi and the start and termination of six-Qi as well as their early or late arrival?

Qibo: What a clever question! In the first-1st year, the initial Qi starts from the first notch under the water level and terminates at 87.5^{th} notch; the second Qi starts from the 87.6^{th} notch and terminates at 75th notch; the third Qi starts from 76th notch and terminates at 62.5^{th} notch; the fourth Qi starts from 62.6^{th} notch and terminates at 50th notch; the fifth Qi starts from 51st notch and terminates at 37.5^{th} notch; the sixth Qi starts from 37.6^{th} notch and terminates at 25th notch. This is the first six-step with the notches of the starting and termination of six-Qi given.

In the second-2nd year, the initial Qi starts from the 26th notch and terminates at 12.5^{th} notch; the second Qi starts from the 12.6^{th} notch and terminates at 100th notch under the water level; the third Qi starts from 1st notch and terminates at 87.5^{th} notch; the fourth Qi starts from 87.6^{th} notch and terminates at 75th notch; the fifth Qi starts from 76th notch and terminates at 62.5^{th} notch; the sixth Qi starts from 62.6^{th} notch and terminates at 50th notch. This is the second six-step with the notches of starting and termination given.

In the third-3rd year, the initial Qi starts from the 51st notch and terminates at 37.5^{th} notch; the second Qi starts from the 37.6^{th} notch and terminates at 25th notch; the third Qi starts from 26th notch and terminates at 12.5^{th} notch; the fourth Qi starts from 12.6^{th} notch and terminates at 100th notch under the water level; the fifth Qi starts from 1st notch and terminates at 87.5^{th} notch; the sixth Qi starts from 87.6^{th} notch and terminates at 75th notch. This is the third six-step with the notches of starting and termination given.

In the fourth-4th year, the initial Qi starts from the 76th notch and terminates at 62.5^{th} notch; the second Qi starts from the 62.6^{th} notch and terminates at 50th notch; the third Qi starts from 51st notch and terminates at 37.5th notch; the fourth Qi starts from 37.6th notch and terminates at 25th notch; the fifth Qi starts from 26th notch and terminates at 12.5th notch; the sixth Qi starts from 12.6th notch and terminates at 100th notch under the water level. This is the fourth six-step with the notches of starting and termination given. The next quadrennium, in the fifth-5th year, the initial Qi starts again from the first notch and the order repeats on endlessly and goes round and begins again.

Emperor: I'd like to know how to calculate the year.
Qibo: What a detailed question! During the first revolution, heavenly Qi starts from the first notch; during the second revolution, heavenly Qi starts from the 26th notch; during the third revolution, heavenly Qi starts from the 51st notch; during the fourth revolution, heavenly Qi starts from the 76th notch; during the fifth revolution, heavenly Qi starts again from the first notch, which is the so-called quadrennium. Hence in the third, seventh or eleventh year, the notches of the start and termination are the same; in the fourth, eighth or twelfth year, the notches of the start and termination are the same; in the fifth, ninth and first[t] year, the notches of the start and termination are the same; in the sixth, tenth and second year, the notches of the start and termination are the same, which will go round and begin again.

Emperor: I'd like to know their functions.
Qibo: With respect to heavenly Qi, the origin of six-Qi should be sought, with respect to earthly Qi, the position of six-Qi to five elements should be sought, and with respect to human body, the Qi interaction should be sought.

Emperor: What is Qi interaction?
Qibo: Heavenly Qi is in the upper and earthly Qi is in the lower, while the Qi interaction is in the middle where the human beings live. It's believed that heavenly Qi dominates above the heaven-pivot while earthly Qi dominates below the heaven-pivot; human-Qi complies and all things come into being in the region where they interact. This is the information concerned.

Emperor: What are the elementary Qi and the middle Qi?
Qibo: The elementary Qi accounts for 30 days with remainder and so does the middle Qi.

Emperor: Why are there the elementary Qi and the middle Qi?
Qibo: It is just to differentiate the heavens and the earth.

Emperor: I'd like to know the details.
Qibo: The elementary Qi is earthly Qi and the middle Qi is heavenly Qi.

Emperor: How about their ascent and descent?
Qibo: The ascent and descent of Qi refer to the interaction of heavenly Qi and earthly Qi.

Emperor: I'd like to know their interaction in detail.
Qibo: Earthly Qi can descend after it ascends to the peak, and it descends because of push of heavenly Qi; heavenly Qi can ascend after it descends to the bottom, and it ascends because of push of earthly Qi. When heavenly Qi is descending, its Qi prevails over the earth; when earthly Qi is ascending, its Qi evaporates into the heaven. So, Qi in the upper and Qi in the lower interact mutually, and since ascending and descending

are the alternating causes for each other, there will be changes occurring accordingly.

Emperor: Good! When the cold Qi meets the damp Qi, the dryness meets the heat and the wind meets the fire, is there any transit?
Qibo: There is domination and retaliation in six-Qi, and their emergence of domination or retaliation may be normal, transformative, functional or alterative; if it is alterative, there will be the evil Qi.

Emperor: What does the evil Qi mean?
Qibo: The growth of things depends on the transformation of Qi while the utmost development of things results from the changes of Qi. The combat between changes and transformations is the source of success and failure. Thus, Qi goes either forward or backward and functions either slowly or swiftly. These four factors cause transformations and changes and bring about wind.

Emperor: Qi can go slowly or rapidly, and forward or backward, by which the wind is then generated, leading to transformations and changes of six-Qi, just because of their exuberance and decline. Success or failure depends on each other dynamically; why is this so?
Qibo: Success or failure lies in the Qi motion, and ceaseless motion can result in all changes.

Emperor: Is there any definite time for it?
Qibo: If there is no generation or transformation, it is the stage of quiescence.

Emperor: Is there anything with no generation or transformation?

Qibo: If there were no going out and coming in, the spirit will vanish; if there were no ascent and descent, the vital establishment will be withered away. Thus, if there were no going out or coming in, there will be no birth, development, maturity, senility and death; if there were no ascent or descent, there will be no generation, growth, transformation, harvest and storage. Hence, none of the visible things have activities such as ascent, descent, going out and coming in. Therefore, the visible things are the world where generation and transformation take place; if the visible things are out of shape, the generation and transformation will vanish. Thus, nothing can exist without going out or coming in and without ascent or descent. The transformations can be differentiated as small or large, and the time can be differentiated as late or early. No matter what it is in view of four conditions, it is important to maintain normality, and abnormality can result in disasters. It's believed that there will be no harm without form, which is the information concerned.

Emperor: Good! Is there anything with no generation and transformation?

Qibo: What a detailed question! It is only the perfect man who can live in the same way as the law of nature.

Emperor: Good.

Chapter 69

Great Theory on Shifting and Interaction of Qi

Yellow Emperor asked: The domination of the five-phase alternates corresponding to weather conditions in a year. Yin and Yang reciprocate in movement to correspond with the changes of cold and summer-heat. Genuine Qi and evil Qi struggle with each other. The internal and the external separate, the six meridians fluctuate, and five Qi deviate excessively or insufficiently, resulting in single predomination and annex. I would like to know its origin. Is there a general rule, and can you explain it to me?
Qibo kowtowed again and said: What an excellent question you have asked! It is a profound theory emphasized by emperors and passed on by teachers in the past. Although I am not intelligent enough, I have heard of this theory.

Emperor: I have heard that if one fails to teach when meeting the proper person, he will miss the chance of passing on the principle. If one passes the principle to an unworthy person, it will be the same as neglecting the precious principle. Although I lack both ability and knowledge and I am not capable enough to learn such a profound theory, I really have sympathy with

the people who are suffering from diseases. I hope that you can remember this theory and pass it on forever. I will take charge of the matter abiding with the rules. What do you think about it?
Qibo: Please allow me to explain it. It is said in *The Upper Set of Classics* that if one knows the principles, he will know the heavens in the upper, the earth in the lower and human beings in the middle, and he will live long.

Emperor: What does it mean?
Qibo: The fundamental thing here is to infer the Qi positions of heavens, earth and humans. When the Qi situates in the heavens, it is of astronomy. When the Qi situates on the earth, it is of geography. When the Qi communicates with human beings, it is of human affairs. So, excessive Qi arrives prior to the season, the insufficient Qi arrives behind the season. The human body is also changing along with it.

Emperor: What is the condition of excessive changes in the transformation of the five-phase?
Qibo: When the yearly wood-motion is excessive, it will lead to the prevalence of wind Qi and invasion of evil into the spleen-earth. People will suffer from diarrhea after indigestion, poor appetite, heavy body, vexation, depression, borborygmus and abdominal fullness, which corresponds to Wood Star in the sky. If the wood-motion is overabundant, it will lead to sudden flare into temper, dizziness and disease of the head. When the earth Qi fails to implement its decree, the wood Qi is overabundant solely. Then clouds are flying, things are fluctuating, leaves and branches are shaking and even falling down, and people will suffer from hypochondriac pain and severe vomiting. If Chongyang pulse (stomach meridian) is

exhausted, the disease is incurable, which corresponds to Metal Star in the sky.

When the yearly fire-motion is excessive, it will lead to the prevalence of summer heat and invasion of evil into the lung-metal. People will suffer from malaria, shortness of breath, cough, panting, hemorrhage, hematochezia, lingering diarrhea, dry throat, deafness and hot sensation in the chest, shoulder and back, which corresponds to Fire Star in the sky. If fire-motion is overabundant, it will lead to thoracic pain, hypochondriac fullness, pain in the chest, back and scapula, pain over the inner side of the arms, body fever, skin pain and acute eczema. When the metal Qi fails to implement its decree, the fire Qi is overabundant solely. Then it will lead to rain, freezing, frost and cold, which corresponds to Water Star in the sky. In the year of Shaoyin and Shaoyang governing the heavens, there is blazing of fire, dry spring, scotching of plants and diseases marked by delirium, mania, cough, panting, hematochezia and hematuria. If Taiyuan pulse (lung meridian) is exhausted, the disease is incurable, which corresponds to Fire Star in the sky.

When the yearly earth-motion is excessive, it will lead to the prevalence of rain and damp and invasion of evil into the kidney-water. People will suffer from abdominal pain, coldness of the limbs, unhappiness, heavy body and dysphoria, which corresponds to Earth Star in the sky. If earth-motion is overabundant, it will lead to muscular atrophy, flaccidity of the feet, frequent convulsion, sole pain, water retention, abdominal fullness, poor appetite and inability to lift the four limbs. During the time when earth-motion changes in domination, water Qi is latent and the transforming Qi of the earth is in domination solely, consequently leading to gushing of the springs, overflowing of the rivers, appearance of fish in the marshland which was once dry, storm, collapse of earth, and fish being found on the land. In terms of human diseases, abdominal fullness, sloppy stool and borborygmus can develop. If Taixi pulse (kidney meridian) is exhausted, the disease is incurable, which corresponds to Wood Star in the sky.

When the yearly metal-motion is excessive, it will lead to the prevalence of dryness and invasion of evil into the liver-wood. People will suffer from hypochondriac and abdominal pain, redness and pain of the eyes, and inability to hear. Constricting and conquering Qi leads to heavy body, dysphoria, chest pain involving the back, hypochondriac fullness and pain involving the lower abdomen, which corresponds to Metal Star in the sky. If metal Qi is overabundant, it will lead to panting, cough and Qi reversal as well as pain in the shoulders, back, buttocks, pudendum, thighs, knees, legs, calf and feet, which corresponds to Fire Star in the sky. If the constricting Qi is severe and the generating Qi is reduced, grass and trees are astringed and the leaves become dry and are falling onto the ground. In terms of human diseases, acute pain, hypochondriac pain, inability to turn the body, cough, Qi reversal, or even hemorrhage can develop. If Taichong pulse (liver meridian) is exhausted, the disease will be incurable, which corresponds to Metal Star in the sky.

When the yearly water-motion is excessive, it will lead to the prevalence of cold and invasion of evil into the heart-fire. People will suffer from body fever, vexation, palpitation, cold limbs, internal and external cold and the cold Qi will arrive earlier than usual, which corresponds to Water Star in the sky. If water-motion is overabundant, it will lead to abdominal distension, shank swelling, panting, cough, night sweating and fearing wind, as well as heavy rain falling and gloomy dusty fog, which corresponds to Earth Star in the sky. During the time when Taiyang governs the heavens, it will lead to falling of rain, ice, snow and frost frequently as well as the changes of all the things due to damp Qi. In terms of human diseases, there develops abdominal fullness, borborygmus, sloppy stool, indigestion, thirst and dizziness. If Shenmen pulse (heart meridian) is exhausted, the disease is incurable, which corresponds to Fire and Water Stars in the sky.

Emperor: Good! What is the result of insufficiency of the five-phase?

Qibo: What an excellent question you have asked! When the yearly wood-motion is insufficient, it will lead to the prevalence of dryness, failure of generating Qi to come in time and slow growth of grass and trees. If the constricting and conquering Qi is overabundant, the strong trunk will be broken, tress and the soft leaves will be withered, which corresponds to Metal Star in the sky. People will suffer from abdominal coldness, hypochondriac pain, lower abdominal pain, borborygmus and sloppy stool. It rains frequently and appears cool, which corresponds to Metal Star in the sky, with crop appearing dark green when reaping. In the year when Yangming governs the heavens, if the generating Qi fails to dominate, grass and trees will flourish again and the transforming Qi is urgent, which corresponds to Metal and Earth Stars in the sky, with green plants withering earlier than usual. Retaliating activity leads to flaming summer-heat, change of dampness into dryness, scorching variation of the soft grass and trees, re-sprouting from the root and simultaneous appearance of flowers and fruits. In terms of human diseases, there develops chill-fever disease, sores, ulceration, prickly heat, carbuncle and acne, which corresponds to Fire and Metal Stars in the sky, with crop appearing white and hard when reaping. Dew falls earlier than usual, constricting and conquering Qi prevails, cold rain damages things and insects eat sweet and yellow crops. In the human body, the spleen-earth is attacked by evil, the action of reddish-Qi dominates over the lung-metal, and white Qi is inhibited. Then crop cannot be reaped and people will suffer from cough and running nose, which corresponds to Fire and Metal Stars in the sky.

When the yearly fire-motion is insufficient and growing Qi cannot be executed, it will lead to the slow growth of plants. If it is extremely cold, Yang Qi will be unable to transform and plants will be damaged, which corresponds to Water Star in the sky. People will suffer from chest pain, hypochondriac fullness and pain, pain of the chest, back, between scapulae and the inner side of the arms, depression, dizziness, stomachache, sudden loss of voice, bloating chest and bulging abdomen, referred pain of the hypochondria, waist and back, or even difficultly in extension and flexion and feeling like separation of the hipbone and the thigh, which corresponds to Fire and Water Stars in the sky, with reddish crops when reaping. Retaliating activity leads to gloomy dusty fog and heavy rain falling. As the black-water Qi is inhibited, sloppy stool, abdominal fullness, anorexia, abdominal cold, borborygmus, acute diarrhea, abdominal pain, and failure of feet to support the body in human beings can develop, which corresponds to Earth and Water Stars in the sky, with grain being blackish and unripe.

When the yearly earth-motion is insufficient, it will lead to the prevalence of wind and difficult execution of transforming Qi, and then grass and trees grow normally, are waving violently in wind, and develop luxuriantly but with no fruit, which corresponds to Earth Star in the sky. People will suffer from diarrhea after indigestion, cholera, heavy body, abdominal pain, shaking and stiffness of sinews and bones, tremor and ache of the muscles and frequent flare of temper. Qi of cold-water will take this advantage and become active, the hibernating insects will hibernate early and people tend to suffer from cold diseases, which corresponds to Earth and Wood Stars in the sky, with crops being yellowish when reaping. Retaliating activity leads to severe constricting Qi that causes withering of great trees as well as sudden pain of the chest and hypochondria involving the lower abdomen and frequent sighing in human beings. Insects eat sweet and yellow crops, Qi invades the spleen, yellow crops are reduced in production, people eat less and food seldom feels tasty, and green crops are damaged, which corresponds to Water and Earth Stars in the sky. In the year when Jueyin governs, running water cannot freeze and hibernating insects appear again. Storing-Qi fails to dominate and white-water Qi becomes dominant, which corresponds to Earth Star in the sky, with people being in good health.

When the yearly metal-motion is insufficient, it will lead to the prevalence of flaming-fire, execution of the generating-Qi and action of growing-Qi. Thus, all things grow exuberantly and dryness permeates through, which corresponds to Fire Star in the sky. Then people will suffer from heaviness of the shoulders and back, stuffy nose and sneezing, hematochezia and acute diarrhea, due to the late astringing-Qi, which corresponds to Metal Star in the sky, with grain being hard and sharp. Retaliating activity results in sudden falling of cold rain, hailstones, frost and snow that kill plants. In terms of human diseases, reversal and rejection of Yin and reverse surging of Yang occur, causing pain in the back of the head involving the vertex with fever, which corresponds to Water and Fires Stars in the sky, with grain being reddish and unripe. People will suffer from oral ulcers and even stomachache.

When the yearly water-motion is insufficient, it will lead to the prevalence of dampness, reverse action and rapid transformation of the growing-Qi, resulting in frequent rain in summer, which corresponds to Earth Star in the sky. People will suffer from abdominal fullness, heavy body, diarrhea, cold ulceration with thin pyorrhea, pain of the waist and thigh, inflexibility of the popliteal fossa, calf, and knees, dysphoria, flaccidity and coldness of feet, pain in the soles, or even swollen dorsum of feet. Since the storing-Qi fails to dominate, kidney-Qi will lose balance, which corresponds to Water Star in the sky, with crops being blackish when reaping. In the year of Taiyin that governs the heavens, cold attacking occurs frequently, insects hibernate early, the earth is covered with hard ice and the sunshine is not strong. Then people will suffer from cold diseases in the lower or even abdominal fullness and dropsy, which corresponds to Earth Star in the sky, with crops being yellowish when reaping. Retaliating activity leads to sudden blow of violent wind, falling grass and withered trees that have lost luster. In terms of human diseases, complexion changes, spasm and pain of sinews and bones, tremor and convulsion of muscles, blurred vision, appearance of fissures and urticarial can develop. If Qi invades the chest, it will cause stomachache and abdominal pain. The yellow-earth Qi is damaged and the crop cannot ripen, which corresponds to the Earth Star in the sky.

Emperor: Good! I'd like to know the time dominated by the five-phase.

Qibo: What an excellent question you have asked! When the yearly wood-motion is insufficient, there is the transformation of gentle breeze sound in spring and the administration of clear and cool fog and dew in autumn. There is the domination of chilly residual cold in spring and the retaliation of flaming heat and scotching in summer. Usually the harm occurs in the east, the disorder occurs in liver and the disease is located in the hypochondria internally and in the joints externally.

When the yearly fire-motion is insufficient, there is obvious transformation of brightness in summer while the administration of serious frost and coldness in winter. If there is the administration of congealing chill and coldness in summer, there will be retaliation of gloomy dust and rain frequently. Usually the harm occurs in the south, the disorder occurs in heart and the disease is located in the chest and hypochondria internally and the meridians and collaterals externally.

When the yearly earth-motion is insufficient, there is the transformation of clouds and moisture in the four seasons, while there will be gentle wind sound in spring. There is storm that is shaking and blowing in the four seasons while there will be the retaliation of constricting and conquering Qi and much rain in autumn. Usually the harm occurs in the four directions, the disorder occurs in spleen internally and in muscles and limbs externally.

When the yearly metal-motion is insufficient, there is order of obvious brightness and depressive steaming Qi in summer and the response of serious congealing and constricting coldness in winter. There are changes such as flaming and blazing heat in summer and the retaliation with hailstone, frost and snow in autumn. Usually the harm occurs in the west, the disorder occurs in lung, and the disease lingers in the chest, hypochondria, shoulders and back internally and in the skin and hair externally.

When the yearly water-motion is insufficient, there is the transformation of moisture and dusty clouds and the response of frequent soft wind. There is the changes of gloomy dust and heavy rain in the four directions and the retaliation in the form of frequent storm that shakes and breaks grass and trees. Usually the harm occurs in the north, disorder occurs in kidney, and the diseases are located in the lumbar spine and bone marrow internally and in the muscles and knees externally.

The movement of five-phase is just like the relationship between the steelyard and the sliding weight. The excess should be inhibited, the insufficient should be supplemented, the normal transformation should be reacted to, and the abnormal change should be adjusted, which is the law of germination, growth, transformation, reaping and storage as well as normal principle of Qi. Abnormal change will cause stagnation in the heavens and on the earth. It's believed that the dynamic and static changes in the heavens and in the earth symbolize mind, while the sequential activity of Yin and Yang represents the alternation of cold and heat, which is the information concerned.

Emperor: You the Master have explained the changes of five-Qi and the reactions of the four seasons in detail. However, the disorder of Qi is caused by some kind of attack, which has no regular rules and often occurs suddenly. How to foretell it?
Qibo: The dynamic changes of Qi don't follow certain rules, but its function, transformation, administration, order, harm and change can be predicted with their respective warning signs.

Emperor: Why is it so?

Qibo: The east generates the wind and the wind generates wood. Its function is to act moderately, its transformation is to promote exuberance, the administration is to spread and bloom, its order is to produce wind, its change is to wave and grow and its harm is to desolate.

The south generates heat and heat generates fire. Its function is to show obviously, its transformation is to grow exuberantly, its administration is to enlighten brightly, its order is to give heat, its change is to flame and its harm is to scorch. The center generates dampness and dampness generates earth. Its function is to steam the damp, its transformation is to enrich and preparation for development, its administration is to tranquilize things, its order is to generate the damp, its change is to cause rain falling and its harm is to collapse the earth. The west generates dryness and dryness generates metal. Its function is to depurate, its transformation is to constrict, its administration is to make things strong and sharp, its order is to dry, its change is to constrict and conquer and its harm is to perish. The north generates coldness and coldness generates water. Its function is to produce coldness, its transformation is to cool and tranquilize things, its administration is to congeal and constrict, its order is to make icy coldness, its change is to make piercing coldness and its harm is to produce ice, snow, frost and hailstone. By these routine phenomena, the movement of the five-phase can be observed, in which there are function and transformation, administration and order, and change and harm. All the things develop in correspondence with such phenomena, and so do human beings.

Emperor: You the Mister have talked about the sign of weather changes in a year, and the excess or insufficiency of

the five-phase corresponds to the five stars in the sky accordingly. But now the variation of the function, transformation, administration, order, harm and change are irregular and often occur suddenly; so, do the five corresponding stars also change accordingly?
Qibo: The five stars move in accord with the movement of the heavens, and so there is no irregular movement, and none of correspondences reverse the celestial movement. The mutative movements result in the changes of Qi shifting, but the five stars won't correspond suddenly. It's believed that normal correspondences are regular but abnormal correspondences are sudden.

Emperor: How about their correspondences?
Qibo: Each moves in accordance with the Qi transformation in that year.

Emperor: What about their movements: slowly, rapidly, reversely or compliantly?
Qibo: If five stars move in the orbit for longer time or even against the orbit, their light is faint, which indicates that they are inspecting their divisions below. When they move away from the orbit, return rapidly, or pass by the orbit, it indicates that they are examining if anything is missing or wrong. When they linger or circle in the orbit and deviate from or approach the orbit, it indicates that they are discussing whether to grant calamities or blessings to the people under their jurisdiction.

The near correspondence shows faint light, while the remote correspondence has large light. If the light from the five stars is one time brighter than usual, the transformation is greater. If the light from the five stars is twice as bright as usual, calamities will occur immediately. If the light from the five stars is one time fainter than usual, its transformation is lighter. If the light from the five stars is twice as faint as usual, it indicates that they are examining whether the behaviors of the people below are good or bad. Blessing will be given to those with merits and calamities will be given to those with faults. Thus, it is shown in the image of stars that the high and remote shining is small, the low and near shining is large. The large shining indicates the date of joy or anger is coming soon, while the small shining indicates the date of calamities or blessings is far from now. When the yearly motion is excessive, the yearly star will deviate from the orbit northwards. When the motion and Qi are in harmony, the five stars will move along their own orbit normally. So, when the yearly motion in a year is excessive, its constrained star will lose its light and be combined by the mother-star. When the yearly motion in a year is insufficient, the shining of the yearly star will be combined by its dominating star. Even a learned person can hardly understand its mystery, since this is such a profound theory that it is difficult to judge its merits. The doctors ignorant of celestial movement foretell something without any proofs just to make the kings feel fearful.

Emperor: How about the correspondence between the movement and the calamities?
Qibo: The correspondence varies according to their transformation concerned, and therefore the yearly motions arrive either excessively or insufficiently, the invasions of the stars are reverse or compliant, the lingering time of the stars is either longer or shorter, the images of the stars are reversal or compliance, the constellations are either dominant or restrained, and the signs of such changes are either kind or evil.

Emperor: How to distinguish the kind or evil images of the stars?
Qibo: These images of the stars indicate happiness or anger, grief or sorrow, luster or dryness, which are the normal signs and should be carefully observed.

Emperor: Is there any difference about the high or low location of the six signs?
Qibo: Though different in high or low location, the indications of the stars are the same, and this is also the case with the human beings.

Emperor: Good! What are the situations regarding their function, transformation, administration and order as well as dynamics or excess or insufficiency states?
Qibo: The function, transformation, administration, order, harm and change cannot be overlapped. The exuberance or decline of the domination or retaliation cannot be increased. The duration of going forward or coming back cannot be exceeded. The ascending and descending activities cannot be missed. All these activities correspond to the movement of five-phase.

Emperor: How do they cause diseases?
Qibo: The function and transformation are the auspicious signs of Qi, the administration and order are the manifestations of Qi, the change and variation are the principles of the retaliation of Qi, and the harm and calamity are the beginning of damage. Correspondence between human Qi and the yearly Qi ensures harmony, while non-correspondence causes diseases. The re-attack by evil will worsen diseases.

Emperor: Good! What you have explained is really a profound and brilliant theory, the discipline of the great sage and the great law of excellent elucidation, which has invaluable function and endless application. I have heard that those having good knowledge of the heavens must have good knowledge about human affairs. The doctors good at discussing ancient things must apply them into the present. The doctors good at knowing Qi must know the activities of all things. The doctors good at interpreting the correspondence must integrate with the transformation of the heavens and the earth, and the doctors good at elucidating transformation and change must elucidate the law of the nature, and nobody but you can explain this profound theory. I will select an auspicious day to store it in the Numinous Room and read it daily. It is named *The Changes of Qi Shifting*, and I won't open the book unless I am sincere enough and I will hand it down to the coming generations.

Chapter 70

Great Theory on Routine Functions of Five Phases

Yellow Emperor: The greater heavens are empty and boundless, and the five-phase moves in endless cycles, in which there are different exuberances and insufficiencies corresponding to benefit and damage. I'd like to know what the balanced Qi is. How is it named and how is it recorded.

Qibo: What a meaningful question! The balanced Qi of the wood tends to distribute and be soft, the fire to ascend and light, the earth to grow and transform, the metal to define and calm, and the water to be quiet and smooth.

Emperor: How about the insufficiency of five-phase?

Qibo: The insufficient wood tends to lose harmony, the insufficient fire to hide brightness, the insufficient earth to degrade the inspection, the insufficient metal to comply and change, and the insufficient water to flow off.

Emperor: How about the excess?

Qibo: The excessive wood tends to germinate early, the excessive fire to burn brightly, the excessive earth to be thick and high, the excessive metal to firm and form, and the excessive water to overflow.

Emperor: As to the triple Qi with different recording marks, I'd like to know their manifestations.
Qibo: What a detailed question you have asked! In the year recording marked with Distribution and Softness, the wood-phase moves around virtuously, Yang is stretching and Yin is distributing, and the transformations of five elements are broadly peaceful. Its Qi is proper, its property is to obey, its function is to bend and stretch, its transformation is to grow and blossom, its categorization is grass and wood, its administration is to disperse, its climate is warm, its action is wind, its correspondence is in liver that fears the coolness, and its opening is at eyes. It corresponds to sesame in grains, to plum in fruits, to kernel in nuts, to spring in seasons, to hairy worm in insects, to dog in animals, to dark green in colors, to sinews in nutrition, to internal straining and sticking fullness in diseases, to sour in flavors, to Jue in scales, to firmness in substance, and to eight in numbers.

In the recording marked with Ascending and Brightness, the normal Yang is governing, the administration of fire-phase is perfect virtuously, and the transformations of five elements are even. Its Qi is high, its property is rapid, its function is to flame and burn, its transformation is to flourish, its categorization is the fire, its administration is to shine, its climate is summer-heat, its action is heat, its correspondence is in heart that fears the coldness, and its opening is at tongue. It corresponds to wheat in grains, to apricot in fruits, to vascular bundles in fruitage, to summer in seasons, to winged worm in insects, to horse in animals, to red in colors, to blood in nutrition, to spasm in diseases, to bitter in flavors, to Zhi in scales, to vessels in substance, and to seven in numbers.

In the recording marked with Earth-up and Transformation, the Qi in the leisurely sky is collaborative, it governs all the directions virtuously, and the transformations of five elements are perfect. Its Qi is peaceful, its property is obedient, its function is either high or low, its transformation is replete, its categorization is the earth, its administration is to calm down, its climate is wet steam, its action is the damp, its correspondence is in spleen that fears the wind, and its opening is at mouth. It corresponds to millet in grains, to jujube in fruits, to flesh in fruitage, to late summer in seasons, to naked worm in insects, to cattle in animals, to yellow in colors, to muscle in nutrition, to lump in diseases, to sweet in flavors, to Gong in scales, to skin in substance, and to five in numbers.

In the recording marked with Definition and Calmness, the Qi astringes without combating and conquering without killing, the transformations of five elements are spacious and bright. Its Qi is clean, its property is sturdy, its function is to scatter and fall, its transformation is to harden and astringe, its categorization is the metal, its administration is vigorous and conquering, its climate is cool and vigorous, its action is to dry, its correspondence is in lung that fears the heat, and its opening is at nose. It corresponds to rice in grains, to peach in fruits, to shell in fruitage, to autumn in seasons, to beetle in insects, to chicken in animals, to white in colors, to skin and hair in nutrition, to cough in diseases, to pungency in flavors, to Shang in scales, to external hardness in substance, and to nine in numbers.

In the recording marked with Quiet and Smooth, the Qi is to store without damage and to administer with smooth execution, and the transformations of five elements are integrated. Its Qi is bright, its property is downward, its function is to irrigate and fertilize, its transformation is to congeal and harden, its categorization is the water, its administration is to run smoothly and continuously, its climate is constrictive and conquering, its action is to cause cold, its correspondence is in kidney that fears the damp, and its opening is at both external genitalia and anus. It corresponds to bean in grains, to chestnut in fruits, to juice in fruitage, to winter in seasons, to scaled worms in insects, to pig in animals, to black in colors, to bone and marrow in nutrition, to the reversal in diseases, to saltiness in flavors, to Yu in scales, to external hardness in substance, and to six in numbers.

So, there is no killing during germination, no damage during growth, no restraining during transformation, no impairment during harvest and no inhibition during storage, which is termed balanced Qi.

The recording marked with Losing Harmony leads to a feature of dominated generating Qi, so that generating Qi fails to administer, transforming Qi is elevated, growing Qi is still and astringing Qi comes earlier, in which cold rain falls from time to time, wind and cloud are rising together, grass and trees flourish later and tend to be dried and withered, the crops ripen quickly, and people tend to have tight skin and full muscles. Its Qi is astringent, its function is gathering, its alteration of body is spasm and flaccidity, its tendency is fright and horror, and its correspondence is in liver. It corresponds to jujube and plum in fruits, to pits and shell in fruitage, to sorghum rice in grains, to sour and pungency in flavors, to white and dark green in colors, to dog and chicken in animals, to hairy worm and beetle in insects, to chilly fog and dew in climate, to Jue and Shang in scales, and to shaking and horror in diseases, mainly due to wood subject to metal transformation. So, the lesser Jue is similar to semi-Shang, the upper Jue is similar to the normal Jue, and the upper Shang is similar to normal Shang. Diseases like flaccid limbs, carbuncle, swelling, sore and ulcer, and parasitic infestation will develop due to the excessive sweetness, due to the evil damaging liver. Since the upper Gong is similar to normal Gong, there will be bleak chill and conquering constriction and then flaming and boiling heat, with disasters occurring in the east serving as retaliation; flying insects, moth, maggot, pheasant and even thunder will appear.

The recording marked with Hiding Brightness makes a feature of dominated growing Qi, so that growing Qi fails to disperse, storing Qi is rising, astringing Qi administers itself, transforming Qi acts in still condition, cold Qi is rising and summer Qi acts feebly. Then all things, depending on the transformation of earthly Qi, can be generated with no growth and yield with no maturation so that they are aging during transformation. Yang Qi is hidden and the insects hibernate early. Its Qi is depressive, its function is drastic, its alteration of body is either overt or insidious, its attack is pain, and its correspondence is in heart. It corresponds to chestnut and peach in fruits, to vascular bundles and juice in fruitage, to bean and rice in grains, to bitter and saltiness in flavors, to black and red in colors, to horse and pig in animals, to winged and scaled worms in insects, to ice, snow and frost and cold in climate, to Zhi and Yu in scales, and to dementia, sorrow and amnesia in diseases, which is due to insufficient fire phase subject to water transformation. So, the lesser Zhi is similar to lesser Yu, and the upper Shang is similar to normal Shang; then evil will damage heart, and there appears congealing chill, piercing cold wind followed by rainstorm, with disasters occurring in the south, which results in torrential rain, roaring thunder, murky clouds and incessant rain.

The recording marked with Degradation makes a feature of reduced growing Qi, transforming Qi fails to execute, generating Qi administers alone, growing Qi is intact, raining is delayed and astringing Qi is even, by which wind and cold are rising together, the grass and woods are sprouting with no fruit or only with empty grain. Its Qi is scattered, its function is quiet and still, its alterations of body are exudative sores, erosive ulcer, carbuncles and swelling, its attack is damp stagnation, and its correspondence is in spleen. It corresponds to plum and chestnut in fruits, to juice and nut in fruitage, to bean and sesame in grain, to sour and sweet in flavors, to dark green and yellow in colors, to cattle and dog in animals, to the naked and hairy worms in insects, to waving and roaring wind with shaking and breaking situation, to Gong and Jue in scales, and to lingering fullness due to earth-phase subject to wood phase. So, the lesser Gong is similar to lesser Jue, the upper Gong is similar to normal Gong, and the upper Jue is similar to normal Jue. Its corresponding diseases are dyspepsia and diarrhea after indigestion due to evil damaging spleen. The waving and roaring wind shakes and pulls the earth and the green plants are withering and scattering. Its disaster is in four directions, its destruction and breakage will be caused by tigers and wolves; when the clear Qi plays its role, generating Qi will be inhibited.

The recording marked with Compliance and Change makes a feature of decreased astringency. The astringing Qi is delayed, the generating Qi is elevated, the growing Qi is combined with transforming Qi virtuously and then fire administration can execute, leading to exuberance of everything. Its Qi is elevated, its function is dry and vigorous, its alterations of body are coughing, vexation, vertigo and reversal, its attacks of diseases are cough and panting, its correspondence is in lung; it corresponds to plum and apricot in fruits, to shell and vascular bundles in fruitage, to sesame and wheat in grains, to bitter and pungency in flavors, to white and red in colors, to chicken and sheep in animals, to beetle and winged worms in insects, to brightness and scorching hot, to Shang and Zhi in scales, and to sneeze, cough, nasal obstruction and bleeding in diseases, due to metal phase subject to fire phase. So, the lesser Shang is similar to lesser Zhi, the upper Shang is similar to normal Shang, and the upper Jue is similar to normal Jue. The evil damages lung, and there appears flaming fire-heat followed by ice, snow, frost and hailstones, and disaster in west as number seven. The scaled worms, pigs and rats are curling up when yearly Qi arrives earlier, leading to great cold.

Recording marked with Flowing Off makes a feature of reversal Yang. The storing Qi fails to rise, the transforming Qi is hyperactive and the growing Qi is distributing widely. Then the hibernating animals fail to hibernate. The soil is moist, the rivers and springs are declining while the grass and wood grow and bloom in an abundant and luxuriant manner. Its Qi is stagnated, its function is to ooze and discharge, its alteration of body are firm and immotile, its attacks of diseases are dryness and withering, and its correspondence is in kidney. It corresponds to jujube and apricot in fruits, to juice and flesh in fruitage, to corn and broomcorn in grains, to sweet and saltiness in flavors, to pig and cattle in animals, to the scaled and naked worms in insects, to dim dusts and gloomy fog in climate, to Yu and Gong in scales and to flaccidity, reversal and firm binding in the lower due to water phase subject to earth phase. So, the lesser Yu is similar to lesser Gong and the upper Gong is similar to the normal Gong, the diseases are urinary retention and constipation due to evil damaging kidney, insufficiency of water motion is the same as the insufficiency of earth motion, the damp earth governing the weather is the same as the normal condition of earth motion. Its disease is retention of urine or difficulty in urination due to the attack of the kidney by evil. There is stagnation of dust and sudden storm, followed by shaking, pulling, breaking and destruction of things, its catastrophe is in one division in the north characterized by caterpillar and fox going out, and the variation is not hiding.

So, taking advantage of insufficient earth, the dominated Qi or dominating Qi is coming unexpectedly and damaging brutally. After that, the disasters will reflect on themselves with mild retaliation due to mild damage and with severe retaliation due to severe damage, which is the constant change of the climate.

The recording marked with Growth is characterized by a feature of early germination; the earth Qi is loose and discharging, the green Qi of grass and trees is emerging, and Yang Qi is distributing widely. Its transformation is germination, its Qi is soothing, its administration is dispersing, its action is free and relaxed, its alteration of body is vertigo and vertex, its normal climate is breeze with gentle sound and the seedlings are shooting out, and its abnormal climate is the blowing wind with vibrating, pulling and breaking phenomena. It corresponds to sesame and rice in grains, to chicken and dog in animals, to plum and peach in fruits, to green, yellow and white in colors, to sour, sweet and pungent in flavors, to spring in seasons, to the meridians of Jueying and Shaoyang of foot, to liver and spleen in solid viscera, to hairy and beetle worms in insects, to hard shell and core in stuff, and to anger in diseases. So, the greater Jue is similar to the upper Shang and the upper Zhi will have Qi reversal, leading to vomiting and diarrhea. If wood Qi cannot execute its normal action, the astringent metal Qi will retaliate, and it looks as if autumn Qi is coming coolly and vigorously, even with descending and conquering Qi. The clear Qi comes drastically and the grass and trees are withering, while the evil will damage liver accordingly.

The recording marked with Bright Burning makes a feature of impressive exuberance; Yin Qi is transformed internally, Yang Qi is blooming externally, flaming summer-heat is spreading and all the things are prosperous. Its transformation is growing Qi, its Qi is upright, its administration is stirring, its action is to show sounds and colors, its alteration is scotching hot with mental disturbance, its normal climate is noisy summer heat with steamy depression and its abnormal climate is intensively hot with boiling heat. It corresponds to wheat and bean in crops, to sheep and pig in animals, to the apricot and chestnut in fruits, to red, white and black in colors, to bitter, pungency and saltiness in flavors, to spring in seasons, to Shaoyin, Taiyang, Jueyin and Shaoyang of hand, to heart and lung in solid viscera, to winged and scaled worms in insects, to vascular bundles in fruitage, and to hysterical laughing, malaria, sores, ulcer, bleeding, dementia and red eye in diseases. So, the upper Yu is similar to normal Zhi, whose Qi is intact and whose disease is convulsion. When the astringent Qi of the upper Zhi is delayed, its administration is violent and then the storing Qi retaliates, leading to congealed chill, and even raining, frost, and hailstone with piercing coldness, and evil damages heart accordingly.

The recording marked with Thick Highness makes a feature of spacious transformation. Its Qi is thick, clear and quiet virtuously, growing compliantly with fullness, and is characterized by internal filling with extreme, and substantial transforming with bumper shape. There appears smoky dust and gloomy mist over the thick earth, heavy rain falling from time to time, and the damp Qi prevailing while the dry Qi is receding. Its transformation is intact, its Qi is ample, its administration is quiet, its action is comprehensive, its alteration of body is the damp accumulation and retention, its normal phenomenon is soft moistness with humid soil, its abnormal phenomenon is booming thunder and heavy downpour, and mountains fall and the earth is split. It corresponds to millet and sesame in grains, to cattle and dog in animals, to jujube and pear in fruits, to yellow, black and blue in colors, to sweet, saltiness and sour in flavors, to late summer in seasons, to foot-Taiyin and foot-Yangming in meridians, to spleen and kidney in solid viscera, to the naked and hairy worms in insects, to flesh and pit in stuff, to abdominal fullness and four limbs failing to raise. Since there appears wind, the evil will damage spleen.

The recording marked with Firm Formation makes a feature of astringency and contraction. Heavenly Qi is clean, earthly Qi is bright, Yang Qi is easy-going, and Yin administers transforming Qi; since dryness exudates the administration, all things can be allowed to mature, and since the astringing Qi is distributing widely, the transforming Qi of late summer fades out. Its transformation is formation, its Qi is fading, its administration is constriction, its action is sharp and vigorous, its alteration of body is acute fracture, ulcer and sores, its normal climate is frost, dew and chill, and its abnormal climate is conquering and withering. It corresponds to rice and millet in grains, to chicken and horse in animals, to peach and apricot in fruits, to white, green and red in colors, to pungency, sour and bitter in flavors, to autumn in seasons, to hand-Taiyin and hand-Yangming in meridians, to lung and liver in solid viscera, to beetle and winged worm in insects, to shell and vascular bundles in fruitage, and bloating chest with lifting of the head during breathing in patients. So, the upper Zhi is similar to normal Shang, whose Qi is intact and whose disease is cough. If administration of metal Qi becomes violent, the big trees fail to bloom and the grass is fragile with a dry leaf tip. It is as if retaliation by the Qi of late summer, the great fire Qi is prevailing with scotching heat, and the vine is withering to death; accordingly the evil will damage lung.

The recording marked with Overflow marks a feature of sealing and storage; cold governs all the transformations, the heavens and the earth are severely congealing, storing Qi administers widely and the growing Qi of fire cannot be arisen. Its transformation is piercingly cold, its Qi is firm, its administration is quiet, its action is flowing and irrigation, its alteration is watery diarrhea and severe vomiting, its common climate is severely congealing and cold fog, its climatic change is ice, snow, frost and hailstone. It corresponds to bean and millet in grains, to pig and cattle in animals, to chestnut and jujube in fruits, to black, red and yellow in colors, to saltiness, bitter and sweet in flavors, to winter in seasons, to foot-Shaoyin and foot-Taiyang in meridians, to kidney and heart in solid viscera, to the scaly and naked worms in insects, to substantial juice in fruitage, and to distension in disease. When in the upper Yu, the growing Qi of fire isn't transformed. If the administration of water is excessive, the transforming Qi of earth is rising greatly and there is intermingled dust and the damp with frequent heavy rain falling; accordingly the evil damages kidney.

It's believed that if any of the five phases run in abnormal way, its dominating Qi will come to retaliate, while if in the normal way, even the dominating Qi will be identified, which is the information concerned.

Emperor: Heavenly Qi is insufficient in the northwest with the cold on the left and the cool on the right, while earthly Qi is insufficient in the southeast with the hot on the right and warm on the left; what is the reason for this?

Qibo: Qi has Yin and Yang aspects and altitude has high and low levels, which reflect the difference of the greater and lesser. The southeast corresponds to Yang. And for Yang, since its essence descends to the lower, the right is hot while the left is warm. The northwest corresponds to Yin. And for Yin, since its essence ascends to the upper, the left is cold while the right is cool. Hence, since the terrain level is either high or low and the climate appears either warm or cool, the climate in the high is cold while the climate in the low is hot. Therefore, those who live in the cold tend to have distension while those who live in the warm tend to have sores. Purgation is applied to cure the distension, while diaphoresis is applied to cure sores, which reflects the constant effect on the opening and closing of interstitial striae as well as the difference between the greater and lesser.

Emperor: How about its effect on the life span?

Qibo: People in the area where Yin-essence is ascending can enjoy a longer life span, while people in the area where Yang-essence is descending have a shorter life span.

Emperor: Good. How to treat these diseases?
Qibo: Due to Qi from the northwest, the diseases are treated by dissipating cold and cooling the internal heat, while due to Qi from the southeast, the diseases are treated by astringing Yang Qi and warming the internal cold, which is another form of so-called treating the same disease with different methods. It's believed that the diseases due to cold Qi or cool Qi can be treated with warmth or the heat as well as bathing with decoction. The diseases due to warm Qi or hot Qi can be treated with warmth or the heat as well as strengthening its interior Qi. The treatment should be identified to the Qi in the proper area and the disease can be calmed down, but the disease with false manifestation can be treated by contrary therapy.

Emperor: Good. But with the same Qi in the same area, there is still different growth, development and life span; what is the reason for this?
Qibo: This is due to the difference between the high or low altitude. The clear high-altitude area is dominated by Yin Qi, while turbid low-altitude area is predominated by Yang Qi. The Yang arrives earlier than the due seasonal time, while the Yin arrives later than the due seasonal time, which is the geographical constant and the law of generation and transformation.

Emperor: Is there any difference of the life span?
Qibo: People living in high altitude tend to enjoy a longer life span, while people living in low altitude tend to have shorter life span. It varies with the differences among different

altitudes, which has less difference of life span due to less difference of altitudes, but has greater difference of life span due to greater difference of altitudes. So, when treating diseases, any doctor has to be aware of the general law of the heavens and the earth, the alternation of Yin and Yang, the earlier and later arrival of Qi, the life span of people, as well as the timing of generation and transformation, by which the physique and Qi mechanism of human body can be identified.

Emperor: Good. In a certain year, one who should have had the disease doesn't contract it, or the Qi which should have had response or action doesn't have it — why?
Qibo: It is controlled by the heavenly Qi, with which the Qi of solid viscera can comply.

Emperor: I'd like to know more details about it.
Qibo: When Shaoyang is governing the heavens, fire Qi is descending, lung Qi is ascending to follow the heavenly Qi, and Qi of white-metal is rising to play a role. Grass and trees are damaged, fire Qi is found to be blazing, metal Qi is changed and consumed, and great summer-heat is prevailing. People then tend to have cough, sneeze, running nose, nose-bleed, nasal obstruction, oral sores, chill, fever and edema. Wind is blowing over the earth and dust-sand is flying; people tend to have heartache, stomachache, and critical reversal with diaphragmatic obstruction, which will occur suddenly.

When Yangming is governing the heavens, the dry Qi is descending, liver Qi is ascending to follow the heavenly Qi, the green Qi is rising and the wood plays a role for erection, which damages the earth, cool chill is coming frequently, and trees are damaged and grass is withered. People then have hypochondriac pain, reddish eyes, tremor, shivering, flaccidity of sinews and failure to stand for a long duration. When violent heat arrives, the earth Qi turns to hot as summer-heat and depressive Yang Qi emerge, which are associated with abnormal urine, chill-fever like malaria, and even heartache. Fire Qi is prevailing, leading to plant withering, flowing water with no freezing and even hibernating insects come out.

When Taiyang is governing the heavens, cold Qi is descending, and heart Qi is ascending to follow the heavenly Qi; fire Qi glows bright and red Qi is rising, leading to metal Qi damage. Cold Qi is rising frequently, its domination makes water freeze and fire Qi ascends brightly. People then tend to have heart vexation, dry throat, frequent thirst, running nose, sneeze, frequent sorrow and yawning; since heat Qi is flowing frantically, cold Qi retaliates and frost falls, which is associated with amnesia and even heartache. The earth is moistened and water overflows. The cold arrives as guest Qi that falls down to add Yin transformation, and damp Qi transforms the things, leading to water retention, anorexia due to middle fullness, numbness of skin and muscles, stagnation of sinews and vessels, and even edema and back carbuncles.

When Jueyin is governing the heavens, the wind Qi is descending, and spleen Qi is ascending to follow heavenly Qi. Since the earthly Qi becomes prominent and earth yellow Qi is rising, the water Qi is damaged and the function of earth is changed. People then tend to have heavy body, flaccid muscles, poor appetite and tasteless mouth. The wind is prevailing in the sky with waving clouds and shaking things, leading to vertigo and tinnitus as diseases. Fire-Qi is burning violently and the earthly Qi becomes hot. The great heat is depleting the fluid with reddish excretions. Hibernating insects are often found to be out and flowing water fails to freeze, and these changes are rapid.

When Shaoyin is governing the heavens, the hot Qi is descending, lung Qi is ascending to follow heavenly Qi, and the Qi of white-metal is rising to play a role by damaging grass and trees. People then tend to have panting, vomiting, chill-fever, sneeze, running nose, and nasal obstruction. Since great summer-heat is prevailing, sores and ulcer can develop with burning sense as well as burning metal and stone. The earth is dry and clean with frequent coolness and coldness, which is associated with hypochondriac pain and frequent sighing. The descending and conquering Qi is prevailing, leading to changes of the grass and trees.

When Shaoyin is governing the heavens, damp Qi is descending and kidney Qi is ascending to follow the heavenly Qi. Qi of black-water is rising to cause change with damaged fire Qi and dusty emergence of clouds and rains. People tend to have discomfort in the chest, impotence, and severe decline of Yang Qi having no rising function. Also, people tend to have the pain of waist and buttocks, difficulty in turning the body, and critical reversal. The earth is about to store Yin, the great cold is coming and insects hibernate early; then people tend to have oppressive distension below the heart, pain in the lower abdomen while the earth is split and ice is hardened, which can sometimes impair dieting and be relieved in terms of the fire over-straining the melt. If the water is increased, its flavor is salty, which can be reduced when the water can flow smoothly.

Emperor: In the same year, there appears fertility or infertility with the different transformation of insects; what Qi is responsible for it?

Qibo: Six-Qi and five kinds of animals have the relationship of dominating and restraining each other, so that the identical Qi leads to exuberance while non-identical Qi leads to reduction, which is the law of the heavens and the earth and the constant of generation and transformation. So, when Jueyin is governing the heavens, the hairy worms are quiescent, the winged worms are reproductive and the beetle worms fail to reproduce; when governing the earth, the hairy worms are reproductive, the naked worms are consumed and the winged worms are sterile. When Shaoyin is governing the heavens, the winged worms are quiescent, the beetle worms are reproductive and the hairy worms fail to reproduce. When governing the earth, the winged worms are reproductive and the beetle worms are sterile. When Taiyin is governing the heavens, the naked worms are quiescent, the scaled worms are reproductive and the winged worms are sterile. When governing the earth, the naked worms are reproductive and the scaled ones are sterile. When Shaoyang is governing the heavens, the winged worms are quiescent, the hairy worms are reproductive and the naked worms are sterile. When governing the earth, the winged worms are reproductive, the beetle worms are consumed and hairy worms are sterile. When Yangming is governing the heavens, the beetle worms are quiescent, the winged worms are reproductive and the beetle worms are sterile. When governing the earth, the beetle worms are reproductive, the hairy worms are consumed and winged worms are sterile. When Taiyang is governing the heavens, the scaled worms are quiescent and the naked worms are reproductive; when governing earth, the scaled worms are consumed and the naked worms are sterile. Whenever six-Qi over-restrains the year phase indicating sterility, its sterile outcome will be more severe. So, six-Qi has the control, while five phases have the generation. The earthly Qi can control the one dominated by itself, while the heavenly Qi dominates the one dominating itself. The heaven controls the color while the earth controls the shape.

The decline and exuberance of five kinds of insects vary with the Qi corresponding to themselves. Hence, there appears fertility or infertility with the different transformation of insects, which is the principle of variation, termed the central dogma. The external central dogma has five types for generation and transformation, and there are five-Qi, five flavors, five colors, five categories and five compatibilities.

Emperor: What is the cause?
Qibo: The internal central dogma is termed spirit mechanism, and without it the vitals cease. The external central dogma is termed Qi accomplishment, and without accomplishment of Qi there is extinguishment of transformation. So, there are different controls, different domination, different generation and different accomplishment. It's believed that if not knowing the superimposition of year phase and six-Qi as well as their similarities and differences, it is not possible to discuss the generation and transformation. This is the information concerned.

Emperor: The genesis of Qi leads to generation and transformation, the spread of Qi leads to formation, the distribution of Qi leads to reproduction, and termination of Qi leads to alteration, which is consistent in essence. However, although all are nourished by five flavors, there is thin or thick generation and transformation, increase or decrease of maturity, and the difference in start and termination; what is the reason?
Qibo: It is controlled by the earthly Qi, and there is no generation with no heavenly Qi and there is no growth without earthly Qi.

Emperor: I'd like to learn the mechanism.

Qibo: The different Qi of the cold, heat, dry and damp is determined by their different transformations. Thus, when Shaoyang is governing the earth, there is no generation of the cold and toxin but pungent flavor; its dominating flavor is the bitter and sour, and its grain is in green and red color. When Yangming governs the earth, there is no generation of the damp toxin but generation of things with the sour flavor and moistness. Its dominating flavors are pungency, bitter and sweet, and its grain is in red or plain. When Taiyang governs the earth, there is no generation of heat toxin as well as things with the bitter flavor; its dominating flavor is plain and salty, and its grain is in yellow or black.

When Jueyin governs the earth, there is no generation of the cool toxin but generation of things with sweet flavor. Its dominating flavor is sour and bitter, its grain is in green or red, its Qi is specific and its flavor is pure. When Shaoyin governs the earth, there is no generation of the cold toxin but generation of things with the pungent flavor. Its dominating flavor is pungency, bitter and sweet, and its grain is in white and red. When Taiyin governs the earth, there is no generation of the dry toxin but generation of things with salty flavor or with heat Qi. Its dominating flavor is sweet and salty, and its grain is in yellow and black. Its Qi is pure and thick so that the salty flavor can be maintained, while its Qi is specific so that the pungent flavor can be transformed, indicating the simultaneous administration by both the metal Qi and earthly Qi.

It's believed that in order to supplement the insufficiency of the upper or the lower, the complying method is applied, while in order to treat the excess of the upper or the lower, the reversal method is applied, which is regulated according to the variation of the cold, heat, exuberance and decline. It's believed that whatever therapies are applied, including treating the upper or the lower as well as treating the internal or external, the etiology should be identified. The body with tolerance to toxic drugs can be treated with a thick one, while the intolerance can be treated with the thin one. This is the information concerned. For the contrary Qi, the disease in the upper is treated in the lower. The disease in the lower is treated in the upper. The disease in the middle is treated round the middle region. The disease due to the heat is treated with the cold and with warm medication. The disease due to the cold is treated with the heat and with cool medication. The disease due to the warm is treated with the cool and with cold medication. The disease due to the cool is treated with the warm and with the heat medication. So, the therapies include resolving the retention or breaking the hardness, vomiting or discharging the evils, and supplementing the insufficiency or purging the excess, and no matter whether the case is new or chronic, the principle of the application is the same.

Emperor: Some disease occurs in the middle with neither excess nor firmness and comes and goes; how to treat it?
Qibo: How detailed your question is! If there is no retention of the disease, its cause should be searched in the solid viscera, so as to supplement the deficiency, dispel the evil with medicinal herbs, maintain with diet, and bathe with decoction for harmonizing both interior and exterior, by which the disease can be cured.

Emperor: There are toxic and non-toxic herbs; is there any regulation for their application?
Qibo: Since there is new or chronic disease, large or small formulae, and toxic or non-toxic herbs, the medication of course has regulations. The medication with strong toxic drugs cannot be stopped till sixty percent of the condition has been improved; with moderate toxic drugs, till seventy percent; with slightly

toxic drugs, till eighty percent; and with non-toxic drugs, till ninety percent. Then the cereal, meat, fruit and vegetable are ingested as dietary therapy to regulate the health, avoiding over-application and damaging the healthy Qi. If the toxin cannot be resolved completely, the therapy mentioned above should be repeated. After identifying the yearly Qi dominantly, the harmony between the nature and human shouldn't be violated, and supplementing therapy is not allowed for the excess and purging therapy for the deficiency. Otherwise, it will impair the life span of humans and cause sequelae. Generally, abetting the evil and losing healthy Qi should be avoided so as to prevent the patient from dying with a lingering disease.

Emperor: Some chronic cases have obtained the smooth Qi but health is still not restored, or the disease has been cured but the patient is still thin and weak; how to deal with it?
Qibo: What a meaningful question you ask! The transformation cannot be replaced and the phasing of four seasons cannot be countered. If the meridians and collaterals have been communicated with, and blood and Qi have been harmonized, its rehabilitation from the insufficiency is just the same to the healthy person. By maintaining and harmonizing body, waiting patiently for time, keeping the genuine Qi, and avoiding deviation, the physique can be strengthened and the vital Qi can be enhanced, which can reach the realm of the sage-king. This is the information concerned. So, the Chief Essentials said that the change of the heavens and the earth cannot be controlled by the manpower, the rule of four seasons cannot be reversed, and maintaining and harmonizing should be applied to wait for the recovery of genuine Qi.

Emperor: Good.

Chapter 71

Great Theory on Normality of Six-Qi

Yellow Emperor asked: There are normal transformations and abnormal changes of six phases of Qi, predomination, anti-predomination, excess and regulation of earthly Qi as well as the sequential transformation of the sweet, bitter, pungent, salty, sour and bland flavors, which I know already. The transformation of five phases will comply with the five elements, reverse heaven-governing Qi, with heavenly Qi but reverse earthly Qi, and with earthly Qi but reverse heavenly Qi; also, the two Qi will or will not harmonize each other. I do not have a clear picture about this. I'm eager to know the laws of heavenly Qi and earthly Qi, in order to harmonize the phasing, regulate the transformation, coordinate the upper and the lower without destroying the rules, and make heavenly Qi ascend and earthly Qi descend without losing their timing and five phasing rotate with no deviation. How to prepare the five flavors and how to comply with and reverse the phasing and Qi changes?

Qibo kowtowed and bowed again to say: What a good question you have asked! This is the law of the heavens and the earth and the source of the changes in nature, and nobody but the saint emperor can study such a profound theory. Though I'm not so intelligent, please allow me to explain it in order to make it last forever without any change.

Emperor: I hope that you the Master can analyze and infer it, follow the categories and orders about heavenly stems or earthly branches and the portion of heaven-governing Qi or earth-governing Qi, differentiate the phases of various Qi, define the normal heaven-governing Qi and earth-governing Qi, discover the changes of the Qi, and clarify the normal conditions. Can I listen to it?

Qibo: Firstly, the year record should be established according to heavenly stems and earthly branches, in order to confirm the phases of metal, wood, water, fire and earth with their rotation rule, as well as the cold, summer-heat, dry, damp, wind and fire when governing the heavens and the earth. Then, the natural changes can be recognized, by which people can regulate their health status and balance their Yin and Yang. Thus, the rules of climate change are easily understood and the rules of Qi phases can be inferred. Please allow me to explain it.

Emperor: What is the year outline in the domination of Taiyang?

Qibo: It is in the year with record of the 5th and 11th.

In the year with record of the Ninth-5th and Ninth-11th, its features are heaven-governing Qi by Taiyang-cold-water, the guest year phase of wood as greater Jue and earth-governing Qi by Taiyin-damp-earth. It is the phase of wind. As for its normal climate, noisy breeze blows over the living things; as for its abnormal change, a gale blows down the trees and rips off the roof; as for its disorder, it will lead to vertigo, tremor, and blurred vision.

Its guest phases in order are greater Jue (the initial phase), lesser Zhi, greater Gong, and lesser Shang, terminating in greater Yu (the final phase), while the host phases are the same as the guest phases.

In the year with record of the Fifth-5th and Fifth-11th (fire is overstrained by Zhi), its features are heaven-governing Qi by Taiyang-cold-water, the guest year phase of fire as Taizheng, and earth-governing Qi by Taiyin-damp-earth. It is the phase of heat. Its normal transformation is summer-warmth and stagnated heat, its abnormal change is flaming fire, and the disease is stagnation of heat evil.

Its guest phases in order are greater Zhi, lesser Gong, greater Shang, lesser Yu and greater Jue (final phase), while its host phases in order are lesser Jue, greater Zhi, lesser Gong, greater Shang and the final phase lesser Yu (the final phase).

In the year with record of the First-5th (year according, also double heaven according) or the First-11th (year according, also double heaven according), its features are heaven-governing Qi by Taiyang-cold-water, the guest year phase of earth as Taihong, and earth-governing Qi by Taiyin-damp-earth. It is the phase of haze. Its normal transformation is soft, moist, heavy and lustrous, and its abnormal change is terrible storm and lightning, and its disease is characterized by heaviness of damp evil in the lower.

Its guest phases in order are the initial phase greater Gong, lesser Shang, greater Yu, lesser Jue and greater Zhi (the final phase), while its host phases in order are greater Jue (the initial phase), lesser Zhi, greater Gong, lesser Shang and the final phase greater Yu (the final phase).

In the year with record of the Seventh-5th and the Seventh-11th, its features are heaven-governing Qi by Taiyang-cold-water, its guest phase of metal as greater Shang, and earth-governing Qi by Taiyin-damp-earth. It is the phase of coolness. Its normal transformation is frost, dew and decline, its abnormal change is desolation and withering, and the disease then is characterized by dryness, stuffiness and fullness in the back and the chest.

The guest phases in order are the initial phase greater Shang, lesser Yu, greater Jue, lesser Zhi and the final phase greater Gong, while the host phases in order are lesser Jue (the initial phase), greater Zhi, lesser Gong, greater Shang and lesser Yu (the final phase).

In the year with record of the Third-5th and Third-11th, its features are heaven-governing Qi by Taiyang-cold-water, its guest year phase is water as Taiyu and earth-governing Qi by Taiyin-damp-earth. It is the phase of heat. Its normal transformation is piercing and freezing cold, its abnormal changes are ice, snow, frost and hailstone, and its disease then is characterized by retention of great cold in the septa of muscles and joints.

The guest phases in order are the initial phase greater Yu, lesser Jue, greater Zhi, lesser Gong and the final phase greater Shang, while the host phases in order are greater Jue (the initial phase), lesser Zhi, greater Gong, lesser Shang and the final phase greater Yu (the final phase).

In any year with heaven-governing Qi of Taiyang-cold-water, its Qi transformation arrives earlier than the due time. The heaven-governing Qi is constricting while earth-governing Qi is calm. Then, the cold Qi governs the sky so that Yang Qi fails to have an effect on the weather. However, the water and the earth collaborate with each other, and correspond with Water Star and Earth Star. Under this condition, it corresponds to the grain in yellow or black, to the governing-Qi in constriction, and to the earth-governing Qi in slow reaction. The cold-water governs widely, the rivers and lakes have no Yang evaporation, and then the fire has to wait for surging. When Shaoyang-minister-fire dominates in the middle, the rain falls in due time and stops after reaching extreme peak. When earth-governing Qi returns to Taiyin-damp-earth, the clouds move to the north, and the damp distributes everywhere to moisten everything. Meanwhile, the cold Qi covers all in the upper, thunder crashes in the lower, and cold and damp Qi are intermingling and lingering. In this kind of climate, people tend to suffer from cold-damp, muscle flaccidity, feeble feet with no contraction, diarrhea and bleeding.

The Qi in the initial phase is warm and prevalent. When Jueyin-wind-wood is promoted and earthly Qi is demoted, grass and trees become exuberant and verdant earlier than their usual time and people are susceptible to epidemic diseases and warm diseases with body fever, headache, vomiting and sores of the skin and muscles. In the second phase, the Qi is quite cool by contrast, and people tend to feel chilly. Grass growth is prevented due to cold, fire Qi is inhibited and people tend to suffer from Qi depression and fullness in the middle. Then coldness begins to emerge. In the third phase, the Qi of Taiyang-cold-water dominates in the heavens, cold Qi is prevailing, and rain is falling. People tend to have the disease due to cold, and the unusual diseases in the interior are carbuncles and gangrene, watery diarrhea, and heart heat with dysphoria, which may be incurable and lead to death if not treated. In the fourth phase, the Qi is characterized by a struggle between wind and damp and transformation of wind turns into rain, so that all living creatures can grow, transform and ripen. Then people tend to suffer from diseases with great heat and shortness of breath, flaccid muscles, feeble feet and bloody and mucous dysentery. In the fifth phase, Qi of Yangming-dry-metal, Yang Qi returns and the grass grows, transforms and ripens. People tend to feel comfortable. In the final phase, Qi of Taiyang-cold-water dominates and Taiyin-damp-earth exerts its effect so that Yin condenses in the sky and a haze covers the wild field. People tend to feel chilly with the cold wind attacking, and those who are pregnant will die.

Hence in any year with heaven-governing Qi of Taiyang-cold-water, the bitter flavor has to be ingested, with the dry treating the damp and with the warm treating the cold, in order to break the depressive Qi, previously enrich the transformation source, inhibit the Qi of the phase, support the thing dominated, and avoid the fulminant Qi leading to diseases. The grain with year-Qi has to be ingested to keep its perfect Qi and avoid deficient Qi to secure the healthy Qi. According to the similarities and differences of Qi compared with the current phase, increased or decreased doses can be decided accordingly. If the phase is the same as the cold-damp, it will be dried for heat transformation, and if the phase is different from the cold-damp, it will be dried for damp transformation. Thus, for the similarities, more doses will be given, and for the difference, fewer doses. In addition, application of cold drug should avoid cold phase, application of cool drug should avoid cool phase, application of warm drug should avoid warm phase, application of heat drug should avoid heat phase; dieting also is based on the same principle. If there are extraordinary conditions, application should be adjusted accordingly, and reversing this principle will lead to diseases, which is called chronomedicine.

Emperor: Good. What is the administration in Yangming year?

Qibo: It is the year with record of 4th and 10th.

In the year with record of the Fourth-4th and Fourth-10th, its features are heaven-governing Qi by Yangming-dry-metal and earth-governing Qi by Shaoyin-monarch-fire with the same predominating and retaliating Qi to the normal Shang. Its year phase is wood as lesser Jue with dominating clarity and retaliating heat.

Its guest phases in order are lesser Jue (the initial phase), greater Zhi, lesser Gong, greater Shang and lesser Yu, while the host phases are the same as the guest initiating in lesser Jue and terminating at lesser Yu.

In the year with record of the Tenth-4th and Tenth-10th, its features are heaven-governing Qi by Yangming-dry-metal and earth-governing Qi by Shaoyin-monarch-fire with the same predominating cold Qi and retaliating rain Qi to the normal Shang. Their year phase is heat, cold in domination and rain in retaliation.

Its guest phases in order are the initial phase lesser Zhi, greater Gong, lesser Shang, greater Yu and lesser Jue, while the host phase in order initiates in greater Jue and terminates in greater Yu (the final phase).

In the year with record of the Sixth-4th and Sixth-10th with the year phase of earth as lesser Gong, its features are heaven-governing Qi by Yangming-dry-metal and earth-governing Qi by Shaoyin-monarch-fire with the same predominating wind Qi and retaliating cool Qi. The Qi of year phase is rain, wind and cool.

Its guest phases in order are the initial phase lesser Gong, greater Shang, lesser Yu, greater Jue and the final phase greater

Zhi, while the host phase in order initiates at lesser Jue (the initial phase) and terminates at lesser Yu (the final phase).

In the year with record of the Second-4th (heaven-identification) and the Second-10th (year identification and triple-year identification) with the year phase of metal as lesser Shang, their features are heaven-governing Qi by Yangming-dry-metal, earth-governing Qi by Shaoyin-monarch-fire with the same predominating Qi and retaliating cool Qi to the normal Shang. Their Qi of year phase is cool, heat and cold.

Its guest phases in order are the initial phase lesser Shang, greater Yu, lesser Jue, greater Zhi and the final phase greater Gong, while the host phase in order initiates in greater Jue (the initial phase) and terminates in greater Yu (the final phase).

In the year with record of the Eighth-10th and Eighth-4th with the year phase of water as lesser Yu, their features are heaven-governing Qi by Yangming-dry-metal, earth-governing Qi Shaoyin-monarch-fire with the same predominating rain Qi and retaliating wind Qi. Their Qi of year phase is cold, rain and wind.

Its guest phases in order are the initial phase lesser Yu, greater Jue, lesser Zhi, lesser Gong and the final phase greater Shang, while the host phase in order initiates in lesser Jue (the initial phase)and terminates in lesser Yu (the final phase).

In any year with heaven-governing Qi of Yangming-dry-metal, its Qi transformation arrives later than the due time. The heaven-governing Qi is urgent, while earth-governing Qi is bright. Then, the Yang Qi governs the sky so that flaming summer-Qi prevails, everything is dry and hard, and gentle wind flows. Wind Qi and dry Qi are weaving and prevail in the intermingling air, so that there is more Yang and less Yin, clouds move to the source of rain, the rain transformation is distributed and then extreme dryness turns into moistness.

Under this condition, it corresponds to the grain in white or red, interval seasonal grains ripen with the excessive Qi, and the reproduction of beetles from the gold (white) Qi and many birds from the fire Qi is inhibited. Metal Qi and fire Qi collaborate and correspond to Metal Star and Fire Star. The administration is urgent, its effect is drastic, hibernating insects are exposed, and flowing water doesn't freeze. People tend to have cough, throat obstruction, episodes of chill and fever, sudden shivers, and urinary retention. If metal Qi is earlier and urgent, hairy worms will die. However, if heat-Qi comes later and is drastic, the beetles will be harmed. The emergence is stirring, the burst of dominating-Qi and retaliating-Qi will disturb the normal as cool Qi and heat are intermingling.

When Qi in the initial phase arrives, earthly Qi is depromoted, Yin-Qi begins to coagulate, air starts to be cool, water is frozen, and there is transformation of cold rain. People tend to have heat and distension in the middle, edema of face and eyes, somnolence, nasal obstruction and bleeding, sneeze, yawning, vomiting, dark urine and even dripping urination. When Qi in the second phase arrives, Yang Qi is distributed. People feel comfortable and everything is flourishing. Then the epidemic disease prevails and people are at risk of sudden death. When Qi in the third phase arrives, heavenly Qi administration is distributed, the cool Qi is prevailing, dry Qi and heat Qi are intermingling, the extreme dry Qi turns into moist, and people tend to have chill and fever. When Qi in the fourth phase arrives, cold rain falls, the diseases are characterized by sudden fainting spells, shivers and delirium, short breath, dry throat with severe thirst involving heart pain, carbuncles and sores, cold malaria, bone flaccidity and bloody stool. When Qi in the fifth phase arrives, the spring Qi prevails unexpectedly in autumn, so grass is flourishing and people live in harmony. When Qi in the final phase arrives, Yang Qi is distributed, the climate turns warm abnormally, the hibernating insects are exposed, and flowing water doesn't freeze. People maintain their health and live a calm life and warm disease occurs if Yang is luxuriant.

Hence in any year with heaven-governing Qi of Yangming-dry-metal, the grain with year-phase-Qi is ingested to secure the healthy Qi and the grain with interval-Qi should be ingested after the evil Qi is removed. In the current year, the salty, the bitter and the pungent flavors should be ingested as sweating, clearing and dispersing therapies. Qi of year phase should be secured without being damaged by evil. The Qi of depression should be broken and the source of dominated Qi should be supported. According to whether there is mild or severe chill and fever, the formulae can be determined. The one identical to heat-Qi is mostly transformed as earthly Qi while that identical to the cool is mostly transformed as heavenly Qi. In addition, application of cool drug should avoid cool phase, application of heat drug should avoid heat phase, application of cold drug should avoid cold phase, application of warm drug should avoid warm phase; dieting also is based on the same principle. If there are extraordinary conditions, application should be adjusted accordingly, and reversing this principle will reverse the principle of the heavens and the earth and disturb the principles of Yin and Yang.

Emperor: Good. What is the administration in Shaoyang year?

Qibo: It is the year with record of the 3rd and 9th.

In the year with record of the Ninth-3rd and Ninth-9th, with the year phase of wood as greater Jue, its features are heaven-governing Qi by Shaoyang-minister-fire and earth-governing Qi by Jueyin-wind-wood. Their year phase is high wind. Their transformations are characterized by agitating whistling and revival, their change by vibrating, pulling, destruction and drawing, and their diseases are vertigo and tremor, sticking pain of hypochondria and fright.

Its guest phases in order are greater Jue (the initial phase), lesser Zhi, greater Gong, lesser Shang and greater Yu, while the host phase in order start at normal Jue and terminate at greater Yu (the final phase).

In the year with record of the Fifth-3rd (year identification) and the Fifth-9th (year identification), with the year phase of fire as greater Zhi, its features are heaven-governing Qi by Shaoyang-minister-fire and earth-governing Qi by Jueyin-wind-wood. Their year phase is summer-heat. Their transformations are noisy agitation whistling and stuffy heat revival, their changes are flaming and boiling heat, and their diseases are heat depression in the upper, bleeding, bloody excretion, and heart pain.

Its guest phases in order are the initial phase greater Zhi, lesser Gong, greater Shang, lesser Yu, and greater Jue, while the host phase in order start at lesser Jue and terminate at lesser Yu (the final phase).

In the year with record of the First-3rd and First-9th, with the year phase of earth as greater Gong, its features are heaven-governing Qi by Shaoyang-minister-fire and earth-governing Qi by Jueyin-wind-wood. The year phase is Yin-rain. Their transformations are soft moist and heavy luster, the changes are shocking and stormy rain, and the diseases are heavy body, edema, retention and oppressive distension.

Its guest phases in order are the initial phase greater Gong, lesser Shang, greater Yu, lesser Jue, and greater Zhi, while the host phase in order starts at greater Jue (the initial phase) and terminates at greater Yu.

In the year with record of the Seventh-3rd and Seventh-9th, with the year phase of metal as greater Shang, its features are heaven-governing Qi by Shaoyang-minister-fire and earth-governing Qi by Jueyin-wind-wood. The year phase is cool. Their transformations feature as fog, dew and clear and cool climate, the changes are constricting and declination, and the diseases are confined to the shoulders, back and chest.

Its guest phases in order are the initial phase greater Shang, lesser Yu, greater Jue, lesser Zhi, and greater Gong, while the host phase in order starts at lesser Jue (the initial phase) and terminates at lesser Yu.

In the year with record of the Third-3rd and Third-9th, with the year phase of water as greater Yu, its features are heaven-governing Qi by Shaoyang-minister-fire and earth-governing Qi by Jueyin-wind-wood. The year phase is cold and constriction. The transformations are compression and piercing cold, and the diseases feature cold and edema.

Its guest phases in order are the initial phase greater Yu, lesser Jue, greater Zhi, lesser Gong, and greater Shang, while the host phase in order starts at greater Jue (the initial phase) and terminates at greater Yu (the final phase).

In any year with heaven-governing Qi of Shaoyang-minister-fire, its Qi transformation arrives earlier than the due time. The heaven-governing Qi is normal while earth-governing Qi is stirring. Wind rises suddenly, the grass and trees are drooping, sand is flying, and minister-fire is prevailing. Yin Qi is moving and Yang Qi is transformed so that rain is falling and fire and wood collaborate each other, which corresponds to Fire Star and Wood Star in the upper. This condition corresponds to the grain in red or dark green, its transformation is severe, and its action is disturbing. Therefore, heaven-wind and earth-heat intermingle and distribute, clouds and air are boiling while Taiyin is moving wildly, cold Qi is coming, and cool air and rain emerge together. Then people tend to have cold in the middle, external sore and ulceration, diarrhea and fullness in the body. An experienced person having the condition, will adapt and not fight against it. With the frequent recurrence, people will have chill and fever time and again, as well as malaria, diarrhea, deafness, blurred vision, vomiting, depression in the upper, edema and uncommon complexion.

When Qi in the initial phase arrives, earthly Qi recedes. Wind-Qi dominates and causes swaying, cold-Qi is gone, the climate is getting quite warm, and grass and trees flourish earlier. Cold-Qi, though coming, fails to reduce the temperature, then warm diseases arise. The diseases are characterized by depression in the upper, bleeding, red eyes, cough with Qi reversal, headache, metrorrhagia, fullness in the hypochondria, and small sores in the skin. When Qi in the second phase arrives, fire Qi as host is depressed instead, white dust flies everywhere, clouds move and are filled with moisture, wind is dominated by damp and then rain is dripping, and people are healthy in general. Its diseases are heat-depression in the upper, cough with Qi reversal, vomiting, sores in the interior, stuffy chest and throat, headache, body fever, confusion and purulent sore. When Qi in the third phase arrives, heavenly Qi is distributed, flaming summer is coming, Shaoyang-minister-fire is over the sky and then rain stops. People tend to have fever in the interior, deafness, blurred vision, bleeding, purulent sore, cough, vomiting, stuffy nose, nosebleed, thirst, sneeze, yawn, throat obstruction, red eyes and even sudden death. When Qi in the fourth phase arrives, the cool Qi comes, the flaming summer is moderated and the dew is being deposited. People are in harmony and the disease is characterized by fullness and heavy body. When Qi in the fifth phase arrives, Yang Qi leaves, coldness comes, the rain falls, the sweat pores are blocked and hard trees wither early. Then people should avoid cold evil, and the wise men prefer to live in airtight houses. When Qi in the final phase arrives, earthly Qi is normal, wind comes, all living things are generated unexpectedly and the thick fog is prevailing. Their diseases are characterized by incontinence, heartache and cough due to failure of Yang Qi storage.

The excessive Qi of year phase and seasonal phase should be inhibited and the dominated Qi be supported. The resultant depression Qi should be broken and its source of transformation be enriched. If violent excess isn't produced, the difficult diseases cannot arise. Therefore in the current year phase, the salty, pungent and sour flavors are better ingested, the draining, discharging, soaking and dispersing therapies are better adopted, and the excess can be adjusted according to cold and warm climate. The year phase, similar to wind-heat, should be given more cold transformation, but if it is different from the wind-heat, it should be given less cold transformation. Application of heat drug should avoid heat phase, application of warm drug should avoid warm phase, application of cold drug should avoid cold phase, application of cool drug should avoid cool phase; dieting also follows the same principle. If there are extraordinary conditions, application should be adjusted accordingly, and reversing this principle will lead to diseases, also called as chronomedicine.

Emperor: Good. What is the administration in Taiyin year?
Qibo: It is the year with record of the 2nd and 8th.

In the year with record of the Fourth-2nd and Fourth-8th, with the year phase of wood as lesser Jue, the features are heaven-governing Qi by Taiyin-damp-earth and earth-governing Qi by Taiyang-cold-water with the same clarity as predominating Qi and heat as retaliating Qi. The year phase is wind with clarity and heat.

Its guest phases in order are lesser Jue (the initial phase), greater Zhi, lesser Gong, greater Shang, and the final phase lesser Yu, while the host phase in order starts at lesser Jue and terminates at lesser Yu.

In the year with record of the Tenth-2nd and Tenth-8th, with the year phase of fire as lesser Zhi, the features are heaven-governing Qi by Taiyin-damp-earth and earth-governing Qi by Taiyang-cold-water with the same predominating cold Qi and retaliating rain Qi. The year phase is heat with cold and rain.

Its guest phases in order are the initial phase lesser Zhi, greater Gong, lesser Shang, greater Yu, and the final phase lesser Jue, while the host phase in order starts at greater Jue and terminates at greater Yu.

In the year with record of the Sixth-2nd (triple heaven-identification) and the Sixth-8th (triple heaven-identification), with the year phase of earth as lesser Gong, the features are heaven-governing Qi by Taiyin-damp-earth and earth-governing Qi by Taiyang-cold-water with the same predominating wind Qi and retaliating clarity Qi to the normal Gong. The year phase is rain with wind and clarity.

Its guest phases in order are the initial phase lesser Gong, greater Shang, lesser Yu, greater Jue, and the final phase lesser Zhi, while the host phase in order starts at lesser Jue (the initial phase) and terminates at lesser Yu.

In the year with record of the Second-2nd and the Second-8th, with the year phase of metal as lesser Shang, the features are heaven-governing Qi by Taiyin-damp-earth and earth-governing Qi by Taiyang-cold-water with the same predominating wind Qi and retaliating clarity Qi in the two years. The year phase is cool with heat and cold.

Its guest phases in order are lesser Shang, greater Yu, lesser Jue, greater Zhi, and the final phase lesser Gong, while the host phase in order starts at greater Jue (the initial phase) and terminates at greater Yu.

In the year with mark of the Eighth-2nd (according year-identification) and the Eighth-8th (according year-identification), with the year phase of water as lesser Yu, the features are heaven-governing Qi by Taiyin-damp-earth, and earth-governing Qi by Taiyang-cold-water with the same predominating rain Qi and retaliating wind Qi in the two years to the normal Gong. The year phase is cold with rain and wind.

Its guest phases in order are the initial phase lesser Yu, greater Jue, lesser Zhi, greater Gong, and the final phase lesser Shang, while the host phase in order starts at lesser Jue (the initial phase) and terminates at lesser Yu.

In any year with heaven-governing Qi of Taiyin-damp-earth, the Qi transformation arrives earlier than the due time. Yin Qi dominates the administration solely and Yang Qi recedes. When big wind arises, heavenly Qi descends, and earthly Qi ascends. There is haze over the wild field and dust arises everywhere, clouds are moving to the south, cold rain falls occasionally, and the crops ripen in the late summer. People tend to have cold and damp-disease, full abdomen, general distension, edema, lump, Qi reversal, cold-pain and spasm. Collaboration of damp and cold evil result in yellow and black dust cloud, prevailing with the Qi intermingling, and corresponds to Earth Star and Water Star in the upper. The administration is constrictive, the action is quiet, and the color corresponds to yellow and black. So, Yin Qi condenses in the upper, cold-Qi accumulates in the lower and cold dominates the fire leading to hailstones. The sun fails to shine and cold air is prevailing. Thus, in the year with excessive Qi, planting crops in the higher altitude is better, while in the year with insufficient Qi planting is best done at lower altitude. In the year with excessive Qi, planting crops is better done late while in the year with insufficient Qi it is better done early. The kind of planting should be based on both the favorable earth condition and Qi transformation. And it is also the case with health maintenance, as the health of people and of grains depend on the interval essence Qi to be ripe.

When Qi in the initial phase arrives, earthly Qi recedes, cold-Qi moves away, spring-Qi is normal, and wind is coming and distributed. When all living things are flourishing, people feel comfortable. When wind and damp is conflicting leading to rain, people tend to have bleeding, sinew and collateral spasm, inflexibility of joints, heavy body and flaccid sinews. When Qi in the second phase arrives, big fire Qi is normal, all things comply with the transformation and people can maintain their fitness. The possible diseases include epidemic warm disease, and people are exposed to the similar illness. Damp and evaporation are conflicting and then rain is falling. When Qi in the third phase arrives, heavenly Qi is distributed, damp-Qi descends, earthly Qi ascends, rain falls, sometimes followed by cold Qi, and people are affected by cold Qi. Then, people tend to have heavy body, edema, and chest and abdominal fullness. When Qi in the fourth phase arrives, fierce fire is coming, damp Qi is steaming, earthly Qi is ascending, heavenly Qi is obstructed, cold wind is at dawn and dusk, evaporation and heat are conflicting, smoky air is condensing over grass and trees, and damp transformation is stationary so that white dew is distributed gloomily indicating the coming of autumn. Then people tend to have interstitial fever, sudden bleeding, malaria, heart and abdominal fullness and heat, abdominal distention and even edema. When Qi in the Fifth phase arrives, cooling Qi is in action, cold dew falls, frost descends early, grass and tree leaves turn yellow and fall, and cold Qi is approaching the human body. Wise men prefer to live in airtight houses. People tend to have disease in the skin and interstitial straie. When Qi in the final phase arrives, cold Qi emerges broadly, damp transformation prevails, frost is accumulated, water is frozen, and the sun fails to shine. People affected by cold Qi tend to have rigidity of joints, waist and buttock pain, and cold Qi and damp Qi are intermingling leading to diseases.

The excessive Qi of year phase and seasonal phase should be inhibited and the dominated Qi in generation and transformation be taken to benefit the Qi of year phase without being damaged. The grain of year phase should be ingested to keep the genuine Qi, and the grain of interval phase be ingested to keep the essential Qi. Therefore in the current year phase, the bitter flavor is better ingested to dry and warm it, and even to disperse and discharge it. Without dispersing and discharging, damp Qi will overflow outward to cause muscle ulceration, chapped skin, exudation and bleeding. Yang fire should be supported to protect the body from severe cold. According to the Qi-identification of phases, the increasing or decreasing of the amount can be determined. The one that is the same as the cold should be given heat transformation, and the one the same as damp should be given dry transformation. The difference is given less amount, while in case of more an increased amount is given. Application of cool drug should avoid cool phase, application of warm drug should avoid warm phase, application of heat drug should avoid heat phase; also, dieting and medication share the same principle. If there are extraordinary conditions, the principle should be adjusted. If reversing this principle, it will lead to diseases.

Emperor: Good. What is the Qi-administration in Shaoyin year?

Qibo: Shaoyin-monarch-fire governs the year with the record of 1st and 7th.

In the year with record of the Ninth-1st and Ninth-7th, with the year phase of wood as greater Jue, its features are heaven-governing Qi by Shaoyin-minister-fire, and earth-governing Qi by Yangming-dry-metal. It is the year phase of high wind. The transformations feature agitating whistling and revival, the change features vibrating, pulling, destruction and drawing, and the diseases feature sticking pain and fullness.

Its guest phases in order are greater Jue (the initial phase), lesser Zhi, greater Gong, lesser Shang and greater Yu, while the host phase in order starts at greater Jue and terminates at greater Yu.

In the year with mark of the Fifth-1st and Fifth-7th, with the year phase of fire as greater Zhi, its features are heaven-governing Qi by Taiyin-damp-earth and earth-governing Qi by Yangming-dry-metal. It is the year phase of flaming summer-heat. The transformations feature annoying shining and depressed heat, and the changes feature flaming and boiling, and the diseases feature heat in the upper and bleeding.

Its guest phases in order are greater Zhi, lesser Gong, greater Shang, lesser Yu and greater Jue, while the host phase in order starts at lesser Jue (the initial phase) and terminates at lesser Yu.

In the year with record of the First-1st and First-7th, with the year phase of earth as greater Gong, its features are heaven-governing Qi by Shaoyin-monarch-fire and earth-governing Qi by Yangming-dry-metal. It is the year phase of Yin-rain. The transformations feature soft moistness and frequent rains, the changes feature shocking and heavy rain, and the diseases feature interior fullness and heavy body.

Its guest phases in order are the initial phase greater Gong, lesser Shang, greater Yu, lesser Jue and greater Zhi, while the host phase in order starts at greater Jue (the initial phase) and terminates at greater Yu.

In the year with record of the Seventh-1st (according heaven-identification) and the Seventh-7th (according heaven-identification), with the year phase of metal as greater Shang, its features are heaven-governing Qi by Shaoyin-monarch-fire and earth-governing Qi by Yangming-dry-metal. It is the year phase of cool and vigorous. The transformations feature fog, dew, and bleak air, the changes feature constricting and withering, and the diseases feature cooling in the lower.

Its guest phases in order are the initial phase greater Shang, lesser Yu, greater Jue, lesser Zhi, and greater Gong, while the host phase in order starts at lesser Jue (the initial phase) and terminates at lesser Yu.

In the year with mark of the Third-1st (year-identification) and the Third-7th, with the year phase of water as greater Yu, its features are heaven-governing Qi by Shaoyin-monarch-fire and earth-governing Qi by Yangming-dry-metal. It is the year phase of cold. Their transformations feature condensing and cool, the changes feature ice, snow, frost and hailstone, and the diseases feature cold in the lower.

Its guest phases in order are the initial phase greater Yu, lesser Jue, greater Zhi, lesser Gong and greater Shang, while the host phase in order starts at greater Jue (the initial phase) and terminates at greater Yu.

In the year under heaven-governing Qi of Shaoyang-minister-fire, its Qi transformation arrives earlier than the due time. Earthly Qi is constricting while heavenly Qi is clarified. Cold intermingles with summer-heat, heat is combined with dry, clouds move to the south, damp transformation begins and the seasonal rain falls. Metal and fire coordinate corresponding Fire Star and Metal Star in the upper. The Qi-administration is clarified, the action is urgent, and the color corresponds to red and white. Water and fire as well as cold and heat conflict in the intercrossed Qi which triggers diseases. Heat disease occurs in the upper, cool disease in the lower, and cold and heat invade the body and struggle against each other in the interior. People tend to have cough, panting, bleeding and bloody discharge, nasal obstruction, sneeze, red eyes, canthal sores, severe cold in the stomach, heart pain, lumbago, big belly, dry pharynx and swelling in the upper.

When Qi in the initial phase arrives, earthly Qi recedes, dryness leaves, cold transformation begins, insects are in hibernation, water is frozen, frost descends again, wind is arriving, and Yang Qi is depressed. People tend to live in airtight house and have rigid joints, and waist and buttock pain. Flaming summer-heat is going to rise and internal or external sores can develop. When Qi in the second phase arrives, Yang Qi is distributed, wind is prevailing, spring Qi is normal and all living things are flourishing. Though cold Qi comes sometimes, people generally manage to stay fit. Their diseases are characterized by blurred vision, red eyes, and Qi depression in the upper leading to heat. When Qi in the third phase arrives, the heaven-governing Qi is distributed, big fire Qi prevails, all living things are in exuberance, and cold Qi comes frequently. People tend to suffer from critical Qi, heartache, alternating bouts of chills and fever, cough with panting and red eyes. When Qi in the fourth arrives, moist and hot summer comes with frequent heavy rains and alternating chill and fever. People tend to suffer from chills and fever, dry pharynx, jaundice, allergic rhinitis, nosebleed and phlegm retention. When Qi in the fifth arrives, there is fright of fire falling but the summer comes expectedly. When Yang is transformed, all living things are generated and developed exuberantly. Most people are healthy and patients tend to have warm disease. When Qi in the final phase arrives, dry-Qi is in action, the rest of the fire Qi is obstructed interiorly leading to swelling in the upper, cough and panting, and even bleeding. Cold Qi is often attacking and there is smoky fog and nebulae. Diseases occur in the interstitial skin or in internal hypochondria involving the lower abdomen with interior cold, indicating that earthly Qi is changing.

The excessive Qi of the phase should be inhibited, the dominated Qi be supported, the depressive emergence be broken, and its source of transformation be enriched without being damaged, leading to diseases. The grain with year-Qi is ingested to perfect its genuine Qi, and grain with interval Qi can be ingested to avoid deficient evil. In the current year, the salty flavor is better ingested to soften it for regulating the upper, and even the bitter flavor to disperse it. The sour flavor is better ingested to secure the lower, and the bitter flavor is used to discharge it. According to the identification, an increased or decreased amount can be determined, the one similar to heavenly Qi should be transformed with the cold and clear, and the one similar to earthly Qi should be transformed with the warm and heat. Application of heat drug should avoid heat phase, application of cool drug should avoid cool phase, application of warm drug should avoid warm phase, application of cold drug should avoid cold phase; dieting also is based on the same principle. If there are extraordinary conditions, application should be adjusted accordingly, and reversing this principle will lead to diseases.

Emperor: Good. What is the administration in Jueyin year?
Qibo: It is the year with record of the 6th and 12th.

In the year with record of the Fourth-6th (heaven-identification) and the Fourth-12th (heaven-identification), with the year phase of wood as lesser Jue, its features are heaven-governing Qi by Jueyin-wind-wood and earth-governing Qi by Shaoyang-monarch-fire, with the same clarity and heat as predominating and retaliating Qi to the normal Jue. It is the year phase of wind with clarity and heat.

Its guest phases in order are lesser Jue (the initial phase), greater Zhi, lesser Gong, greater Shang and lesser Yu, while the host phase in order starts at lesser Jue and terminates at lesser Yu.

In the year with record of the Tenth-6th (according year-identification) and the Tenth-12th (according year-identification), with the year phase of fire as lesser Zhi, its features are heaven-governing Qi by Jueyin-wind-wood and earth-governing Qi by

Shaoyang-monarch-fire, with the same cold and rain as predominating and retaliating Qi to the normal Jue. It is the year phase of heat with cold and rain.

Its guest phases in order are the initial phase lesser Zhi, greater Gong, lesser Shang, greater Yu and lesser Jue, while the host phase in order starts at greater Jue (the initial phase) and terminates at greater Yu.

In the year with record of Sixth-6th and the Sixth-12th, with the year phase of fire as lesser Zhi, its features are heaven-governing Qi by Jueyin-wind-wood and earth-governing Qi by Shaoyang-monarch-fire, with the same cold and rain as predominating and retaliating Qi to the normal Jue. It is the year phase of rain with cold rain and clear wind.

Its guest phases in order are the initial phase lesser Gong, greater Shang, lesser Yu, greater Jue, and lesser Zhi, while the host phase in order starts at lesser Jue (the initial phase) and terminates at lesser Yu.

In the year with record of the Second-6th and the Second-12th, with the year phase of metal as lesser Shang, its features are heaven-governing Qi by Jueyin-wind-wood and earth-governing Qi by Shaoyang-monarch-fire, with the same heat and cold as predominating and retaliating Qi to the normal Jue. The year phase is cool with heat and cold.

Its guest phases in order are the initial phase lesser Shang, greater Yu, lesser Jue, greater Zhi, and lesser Gong, while the host phase in order starts at greater Jue (the initial phase) and terminates at greater Yu.

In the year with record of the Eighth-6th and Eighth-12th, with the year phase of metal as lesser Yu, its features are heaven-governing Qi by Jueyin-wind-wood and earth-governing Qi by Shaoyang-monarch-fire, with the same wind and rain as predominating and retaliating Qi. It is the year phase of cold with rain and wind.

Its guest phases in order are the initial phase lesser Yu, greater Jue, lesser Zhi, greater Gong and lesser Shang, while the host phase in order starts at lesser Jue (the initial phase) and terminates at lesser Yu.

In any year with Jueyin-wind-mood to govern heavenly Qi, Qi transformation moves later than the due time, which is the same as the year of normal Jue, and heavenly Qi transformation is the same as the year phase. When heavenly Qi is stirring, earthly Qi is normal, wind arises in the high and in the distant followed by flaming heat from the earth, clouds move to the south, and damp transformation prevails, in which wind and fire coordinate corresponding to Wood Star and Fire Star. The Qi-administration is disturbing, the action is rapid, the grain colors correspond to dark green and red, and the grain obtain the interval Qi to become ripe. The damage includes striated and winged insects. Wind, dry, fire and heat dominate and retaliate alternatively, the hibernating insects come out, and water flows with no freezing. Heat disease develop in the lower and wind disease in the upper. Wind and dry dominate and retaliate mutually, reflecting in the body.

When Qi the initial phase arrives, cold begins to constrict, the killing Qi is just coming, and people tend to have cold in the lower on the right. When Qi in the second phase arrives, cold Qi is lingering, snow is falling and water is frozen, killing cold air arises, frost is seen, the grass tip is withering, and cold rain often falls. When Yang-Qi is transformed back, people tend to have heat in the middle. When Qi in the third phase arrives, heavenly Qi is distributed and wind often arises. People tend to have watering of eyes, tinnitus and vertigo.

When Qi in the fourth phase arrives, moist summer-heat, damp and heat conflict in upper interval on the left and then people tend to have jaundice and edema. When Qi in the fifth phase arrives, dry and damp dominate alternatively, deep Yin is distributed, cold Qi invades the body and wind and rain prevail. When Qi in the final phase arrives, fierce fire governs the action, Yang begins to be transformed greatly, hibernating insects come out, water flows with no freezing, earthly Qi emerges greatly, grass begins to grow, and people feel comfortable and tend to have epidemic warm diseases.

The excessive Qi of the phase should be inhibited and the dominated Qi be supported, and the Qi of year phase be supported without being damaged. In the current year, it is better to use pungent flavor to adapt to heavenly Qi and to use the salty flavor to adapt to earthly Qi, in which fierce fire cannot be violated without reason. Application of warm drug should avoid warm phase, application of heat drug should avoid heat phase, application of cool drug should avoid cool phase, application of cold drug should avoid cold phase; dieting is also based on the same principles. If there are extraordinary conditions, application should be adjusted accordingly, and violating this principle will lead to diseases.

Emperor: Good. Your explanation has made things clear, but how to know whether it corresponds or not?

Qibo: What a good question you have asked! The six phases of Qi rotate with a certain order and terminate at a certain position, so usually in the morning on the first day of the first month of the lunar year. After observation of the position, we can know the condition of the phase. If the excessive phase arrives earlier, the insufficient phase arrives later than the due time, which is the law of nature and the constant of the weather. If the phase is neither excessive nor insufficient, it is called normal year whose Qi arrives in due time.

Emperor: Dominating Qi and anti-dominating Qi always exist. As disastrous climate changes frequently occur, how to forecast them?
Qibo: Abnormal transformation of Qi is disastrous climate change.

Emperor: How are the start and the termination of heaven-governing Qi and earth-governing Qi?
Qibo: How careful your question is! It is related with the law of natural climate. The change of natural climate starts from the upper heaven and terminates at the lower earth. In the first half year, heavenly Qi governs, and in the last half year, earthly Qi governs. When the upper and the lower interact with each other, the final outcome will control the climate in the phase, by which the outline of climate changes in a year is disclosed. Since you've understood the phasing position, you can know the climatic phase, which is called seasonal phase.

Emperor: I'm responsible for this and will carry out these rules, but sometimes they do not accord with rules of climate changes; why is this so?
Qibo: The climatic Qi has the conditions of excess or insufficiency and the transformation has the conditions of luxuriance or declination, which is in accordance with the general seasonal transformation.

Emperor: I'd like to know what the identification between phase and Qi is.

Qibo: Wind-warm accords with climatic transformation in spring. Heat fumigation and dull fire accord with the climatic transformation in summer; the dominating Qi accords with anti-dominating Qi; dryness, lucidity, smoke and dew accord with the climatic transformation in autumn; clouds, rain, gloom and dust accord with the climatic transformation in late summer; and cold, frost, snow and ice accord with the climatic transformation in winter; this is the general transformation of five phases and six phases of Qi between the heavens and the earth, and also the constant of luxuriance and declination.

Emperor: If the transformation of five phases accords with heavenly Qi, it is termed heavenly accordance, and I know it. I'd like to know what the earthly Qi accordance is.
Qibo: There are three conditions of excessive phasing Qi according to heavenly Qi, or of insufficient phasing Qi according to heavenly Qi. There are three conditions of excessive phasing Qi according to earthly Qi, or of insufficient phasing Qi according to earthly Qi. Totally, there are 24 years with corresponding transformations.

Emperor: I'd like to know how to name these conditions?
Qibo: In the year with record of the First-5th and First-11th, its year phase is greater Gong with Taiyin-damp-earth as adding from the lower. In the year with record of Ninth-3rd and Ninth-9th, its year phase is greater Jue with Jueyin-wind-wood as adding from the lower. In the year with record of the Seventh-1st and Seventh-7th, its year phase is greater Shang with Yangming-dry-metal as adding from the lower. There are three such conditions. In the year with record of Tenth-6th and Tenth-12th, its year phase is lesser Zhi with Shaoyang-minister-fire as adding from the lower. In the year with record

of the Eighth-2nd and Eighth-8th, its year phase is lesser Yu with Taiyang-damp-earth as adding from the lower. In the year with record of Ninth-4th and Ninth-10th, its year phase is lesser Zhi as adding from the lower. There are also three such conditions. In the year with record of Fifth-1st and the Fifth-7th, the year phase is greater Zhi with Shaoyin-monarch-fire as falling from the upper. In the year with record of the Fifth-3rd and the Fifth-9th, the year phase is greater Zhi with Shaoyang-minister-fire as falling from the upper. In the year with record of the Third-5th and the Third-11th, its year phase is greater Yu with Taiyang-damp-earth as falling from the upper. There are three such conditions. In the year with record of the Fourth-6th and the Fourth-12th, its year phase is lesser Jue with Jueyin-wind-wood as falling from the upper. In the year with record of the Second-4th and the Second-10th, its year phase is lesser Shang with Yangming-dry-metal as falling from the upper. In the year with record of the Sixth-2nd and Sixth-8th, its year phase is lesser Gong with Taiying-damp-earth as falling from the upper. There are also three such conditions. Except these 24 years, other years have no adding or falling of climatic Qi as adding from the lower or the upper.

Emperor: What does adding mean?
Qibo: Adding the excessive year phase to earthly Qi is termed according heaven-identification, and adding the insufficient year phase to earthly Qi is termed according year-identification.

Emperor: What does falling mean?
Qibo: Either excessive or insufficient Qi of the year phase falling on heavenly Qi is termed heaven-identification. Since the change of Qi transformation in the year phase is either

excessive or insufficient, the state of disease is expressed differently and the prognosis of life or death is earlier or later.

Emperor: You have mentioned that usage of cold drug should avoid cold phase while usage of heat drug should avoid the heat phase, but I haven't understood the reason. I'd like to know what avoiding means.
Qibo: Using heat drug offends no heat of the phase while using cold drug offends no cold of the phase. Complying with it leads to harmony, while reversing it leads to diseases; so, the dominating Qi of the current phase shouldn't be offended but be avoided, which is called the current Qi for six-phase.

Emperor: How to use the warm and cool drugs?
Qibo: When the dominating Qi is in the heat phase, the heat-drug should be used without offence. When the dominating Qi is in the cold phase, the cold-drug should be used without offence. When the dominating Qi is in the cool phase, the cool-drug should be used without offence. When the dominating Qi is in the warm phase, the warm-drug should be used without offence. When the interval Qi is the same as the host Qi, no offence is allowed. And when the internal Qi is different from the host Qi, slight offence is allowed. They are the four contraindications which should be observed.

Emperor: Good! How about the permissible offence?
Qibo: When the guest heavenly Qi offends the host Qi in the current phase, the host Qi can be complied with. When the guest Qi overcomes host Qi, it can be offended aiming at balance without excess, which is evil Qi domination reversely. It's believed that if there is no offence of heavenly Qi, there is no reversal of earthly Qi with proper climate, no help for

dominating guest Qi, and no support for anti-dominating-Qi, which is called the ideal treatment.

Emperor: Good! Are there any constants for five phases in the year with the specific recording mark?
Qibo: Please let me explain the array.

In the year with record of the First-1st and First-7th, in the upper is Shaoyin-monarch-fire to govern the heaven, in the middle is earth year phase as greater Gong and in the lower is Yangming-dry-metal to govern the earth. The order of heat transformation in the upper is the second, the order of rain transformation of the year phase is the fifth, and the order of dry transformation in the lower is the fourth, which is called the days having normal transformation. The disease by the upper cause is better treated with the salty and cold drugs, the disease by the middle phase is better treated with the bitter and warm drugs, and the disease by the lower cause is better treated with the sour and warm drugs, which is called the proper indication of drugs and diet.

In the year with record of the Second-2nd and the Second-8th, in the upper is Taiyin-damp-earth to govern the heaven, in the middle is metal year phase as lesser Shang, and in the lower is Taiyang-cold-water to govern the earth. The heat transformation in domination and cold transformation in anti-domination are the same, which is called the days having evil-Qi transformation with the calamity in the seventh palace (west). The order of damp transformation in the upper is the fifth, the order of clarity transformation of the year phase is the fourth, and the order of cold transformation in the lower is the sixth, which is called the days having normal transformation. The disease by the upper cause is better treated with the bitter and warm drugs, the disease by the middle cause is better treated with the sour drugs for moderation, and the disease by the lower cause is better treated with the sweet and warm drugs, which is called the proper indication of drugs and diet.

In the year with record of the Third-3rd and Third-9th, in the upper is Shaoyang-minister-fire to govern the heaven, in the middle is water year phase as greater Yu, and in the lower is Jueyin-wind-wood to govern the earth. The order of fire transformation in the upper is the second, the order of cold transformation of the year phase is the sixth, and the order of wind transformation in the lower is the third, which is called the days having normal transformation. The disease due to the upper cause is better treated with the salty and cold drugs, the disease by the middle phase is better treated with the salty and warm drugs, and the disease by the lower cause is better treated with the pungent and warm drugs, which is called the proper indication of drugs and diet.

In the year with record of the Fourth-4th and Fourth-10th, in the upper is Yangming-dry-metal to govern the heaven, in the middle is wood year phase as lesser Jue, and in the lower is Shaoyin-monarch-fire to govern the earth. The clarity transformation in domination and heat transformation in anti-domination are the same, which is called the days having evil-Qi transformation with the calamity in the third palace (east). The order of dry transformation in the upper is the ninth, the order of wind transformation of the year phase is the third, and the order of heat transformation in the lower is the seventh, which is called the days having normal transformation. The disease by the upper cause is better treated with the bitter and slightly warm drugs, the disease by the middle cause is better treated with the pungent drugs for moderation, and the disease by the lower cause is better treated with the salty and cold drugs, which is called the proper indication of drugs and diet.

In the year with record of the Fifth-5th and Fifth-11th, in the upper is Taiyang-cold-water to govern the heaven, in the middle is fire year phase as greater Zhi, and in the lower is Taiyin-damp-earth to govern the earth. The order of cold transformation in the upper is the sixth, the order of heat transformation of the year phase is the seventh, and the order of damp transformation in the lower is the fifth, which is called the days having normal transformation. The disease by the upper cause is better treated with the bitter and warm drugs, the disease by the middle cause is better treated with the sweet drugs for moderation, and the disease by the lower cause is better treated with the sweet and warm drugs, which is called the proper indication of drugs and diet.

In the year with mark of the Sixth-6th and Sixth-12th, in the upper is Jueyin-wind-wood to govern the heaven, in the middle is earth year phase as lesser Gong, and in the lower is Shaoyang-minister-fire to govern the earth. The wind transformation in domination and clarity transformation in anti-domination are the same, which is called the days having evil-Qi transformation with the calamity in the fifth palace (center). The order of wind transformation in the upper is the third, the order of damp transformation of the year phase is the fifth, and the order of fire transformation in the lower is the seventh, which is called the days having normal transformation. The disease by the upper cause is better treated with the pungent and cool drugs, the disease by the middle cause is better treated with the sweet drugs for moderation, and the disease by the lower cause is better treated with the salty and cold drugs, which is called the proper indication of drugs and diet.

In the year with record of the Seventh-7th and Seventh-1st, in the upper is Shaoyin-monarch-fire to govern the heaven, in the middle is metal year phase as greater Shang and in the lower is Yangming-dry-metal to govern the earth. The order of heat transformation in the upper is the seventh, the order of clarity transformation of the year phase is the ninth, and the order of dry transformation in the lower is the ninth, which is called the days having normal transformation. The disease by the upper cause is better treated with the salty and cold drugs, the disease by the middle cause is better treated with the pungent and warm drugs, and the disease by the lower cause is better treated with the sour and warm drugs, which is called the proper indication of drugs and diet.

In the year with record of the Eighth-8th and the Eighth-2nd (according year identification), in the upper is Taiyin-damp-earth to govern the heaven, in the middle is water year phase as lesser Yu, and in the lower is Taiyang-cold-water to govern the earth. The rain transformation in domination and wind transformation in anti-domination are the same, which is called the days having evil-Qi transformation with the calamity in the first palace (north). The order of rain transformation in the upper is the fifth, the order of cold transformation of the year phase is the first, and the order of cold transformation in the lower is the first, which is called the days having normal transformation. The disease by the upper cause is better treated with the bitter and warm drugs, the disease by the middle cause is better treated with the bitter drugs for moderation, and the disease by the lower cause is better treated with the bitter and warm drugs, which is called the proper indication of drugs and diet.

In the year with record of the Ninth-9th and the Ninth-3rd (according heaven identification), in the upper is Shaoyang-minister-fire to govern the heaven, in the middle is wood year phase as greater Jue, and in the lower is Jueyin-wind-wood to govern the earth. The order of fire transformation in the upper is the second, the order of wind transformation of the year phase is the eighth, and the order of dry transformation in the lower is the eighth, which is called the days having normal transformation. The disease by the upper cause is better treated with the salty and cold drugs, the disease by the middle cause is better treated with the sour drugs for moderation, and the disease by the lower cause is better treated with the pungent and cool drugs, which is called the proper indication of drugs and diet.

In the year with record of the Tenth-10th and the Tenth-4th (according year identification), in the upper is Yangming-dry-metal to govern the heaven, in the middle is fire year phase as lesser Zhi, and in the lower is Shaoyin-monarch-fire to govern the earth. The cold transformation in domination and rain transformation in anti-domination are the same, which is called the days having evil-Qi transformation with the calamity in the ninth palace (south). The order of dry transformation in the upper is the fifth, the order of heat transformation of the year phase is the second, and the order of heat transformation in the lower is the second, which is called the days having normal transformation. The disease by the upper cause is better treated with the bitter and slightly warm drugs, the disease by the middle cause is better treated with the salty and cold drugs, and the disease by the lower cause is better treated with the salty and cold drugs, which is called the proper indication of drugs and diet.

In the year with record of the First-11th and the First-5th (year identification & according heaven identification), in the upper is Taiyang-cold-water to govern the heaven, in the middle is earth year phase as greater Gong, and in the lower is Taiyin-damp-earth to govern the earth. The order of cold transformation in the upper is the sixth, the order of damp transformation of the year phase is the fifth, and the order of damp transformation in the lower is the fifth, which is called the days having normal transformation. The disease by the upper cause is better treated with the bitter and heat drugs, the disease by the middle cause is better treated with the bitter and warm drugs, and the disease by the lower cause is better treated with the bitter and warm drugs, which is called the proper indication of drugs and diet.

In the year with record of the Second-12th and the Second-6th, in the upper is Jueyin-wind-wood to govern the heaven, in the middle is metal year phase as lesser Shang, and in the lower is Shaoyin-minister-fire to govern the earth. The heat transformation in domination and cold transformation in anti-domination are the same, which is called the days having evil-Qi transformation with the calamity in the seventh palace (west). The order of wind transformation in the upper is the eighth, the order of clarity transformation of the year phase is the fourth, and the order of fire transformation in the lower is the second, which is called the days having normal transformation. The disease by the upper cause is better treated with the pungent and cool drugs, the disease by the middle cause is better treated with the sour drugs for moderation, and the disease by the lower cause is better treated with the salty and cold drugs, which is called the proper indication of drugs and diet.

In the year with record of Third-1st and Third-7th, in the upper is Shaoyin-monarch-fire to govern the heaven, in the middle is water year phase as greater Yu, and in the lower is Yangming-dry-metal to govern the earth. The order of heat transformation in the upper is the second, the order of cold transformation of the year phase is the sixth, and the order of clarity transformation in the lower is the fourth, which is called the days having normal transformation. The disease by the upper cause is better treated with the salty and cold drugs, the disease by the middle cause is better treated with the salty and warm drugs, and the disease by the lower cause is better treated with the sour and warm drugs, which is called the proper indication of drugs and diet.

In the year with record of the Fourth-2nd and the Fourth-8th, in the upper is Taiyin-damp-earth to govern the heaven, in the middle is wood year phase as lesser Jue, and in the lower is Taiyang-cold-water to govern the earth. The clarity transformation in domination and heat transformation in anti-domination are the same, which is called the days having evil-Qi transformation with the calamity in the third palace (east). The order of rain transformation in the upper is the fifth, the order of wind transformation of the year phase is the third, and the order of cold transformation in the lower is the first, which is called the days having normal transformation. The disease by the upper cause is better treated with the bitter and warm, the disease by the middle cause is better treated with the pungent and warm drugs, and the disease by the lower cause is better treated with sweet and warm drugs, which is called the proper indication of drugs and diet.

In the year with record of the Fifth-3rd and the Fifth-9th, in the upper is Shaoyang-minister-fire to govern the heaven, in the middle is fire year phase as greater Zhi, and in the lower is Jueyin-wind-wood to govern the earth. The order of fire transformation in the upper is the seventh, the order of fire transformation of the year phase is the seventh, and the order of wind transformation in the lower is the third, which is called the days having normal transformation. The disease by the upper cause is better treated with the salty and cold drugs, the disease by the middle cause is better treated with the sweet drugs for moderation, and the disease by the lower cause is better treated with the pungent and cool drugs, which is called the proper indication of drugs and diet.

In the year with record of the Sixth-4th and the Sixth-10th, in the upper is Yangming-dry-metal to govern the heaven, in the middle is earth year phase as lesser Gong, and in the lower is Shaoyin-monarch-fire to govern the earth. The wind transformation in domination and clarity transformation in anti-domination are the same, which is called the days having evil-Qi transformation with the calamity in the fifth palace (center). The order of clarity transformation in the upper is the ninth, the order of rain transformation of the year phase is the fifth, and the order of heat transformation in the lower is the seventh, which is called the days having normal transformation. The disease by the upper cause is better treated with the bitter and slightly warm drugs, the disease by the middle cause is better treated with the sweet drugs for moderation, and the disease by the lower cause is better treated with the salty and cold drugs, which is called the proper indication of drugs and diet.

In the year with record of the Seventh-5th and the Seventh-11th, in the upper is Taiyang-cold-water to govern the heaven, in the middle is metal year phase as greater Shang, and in the lower is Taiyin-damp-earth to govern the earth. The order of cold transformation in the upper is the first, the order of clarity transformation of the year phase is the ninth, and the order of rain transformation in the lower is the fifth, which is called the days having normal transformation. The disease by the upper cause is better treated with the bitter and warm drugs, the disease by the middle cause is better treated with the pungent and warm drugs, and the disease by the lower cause is better treated with the sweet and warm drugs, which is called the proper indication of drugs and diet.

In the year with record of the Eighth-6th and the Eighth-12th, in the upper is Jueyin-wind-wood to govern the heaven, in the middle is water year phase as lesser Yu, and in the lower is Shaoyang-minister-fire to govern the earth. The rain transformation in domination and wind transformation in anti-domination are the same, which is called the days having evil-Qi transformation with the calamity in the first palace (north). The order of wind transformation in the upper is the third, the order of cold transformation of the year phase is the first, and the order of fire transformation in the lower is the seventh, which is called the days having normal transformation. The disease by the upper cause is better treated with the pungent and cool drugs, the disease by the middle cause is better treated with the bitter drugs for moderation, and the disease by the lower cause is better treated with the salty and cold drugs, which is called the proper indication of drugs and diet.

In the year with record of the Ninth-7th and the Ninth-1st, in the upper is Shaoyin-monarch-fire to govern the heaven, in the middle is wood year phase as greater Jue, and in the lower is Yangming-dry-metal to govern the earth. The order of heat transformation in the upper is the second, the order of wind transformation of the year phase is the eighth, and the order of clarity transformation in the lower is the fourth, which is called the days having normal transformation. The disease by the upper cause is better treated with the salty and cold drugs, the disease by the middle cause is better treated with the sour and cool drugs, and the disease by the lower cause is better treated with the sour and warm drugs, which is called the proper indication of drugs and diet.

In the year with record of the Tenth-8th and the Tenth-2nd, in the upper is Taiyin-damp-earth to govern the heaven, in the middle is fire year phase as lesser Zhi, and in the lower is Taiyang-cold-water to govern the earth. The cold transformation in domination and rain transformation in anti-domination are the same, which is called the days having evil-Qi transformation with the calamity in the ninth palace (north). The order of rain transformation in the upper is the fifth, the order of fire transformation of the year phase is the second, and the order of cold transformation in the lower is the first, which is called the days having normal transformation. The disease by the upper cause is better treated with the bitter and warm drugs, the disease by the middle cause is better treated with the salty and warm drugs, and the disease by the lower cause is better treated with the sweet and warm drugs, which is called the proper indication of drugs and diet.

In the year with record of the First-9th and the First-3rd, in the upper is Shaoyang-minister-fire to govern the heaven, in the middle is earth year phase as greater Gong, and in the lower is Jueyin-wind-wood to govern the earth. The order of fire transformation in the upper is the second, the order of rain transformation of the year phase is the fifth, and the order of wind transformation in the lower is the eighth, which is called the days having normal transformation. The disease by the upper cause is better treated with the salty and cold drugs, the disease by the middle cause is better treated with the salty drugs for moderation, and the disease by the lower cause is better treated with the pungent and cool drugs, which is called the proper indication of drugs and diet.

In the year with record of the Second-10th and the Second-4th, in the upper is Yangming-dry-metal to govern the heaven, in the middle is metal year phase as lesser Shang, and in the lower is Shaoyin-monarch-fire to govern the earth. The heat transformation in domination and cold transformation in anti-domination are the same, which is called the days having evil-Qi transformation with the calamity in the seventh palace (west). The order of dry transformation in the upper is the fourth, the order of clarity transformation of the year phase is the fourth, and the order of heat transformation in the lower is the second, which is called the days having normal transformation. The disease by the upper cause is better treated with the bitter and slightly warm drugs, the disease by the middle cause is better treated with the bitter and cold drugs, and the disease by the lower cause is better treated with the salty and cold drugs, which is called the proper indication of drugs and diet.

In the year with record of the Third-11th and the Third-5th, in the upper is Taiyang-cold-water to govern the heaven, in the middle is water year phase as greater Yu, and in the lower is Taiyin-damp-earth to govern the earth. The order of cold transformation in the upper is the sixth, the order of cold transformation of the year phase is the sixth, and the order of rain transformation in the lower is the fifth, which is called the days having normal transformation. The disease by the upper cause is better treated with the bitter and warm drugs, the disease by the middle cause is better treated with the salty and warm drugs, and the disease by the lower cause is better treated with the sweet and warm drugs, which is called the proper indication of drugs and diet.

In the year with record of the Fourth-12th and the Fourth-6th, in the upper is Jueyin-wind-wood to govern the heaven, in the middle is wood year phase as lesser Jue, and in the lower is Shaoyang-minister-fire to govern the earth. The clarity transformation in domination and heat transformation in anti-domination are the same, which is called the days having evil-Qi transformation with the calamity in the third palace (east). The order of wind transformation in the upper is the third, the order of wind transformation of the year phase is the third, and the order of fire transformation in the lower is the seventh, which is called the days having normal transformation. The disease by the upper cause is better treated with the pungent and cool drugs, the disease by the middle cause is better treated with the pungent drugs for moderation, and the disease by the lower cause is better treated with the salty and cold drugs, which is called the proper indication of drugs and diet.

In the year with record of the Fifth-1st and the Fifth-7th, in the upper is Shaoyin-monarch-fire to govern the heaven, in the middle is fire year phase as greater Zhi, and in the lower is Yangming-dry-metal to govern the earth. The order of heat transformation in the upper is the seventh, the order of heat transformation of the year phase is the seventh, and the order of clarity transformation in the lower is the ninth, which is called the days having normal transformation. The disease by the upper cause is better treated with the salty and cold drugs, the disease by the middle cause is better treated with the sweet and cold drugs, and the disease by the lower cause is better treated with the sour and warm drugs, which is called the proper indication of drugs and diet.

In the year with record of the Sixth-2nd and the Sixth-8th, in the upper is Taiyin-damp-earth to govern the heaven, in the middle is earth year phase as lesser Gong, and in the lower is Taiyang-cold-water to govern the earth. The wind transformation in domination and clarity transformation in anti-domination are the same, which is called the days having evil Qi transformation with the calamity in the fifth palace (center). The order of rain transformation in the upper is the fifth, the order of rain transformation of the year phase is the fifth, and the order of cold transformation in the lower is the first, which is called the days having normal transformation. The disease by the upper cause is better treated with the bitter and warm drugs, the disease by the middle cause is better treated with the sweet drugs for moderation, and the disease by the lower cause is better treated with the sweet and warm drugs, which is called the proper indication of drugs and diet.

In the year with record of the Seventh-3rd and the Seventh-9th, in the upper is Shaoyang-minister-fire to govern the heaven, in the middle is metal year phase as greater Shang and in the lower is Jueyin-wind-wood to govern the earth. The order of fire transformation in the upper is the seventh, the order of clarity transformation of the year phase is the ninth, and the order of wind transformation in the lower is the third, which is called the days having normal transformation. The disease by the upper cause is better treated with the salty and cold drugs, the disease by the middle cause is better treated with the pungent and warm drugs, and the disease by the lower cause is better treated with the pungent and cool drugs, which is called the proper indication of drugs and diet.

In the year with record of the Eighth-4th and the Eighth-10th, in the upper is Yangming-dry-metal to govern the heaven, in the middle is water year phase as lesser Gong, and in the lower is Shaoyin-monarch-fire to govern the earth. The rain transformation in domination and wind transformation in anti-domination are the same, which is called the days having evil-Qi transformation with the calamity in the first palace (north). The order of clarity transformation in the upper is the ninth, the order of cold transformation of the year phase is the first, and the order of heat transformation in the lower is the seventh, which is called the days having normal transformation. The disease by the upper cause is better treated with the bitter and slightly warm drugs, the disease by the middle cause is better treated with the bitter drugs for moderation, and the disease by the lower cause is better treated with the salty and cold drugs, which is called the proper indication of drugs and diet.

In the year with record of the Ninth-5th and the Ninth-11th, in the upper is Taiyang-cold-water to govern the heaven, in the middle is wood year phase as greater Jue and in the lower is Taiyin-damp-earth to govern the earth. The order of cold transformation in the upper is the sixth, the order of wind transformation of the year phase is the eighth, and the order of rain transformation in the lower is the fifth, which is called the days having normal transformation. The disease by the upper cause is better treated with the bitter and warm drugs, the disease by the middle cause is better treated with the sour drugs for moderation, and the disease by the lower cause is better treated with the sweet and warm drugs, which is called the proper indication of drugs and diet.

In the year with record of the Tenth-6th and the Tenth-12th, in the upper is Jueyin-wind-wood to govern the heaven, in the middle is fire year phase as lesser Zhi, and in the lower is Shaoyang-cold-water to govern the earth. The cold transformation in domination and rain transformation in anti-domination are the same, which is called the days having evil Qi transformation with the calamity in the ninth palace (south). The order of wind transformation in the upper is the eighth, the order of fire transformation of the year phase is the second, and the order of fire transformation in the lower is the second, which is called the days having normal transformation. The disease by the upper cause is better treated with the pungent and cool drugs, the disease by the middle cause is better treated with the salty drugs for moderation, and the disease by the lower cause is better treated with the salty and cold drugs, which is called the proper indication of drugs and diet.

In the years with definite record of five-phase and seasonal six-Qi, both the normal or abnormal and dominating or anti-dominating transformations have their own constant which must be observed. Therefore, in order to know the key of climate changes, the year record should be mastered, which can help settle the answer to the question, as otherwise it will be far off the mark; this is the information concerned.

Emperor: Good! Does the Qi of five phases also have the year with the anti-dominating-Qi?
Qibo: When the Qi of five phases stagnates extremely, it will take a certain amount of time to emerge.

Emperor: How can it emerge?
Qibo: Five phases have their excessive Qi and insufficient Qi, and the emergence of anti-dominating Qi is different.

Emperor: I'd like to know the details.
Qibo: Excess of anti-dominating Qi leads to sharp emergence, while insufficiency of anti-dominating Qi leads to slow emergence. The sharp emergence causes severe diseases, while slow emergence causes moderate diseases.

Emperor: What are the numbers denoting excess and insufficiency?
Qibo: The excessive Qi has the number denoting development, while the insufficient Qi has the number denoting generation. However, the number of earth phase always has the sole number denoting generating.

Emperor: What about the emergence?
Qibo: When the Qi of earth depression emerges out, the rocky mountains are shaken, thunder is crashing in the air intermingling, yellow and black dust is whirling and turning into white gas, the sharp rain is falling down onto the valleys, beating on the rocks and splashing back into the sky, the flood is inundating the field, the rivers are overflowing wildly, and scatty rocks are lying like animals. After the emergence of anti-domination Qi, the Qi of damp-earth is spreading and turning into timely rain. All the living things begin to germinate, grow, transform and ripen. Then people tend to suffer from heart fullness, abdominal distension, intestinal rumbling with frequent defecation, even heartache, hypochondria distension, vomiting, cholera, retention of fluid, watery diarrhea, general edema and

heavy body. When the clouds are moving to the rain source, rosy clouds surround the rising sun at dawn, and dust fog is floating among the mountains. The emerging out of earthly Qi is in the fourth seasonal Qi. The clouds are flying throughout the mountains, on and off, or in and out. It is the omen of earth depression emergence.

When the Qi of metal depression emerges out, the sky is clear, the earth is bright, the wind is cool, the airstream is swift and the cool Qi is rising. Then the smoky clouds are floating over the trees and grass, the dry-Qi is prevailing, and the gloomy fog is coming up over and over again. When the breaking Qi in autumn is approaching, the trees and grass are withering and there is a metal whistling sound in the air. Then people tend to suffer from cough and Qi reversal, heart fullness and hypochondria distention referred to the lower abdomen, frequent acute pain, failure to turn the body, dry pharynx, dusty face and bad complexion. In nature, the earth is covered with hoarfrost, and the emergence of metal stagnation is in the fifth seasonal Qi. In the evening, white dew falls and there is a sad whistling sound in the woods, which is the omen of metal depression emergence.

When the Qi of water depression emerges, Yang Qi recedes while Yin Qi suddenly emerges, and the great cold arrives, in which rivers and lakes are frozen, cold air turns into frost and snow, even into yellow gloomy nebulae spanning among intermingling air, which becomes frost and the indication of depression can be seen with the water. Then people tend to catch cold invasion and suffer from heartache, waist and buttock pain, rigid large joints with difficulty in extending and flexing, frequent feeling of extreme cold, hard lumps and full abdomen. In nature, the sun fails to shine, a deep haze covers the sky and white dust is whirling everywhere. The emergence of water depression is between the phases of monarch-fire and minister-fire. The sky is deep and dark and Qi is like scattered hemp, fades in and then fades out with black and yellowish color, which is the omen of emergence of water depression.

When the Qi of wood depression emerges, the gloomy sky is full of dust, clouds with other things are moving frantically and s great gale is blowing, which rips roofs, breaks trees and destroys all the plants. Then people tend to suffer from the pain of the stomach and heart area sticking the hypochondria, obstruction of the throat, difficulties in swallowing and drinking, even tinnitus with vertigo, blurred vision with difficulty in recognition, and regular sudden syncope. There is dark dust whirling in the sky, with a monotonous color over the sky and mountains, the turbid air turning yellow and black with stagnation, and the horizontal clouds giving no bursts of rain. The emergence of wood depression is irregular. In the plain, grass is drooping, soft leaves turn over, whistling sounds are heard in the pines, and tigers are growling in mountain caves, which is the omen of emergence of wood depression.

When Qi of fire depression emerges out, there are expansive nebulae over the sky screening the sunshine, and flaming fire is prevailing and great summer-heat arrives. Then mountains and lakes are scorched, trees are oozing sap, smoke is curling up from the houses, earth exposes the hoarfrost, the static water is being dried up, the wild grass is withering with yellow color, hot wind blowing results in the ambiguous speech, and damp-transformation is delayed. Then people tend to suffer from breathlessness, sores and swelling, the distension and discomfort of hypochondria, abdomen, chest, back, the face, head and four limbs, ulcers and prickly heat, spasm of sinews and bone pain, joint pain and jerking, watery diarrhea and warm malaria, acute abdominal pain, continuous bleeding, red eyes and hot heart, vexation and dysphoria, and sudden death in those at high risk. At the end of time measurement in a day, great heat is covering and the sweat is leaking out of the pores in the body. The emergence of fire depression is fourth. Stirring is followed by calmness, extreme Yang is converted into Yin, and damp-transformation is distributed and implemented. Then flowers are blossoming when water is frozen, the mountains are covered with snow and ice, and flaming Yang is seen rising from lakes in the south, which is the omen of emergence of fire depression.

The reaction of depression in five phases is bound to show indications followed by emergence that all is depressed in the extreme till bursting out. The emergence of wood depression has no regular time, the one of water depression emerges around the periods of monarch fire and minister fire. After careful observation of climatic Qi changes in the current phase, the diseases can be predicted. If the rules of seasonal phases are lost or year phase is reversed, the five-phase of seasonal Qi cannot rotate normally, and the administration of growth, transformation, harvesting and storage in the nature has no constant.

Emperor: The emergence of water depression leads to hailstone and snow, the emergence of earth depression leads to heavy rain, the emergence of wood depression leads to destruction and breakage, the emergence of metal depression leads to clarity, and the emergence of fire depression leads to hot air and gloom. What is the cause behind the climatic changes?

Qibo: Qi of five phases is either excessive or insufficient, and the emergence is either moderate or drastic. The moderate emergence influences the Qi of the current phase while the drastic one affects its successive Qi, by which the climatic changes can be predicted.

Emperor: Good! Why will the emergence of five phases of Qi not occur in the proper phase?
Qibo: This is due to the difference of timing.

Emperor: Are there any days when this difference occurs?
Qibo: The difference appears about 30 days before and after the time of burst.

Emperor: Why will Qi of the current seasonal phase arrive earlier or later?
Qibo: If the Qi in the phase is excessive, it will arrive earlier; if insufficient, it will arrive later; both of these are normal.

Emperor: What is the condition of the arrival of the Qi in due time?
Qibo: There is no excess or insufficiency, indicating the Qi arriving in due time; otherwise it will lead to calamity.

Emperor: Good! Why does Qi have its transformation not in the due time?
Qibo: The excessive Qi will dominate in its own phase while the insufficient Qi will abdicate its domination to the Qi that restrains itself.

Emperor: The Qi in four seasons will arrive earlier or later, higher or lower, and left or right, and how to predict it?

Qibo: The Qi of the phases rotates reversely or smoothly and arrives slowly or quickly, so that excessive Qi will transform earlier and insufficient Qi will transform later.

Emperor: I'd like to know how Qi rotates.
Qibo: Spring Qi moves towards the west, summer Qi towards the north, autumn Qi towards the east, and winter Qi towards the south. So, spring Qi starts from the lower, autumn Qi from the upper, summer Qi from the center, and winter Qi from the exterior. Also, spring Qi starts from the left, autumn Qi from the right, summer Qi from the back and winter Qi from the front. These are the normal movements of Qi in four seasons. Thus, high in the space is often winter Qi and down in the land is often spring Qi, and these variations in movement must be carefully observed.

Emperor: Good.

Yellow Emperor: Five-phase and six-Qi are reflected in the climatic phenomena; how are the six normal and abnormal changes of six seasons?
Qibo: The normal seasonal six-Qi involves the transformation and change, domination and retaliation, or benefits and harms; which one do you want to know?

Emperor: I would like to know all of them.
Qibo: Please allow me to explain it. It is all concerned with the emergence of Qi. The arrival of Jueyin carries peace, Shaoyin carries warmth, Taiyin carries dust and moisture, Shaoyang carries flaming summer-heat, Yangming carries cool and vigor, and Taiyang carries cold air, which is the essential of Qi transformation in four seasons.

The arrival of Jueyin turns into the source of wind to act as germination and growth, Shaoyin into the fire source to act as comfort and prosperity, Taiyin into rain source to act as development and growing-up, Shaoyang into heat source to act as external movement, Yangming into decline source to act as maturation, and Taiyang into cold source to act as reaping and storage, which is the constant of executive transformation.

When Jueyin arrives, it turns into growth and wind floating. When Shaoyin arrives, it turns into exuberance and formation. When Taiyin arrives, it turns into transformation, cloud and rain. When Shaoyang arrives, it triggers growth and prosperity. When Yangming arrives, it triggers storage and sealment, which is the constant of Qi transformation.

When Jueyin arrives, it produces wind and finally turns into declination. When Shaoyin arrives, it produces heat and finally turns into cold. When Taiyin arrives, it produces damp and finally turns into heavy rain. When Shaoyang arrives, it produces fire and finally turns into vapor and damp. When Yangming arrives, it produces dryness and finally turns into cool. When Jueyin arrives, it produces cold and finally turns into warmth. It is the constant of normal transformation.

The arrival of Jueyin indicates transformation of hairy worms, the arrival of Shaoyin indicates transformation of winged worms (birds), the arrival of Taiyin indicates transformation of naked worms, the arrival of Shaoyang indicates transformation of winged worms, the arrival Yangming indicates transformation of shell worms (beetles), and the arrival of Taiyang indicates transformation of scaled worms (snakes), which is the constant of worm transformation.

The arrival of Jueyin means generation, the arrival of Shaoyin means exuberance, the arrival of Taiyin means moisturization, the arrival of Shaoyang means prosperity, the arrival of Yangming means hardening, and the arrival of Taiyang means storage, which is the constant of administrative transformation.

When Jueyin arrives, there is gale and very cool air. When Shaoyin arrives, there is stirring heat and cold Qi. When Taiyin arrives, there is thunder and stormy rain. When Shaoyang arrives, there is whirling wind, flaming fire and hoarfrost. When Yangming arrives, there is reduction of temperature and cooling. And when Taiyang arrives, there is cold snow and white dust. These are the constants of climatic changes.

The arrival of Jueyin has the features of stirring, agitating, swaying and shaking. The arrival of Shaoyin features in high bright flame and brownish atmosphere. The arrival of Taiyin features in haze and white dust. The arrival of Shaoyang features in glowing light and red clouds with brownish atmosphere. The arrival of Yangming features in smoky dust, frost, vigor and plaintive sound. And the arrival of Taiyang features in hardness, sharpness and erectness. These are the constants of administrative transformation.

In the period of Jueyin, people tend to have abdominal spasm. In Shaoyin, people tend to have sores, rash and fever. In Taiyin, people tend to have fluid retention and Qi obstruction. In Shaoyang, people tend to suffer from sneeze, vomiting as well as sore. In Yangming, people tend to have edema and deficiency. And in Taiyang, people tend to have inflexibility of joints. They are the common diseases in these periods.

In the period of Jueyin, people tend to have sticking pain in hypochondria. In Shaoyin, people tend to have fright, confusion, fearing cold, chills and delirium. In Taiyin, people tend to have accumulative fullness. In Shaoyang, people tend to have fright, dryness, blurred vision and drastic diseases. In Yangming, people tend to have rhinitis and the diseases of the buttocks, groin, knees, thigh, fibula, leg and feet. In Taiyang, people tend to have lumbago. They are the common diseases in these periods.

In the period of Jueyin, people tend to have muscular spasm contraction. In Shaoyin, people tend to have depression, delirium and nosebleed. In Taiyin, people tend to have milled fullness, cholera, vomiting and diarrhea. In Shaoyang, people tend to have throat obstruction, tinnitus and severe vomiting. In Yangming, people tend to have chapped skin. In Taiyang, people tend to have night sweating and convulsion. They are the common diseases in these periods.

In the period of Jueyin, people tend to have hypochondriac pain, vomiting and diarrhea. In Shaoyin, people tend to have excessive words and laughing. In Taiyin, people tend to have heavy body and edema. In Shaoyang, people tend to have fulminating diarrhea, cramp, convulsion and sudden death. In Yangming, people tend to have rhinitis and sneeze. And in Taiyang, people tend to have diarrhea, constipation and dysuria. They are the common diseases in these periods.

In all these twelve changes, the relationship between nature and the six phases of Qi is expressed as the essential reaction to essential influence, as transformative reaction to transformative influence, as dominative reaction to dominative influence, and as efficient reaction to efficient influence. The relationship between the six phases of Qi and the diseases is expressed as the higher position to disease in the higher, as the lower to the lower, the back to the back, the front to the front, the center to the center, and the external to the external, which are all the constants. So, the wind predomination leads to stirring, heat predomination to puffiness, dry predomination to dryness, cold predomination to edema, and damp predomination to watery diarrhea and even dysuria and edema. The focus varies with the positions of six phases of Qi. And the changes can be predicted.

Emperor: I'd like to know the action of six phases of Qi.
Qibo: Six phases of Qi act on the dominated Qi for different transformation. Then rain transformation of Taiyin acts on Taiyang, cold transformation of Taiyang on Shaoyin, heat transformation of Shaoyin on Yangming, dry transformation on Jueyin, and wind transformation on Taiyin, which varies with its own phase to play its role.

Emperor: How do six phases of Qi get their phase respectively?
Qibo: When they get their phases respectively, there appears normal transformation.

Emperor: I'd like to listen to their positions.
Qibo: When the positions of six phases of Qi are recognized, the direction and the Qi of dominating month can be known.

Emperor: What is the excess or insufficiency of the six phases of Qi?
Qibo: Excess and insufficiency of Qi are different in that the excessive arrives slowly and stays for a long time while the insufficient arrives suddenly and recedes quickly.

Emperor: What is the excess or deficiency of heaven-governing Qi and earth-governing Qi?
Qibo: When heavenly Qi is insufficient, earthly Qi ascends accordingly. When earthly Qi is insufficient, heavenly Qi

descends accordingly while Qi of year phase moves between two Qi, often preceding it. There is contradiction if the Qi of year phase doesn't dominate the seasonal Qi, and there is harmony if the Qi of year phase is the same as the seasonal Qi. If there is variation with the outcome of intermingling of Qi, various diseases will develop. Therefore if the upper dominates, heavenly Qi descends while if the lower dominates, earthly Qi ascends, the extent of which varies with the difference between the two. The smaller the milder, the larger the more severe, even leading to transposition. If the transposition is obvious, paroxysm of diseases will develop. It's said in the book *The Chief Essentials* that 'The more severe has five portions in its own while the mild has seven portions in its own'.

Emperor: Good! You mentioned that usage of heat drugs should avoid the heat and use of cold drugs should avoid the cold. How can I not avoid the heat or cold when using drugs?
Qibo: How carefully you ask the question! Relieving the evil from the exterior needn't avoid the heat while attacking the interior needn't avoid the cold.

Emperor: If I don't adopt relieving or attacking therapy and still use the heat or the cold correspondingly, what will happen?
Qibo: The cold or heat will emerge as internal evil, and the illness will become more severe.

Emperor: I want to know what the outcome is when healthy people were treated in this way.
Qibo: The person with no illness will get disease while the one with illness will suffer from a more severe disease.

Emperor: How does the person with no illness get the disease?
Qibo: Not avoiding the heat phase will lead to the arrival of heat, while not avoiding the cold will lead to the arrival of cold. When cold is arriving, hard lump, full abdomen, acute pain, and diarrhea develop. When heat is arriving, body fever, vomiting, cholera, carbuncle and sores, dizziness, depression, diarrhea, convulsion, swelling, distension, vomiting, stuffy nose, nosebleed, headache, joint deformity, muscular pain, bleeding, bloody stool, dripping urination and urinary retention can be seen as manifestations.

Emperor: How to treat these diseases?
Qibo: The dominating Qi in the current phase should be complied with while the violating Qi to the current phase should be dominated.

Yellow Emperor: Can the drastic drugs be used to treat pregnant women?
Qibo: If there is disease, it causes no harm to pregnant woman, and also no harm to the fetus.

Emperor: What is the reason for this condition?
Qibo: The severe accumulation or large lumps can be attacked by drastic drugs, which should be stopped when the condition is relieved partly, otherwise it will result in death.

Emperor: Good! How to treat the severe disease due to Qi depression?
Qibo: The disease with wood depression should be smoothed, the disease with fire depression should be dispersed, the disease with earth depression should be discharged, the disease with metal depression should be subdued, and the disease with

water depression should be regulated, and then the Qi should be adjusted with inhibitive drugs, which pertains to the dispersing therapy.

Emperor: How about the diseases with complicated Qi?
Qibo: If there is complicated Qi, there is no contraindication. That is to say, when the host Qi is insufficient, the guest Qi can dominate.

Emperor: What a brilliant theory of the sage! About the broad transformation between the heavens and the earth, the pace of the rotation, principles of Qi intermingling, the rule of Yin and Yang administration, the action of cold and summer-heat, nobody but you can master it! Please allow me to store it in the Numinous Orchid Room with title *Official Record of Six Phases of Qi*. I dare not to record it without bathing and fasting first, and then I will write it down carefully as it has to be inherited carefully and passed down generations.

Chapter 72

Acupuncture Therapy for Abnormal Qi-Phase

The original text has been lost.*

---

*The original text has been lost since the Tang Dynasty version edited and annotated by Wang Bing. An article said to be Chapter 72 is provided in Appendix A of this book.

Chapter 73

Root of Diseases

The original text has been lost.*

*The original text has been lost since the Tang Dynasty version edited and annotated by Wang Bing. An article said to be Chapter 73 is provided in Appendix B of this book.

Chapter 74

Great Theory on Crucial Principles

Yellow Emperor asked: There is shifting and integration of five-Qi with alternative excess and deficiency, and I know this. There is respective administration of six-Qi to govern the heavens and the earth; how is the situation when the Qi arrives?
Qibo kowtowed again and answered: What a clear question you've asked! This is the general law of the heavens and the earth and correspondence between humans and nature.

Emperor: I'd like to know how bright integration with the upper Qi and profound integration with the lower Qi are.
Qibo: It is administered by the law of nature which also puzzles doctors.

Emperor: I'd like to know its details.
Qibo: When Jueyin governs the heavens, Qi is transformed into wind; when Shaoyin governs the heavens, Qi is transformed into heat; when Taiyin governs the heavens, Qi is transformed into damp; when Shaoyang governs the heavens, Qi is transformed into fire; when Yangming governs the heavens, Qi is transformed into the dry; and when Taiyang governs the heavens, Qi is transformed into the cold. According to the

visceral correspondence, the disease is named after the concerned viscera.

Emperor: How is transformation concerned with earthly Qi?
Qibo: It is the same as the heaven-governing Qi, and so is the interval Qi.

Emperor: What does the interval Qi mean?
Qibo: The Qi responsible for the phases on the left and the right is called interval Qi.

Emperor: How to differentiate among them (the interval Qi and the heaven-governing Qi and earth-governing Qi)?
Qibo: The heaven-governing Qi and the earth-governing Qi dominate the Qi of the year, while the interval Qi is responsible for the phases of a year.

Emperor: Good. How is the situation with the host Qi in a year?
Qibo: Jueyin, when governing the heavens, turns into wind transformation; governing the earth, into the sour transformation; governing the year phase, into the green; and governing the interval, into active transformation. Shaoyin, when governing the heavens, turns into heat transformation; governing the earth, into the bitter transformation with no Qi of year phase; governing the interval, into burning transformation. Taiyin, when governing the heavens, turns into damp transformation; governing the earth, into the sweet transformation; governing Qi of year phase, into yellow transformation; and governing the interval, into softening transformation.

Shaoyang, when governing the heavens, turns into fire transformation; governing the earth, into the bitter transformation; governing the Qi of year phase, into red transformation; and governing the interval, into bright transformation. Yangming, when governing the heavens, turns into dry transformation; governing the earth, into the pungent transformation; governing the Qi of year phase, into plain transformation; and governing the interval, into the clarity transformation. Taiyang, when governing the heavens, turns into cold transformation; governing the earth, into the salty transformation; governing the Qi of the year phase, into the black transformation; and governing the interval, into the storage transformation. Therefore for treating any disease, the respective administration of six-Qi transformation, the generation of five-flavor and five-complexion, and the preference of five solid-viscera should be understood, and then the relationship of the excess or deficiency Qi and the pathogenesis can be analyzed.

Emperor: When Jueyin governs the earth, the sour transformation is preceded, and I know this. How about the movement of wind transformation?
Qibo: The wind prevails over the earth, indicating its root, and other Qi is the same as the wind. Originating from the heavens, it is the Qi of the heavens; originating from the earth, it is the Qi of the earth. When heavenly Qi and earthly Qi are integrated, there appears the six-Qi, and all the things are created. It's believed that the optimal Qi should be carefully observed so that no pathogenesis can be missed, which is the information concerned.

Emperor: How to select the main drugs for the disease?

Qibo: The drugs are selected according to the Qi of year phase, and there will be no missing ones.

Emperor: Why should the drugs be selected firstly according to the Qi of year phase?
Qibo: Because they can absorb the specific essence from the heavens and the earth.

Emperor: How about the drugs bearing Qi of six-Qi?
Qibo: The drugs bearing Qi of six-Qi are the same as the drugs bearing the Qi of year phase, and there is excess and deficiency in them.

Emperor: How about the drugs that don't bear the Qi of year phase?
Qibo: Their quality is poor and can share the same texture with different grades. There are light or heavy flavors, stirring or calm property, more or less effect, and transient or profound action, and this is the information concerned.

Emperor: The Qi of yearly-phase may damage the solid viscera; how is this explained?
Qibo: The damage will result from being dominated, which is the key.

Emperor: How about the treatment?
Qibo: If the upper excessive Qi dominates the lower, it is balanced by its dominating Qi; if the external excessive Qi dominates the internal, it is treated by its dominating Qi.

Emperor: Good. How to treat the disease in a harmonious year?

Qibo: The aspect of Yin and Yang should be carefully observed and then regulated, aiming at balance. The conventional disease can be treated with the contrary method, while the unconventional disease can be treated with the non-contrary method.

Emperor: You have mentioned that the aspect of Yin and Yang should be carefully observed and then regulated; it's said in the medical literature that the pulses of Renying and Cunkou correspond with each other, just like drawing two pieces of rope with the same length, which is termed normal pulse. How about the Cunkou pulse where Yin is located?
Qibo: It can be observed through differentiating the administration of the south or the north.

Emperor: I'd like to know the details now.
Qibo: In the year of north-administration, Shaoyin in the earth has no correspondence on the Cunkou pulse, Jueyin in the earth has no correspondence on the right pulse, and Taiyin in the earth has no correspondence on the left pulse; in the year of south administration, Shaoyin governing heavens has no correspondence on the Cunkou pulse, Jueyin governing heavens has no correspondence on the right pulse, and Taiyin governing heavens has no correspondence on the left pulse. Whatever has no correspondent pulse can be observed in an opposite way.

Emperor: How about the pulse in Chi region?
Qibo: In the year of the north-administration, the triple Yin in the lower have no correspondence on the Cun pulse while the triple Yin in the upper have no correspondence on the Chi pulse. In the year of the south-administration, the triple Yin in the heavens have no correspondence on the Cun pulse while

the triple Yin in the earth have no correspondence on the Chi pulse. The left and the right pulses are the same. It's believed that knowing the key means catching everything while not knowing the key means catching nothing, which is the information concerned.

Emperor: Good. Qi of the heavens and the earth will excessively affect the interior; how is this so?
Qibo: In the year when Jueyin governs the earth, the domination of the wind excess leads to gloomy earthly Qi, dim wild field and early ripening of grass. Then people tend to have continuous chill, frequent stretching and yawning, heartache with sticking fullness, internal straining in hypochondria, anorexia, obstruction of pharynx and diaphragm, vomiting after eating, abdominal distension, frequent hiccups, being relaxed and feeling a sense of alleviation after defecation or flatus, and heavy body.

In the year when Shaoyin governs the earth, the domination of excessive heat leads to blazing air over the rivers and lakes and brightness in the dim places. People then tend to have frequent rumbling, Qi surging reversely up to the chest, panting, inability to stand for long, chill-fever disease, skin pain, blurred vision, toothache, swollen cheek, fearing cold and fever like malaria, pain in the lower abdomen, and bulging belly. Also, the hibernating insects are exposed.

In the year when Taiyin governs the earth, grass is flourishing early, the domination of damp leads to dusty rocky valleys, and the yellow turns into black over the earth indicating the mixture with the extreme Yin of water. Then people tend to have fluid retention, heartache, deafness with dizziness, swollen pharynx, throat obstruction, genital disease with bleeding, pain and swelling in the lower abdomen, urinary retention, headache due to Qi surging, bulging eyes, pulled neck, feeling of a broken waist, thigh failing to flex, popliteal fossa rigidity, and calf cramp.

In the year when Shaoyang governs the earth, the domination of the excessive fire leads to flaming brightness over the wild field and alternative chill-fever. People then tend to have acute diarrhea with mucus and blood, pain in the lower abdomen, dark urine and even stool blood, and Shaoyin it is also characterized by similar findings.

In the year when Yangming governs the earth, the domination of the dry leads to fog, coolness and gloom. People then tend to have frequent vomiting with bitter water, frequent sighing, inability to turn over due to heartache and hypochondriac pain, and even dry pharynx, dusty complexion, lusterless skin and feverish feeling in the exterior of feet.

In the year when Taiyang governs the earth, the domination of excessive cold leads to severe bleakness and constriction. People then tend to have pain in the lower abdomen involving the scrotum, referred to the waist and spine, heartache due to up-surging Qi, bleeding, swelling, sore throat and swollen chin.

Emperor: Good. How about the treatment?

Qibo: During Qi governing the earth and the excessive wind invading the interior, the disease can be treated with the pungent and the cool, assisted with the bitter, moderated with the sweet and dispersed with the pungent; for the excessive heat invading the interior, the disease can be treated with the salty and the cold, assisted with the sweet and the bitter, astringed with the sour and dispersed with the bitter; for the excessive damp invading the interior, the disease can be treated with the bitter and the heat, assisted with the sour and the bland, dried with the bitter and discharged with the bland; for the excessive fire invading the interior, the disease can be treated with the salty and the cold, assisted with the bitter and the pungent, astringed with the sour and dispersed with the bitter; for the excessive dry invading the interior, the disease can be treated with bitter and the warm, assisted with the sweet and the pungent, and purged with the bitter; for the excessive cold invading the interior, the disease can be treated with the sweet and the heat, assisted with the bitter and the pungent, purged with the salty, moistened with the pungent and hardened with the bitter.

Emperor: Good. How about the changes of Qi governing the heavens?

Qibo: When Jueyin governs the heavens, the domination of excessive wind leads to dusty and dim sky, wind blowing clouds, the coldness rising from the spring Qi, and flowing water with no freezing. People then tend to have stomach pain involving heart, sticking pain up to the hypochondria, obstruction of diaphragm, anorexia, stiff tongue, vomiting after eating, cold diarrhea, abdominal distension, sloppy diarrhea, abdominal lump and urinary retention; the hibernating insects are exposed. The disease originates from spleen, and the exhaustion of Chongyang pulse indicates the incurable disease and death.

When Shaoyin governs the heavens, the domination of excessive heat leads to arrival of depressive heat and the fire Qi prevailing in the administration. People then tend to have vexing heat in the chest, dry throat, fullness in the right armpit, skin pain, chill-fever disorder with cough and panting; with coming heavy rain, hemoptysis, blood stool, nasal obstruction, nosebleed, sneeze, vomiting and urine with dark color, and even sores, edema, pain in the shoulders, back, upper arm and supraclavicular fossa, heartache and lung distension, bulging abdomen with distension and fullness, and cough and panting. The disease originates from lung, and the exhaustion of Chize pulse indicates incurable disease and death.

When Taiyin governs the heavens, the domination of damp leads to heavy cold sky with spreading dark cloud, rain changing the dryness of grass and trees, as well as edema, bone pain, Yin-impediment, which means having no obvious pressure pain point after pressing, pain in the waist, spine, neck and head, occasional dizziness, difficulty in defecation, impotence, hunger but anorexia, cough and spitting with blood, and feeling of having the heart in the mouth. The disease originates from kidney, and the exhaustion of Taixi pulse indicates the incurable disease and death.

When Shaoyang governs the heavens, the domination of excessive fire leads to the warm Qi prevailing and restless status during the metal administration. People then tend to have headache, fever and fearing cold turning into malaria, heat surging on with skin pain, yellowish and reddish urine turning into water retention, edema of body and face, abdominal fullness, breathing with raised head, acute diarrhea with mucus and blood, sores, hemoptysis, vexation, vexing heat feeling in the chest, and even nasal obstruction and nosebleed. The disease originates from lung, and the exhaustion of Tianfu indicates the incurable disease and death.

When Yangming governs the heavens, the domination of the dry leads to late flourishing of trees, late growth of grass and internal changes of bone. People then tend to have pain in the left armpit and hypochondria, cold in the middle turning into malaria, cough, rumbling in the abdomen due to drastic coldness of the changing climate; the remaining trees are withering with the rotten bush in the lower and wilted grass leaves. People also tend to have sharp pain in the heart and hypochondria, inability to turn over, dry throat, dusty complexion, lumbago, hernia in males and pain in lower abdomen in female, blurred vision, canthal sore, ulcer, sores, acne and carbuncles; hibernating insects are exposed. The disease originates from liver, and the exhaustion of Taichong pulse indicates the incurable disease and death.

When Taiyang governs the heavens, the domination of the cold leads to the reversal arrival of cold Qi with water freezing, and blood change in the middle turning into carbuncle and ulcer. People then tend to have reversal heartache, vomiting blood, bloody stool, nasal obstruction and nosebleed, and frequent vertigo and syncope. There is hot blazing fire and pouring rain and even hailstones. There is also fullness of the chest and abdomen, feverish feeling in hands, elbow spasm, swollen armpit, severe palpitation with feeling of heart pounding, discomfort of the chest, hypochondria and stomach, reddish complexion and yellowish eyes, frequent hiccup, dry throat, and even blackish complexion, and thirst with desire to drink water. The disease originates from heart, and the exhaustion of Shenmen pulse indicates incurable disease and death. Thus, the so-called dynamic pulse-Qi can indicate the outcome of viscera.

Emperor: Good. How to treat it?

Qibo: As the Qi governing the heavens, the disease due to domination of excessive wind can be treated with the pungent and the cool, assisted with the bitter and sweet, moderated with the sweet and purged with the sour. The disease due to domination of excessive heat can be treated with the salty and the cold, assisted with the bitter and the sweet, and astringed with the sour. The disease due to domination of excessive damp can be treated with bitter and the heat, assisted with the sour and the pungent, dried with the bitter and discharged with the bland. The disease due to more damp ascending with heat can be treated with the bitter and the warm, and assisted and astringed with the sour till inducing sweating. The disease due to domination of excessive fire can be balanced with the sour and the cold, assisted with the bitter and the sweet, astringed with the sour, dissipated with the bitter and restored with the sour. The disease due to excessive heat shares the same treatment. The disease due to domination of excessive dry can be balanced with the bitter and the moist, assisted with the sour and the pungent and purged with the bitter. The disease due to domination of excessive cold can be balanced with the pungent and the heat, assisted with the sweet and the bitter, and purged with the salty.

Emperor: Good. If evil Qi dominates reversely, how to treat it?
Qibo: When wind governs the earth but is reversely dominated by the cool, the disease can be treated with the sour and the warm and assisted with the bitter and the sweet and balanced with the pungent. When heat governs the earth but is reversed by the cold, the disease can be treated with the sweet and the heat, assisted with the bitter and the pungent, and balanced with the salty. When the damp governs the earth but is reversely dominated by the heat, the disease can be treated with the bitter and the cold, assisted with the salty and the sweet, and balanced with the bitter. When the fire governs the earth but is

reversely dominated by the cold, the disease can be treated with the sweet and the heat, assisted with the bitter and the pungent, and balanced with the salty. When the dry governs the earth but is reversely dominated by the heat, the disease can be treated with the even cold, assisted with the bitter and the sweet, and balanced with the sour, aiming at the harmony. When the cold governs the earth but is reversely dominated by the heat, the disease can be treated with the salty and the cold, assisted with the sweet and pungent, and balanced with the bitter, aiming at the harmony.

Emperor: If Qi governing the heavens is dominated by the evil, how about the treatment?
Qibo: When the wind is transformed in the heavens but is reversely dominated by the cool, the disease can be treated with the sour and the warm, and assisted with the sweet and the bitter. When the heat is transformed in the heavens but is reversely dominated by the cold, the disease can be treated with the sweet and the warm and assisted with the bitter, sour and pungent. When the damp is transformed in the heavens but is reversely dominated by the heat, the disease can be treated with the bitter and the cold and assisted with the bitter and the sour. When the fire is transformed in the heavens which are dominated by the cold, the disease can be treated with the sweet and the heat and assisted with the bitter and the pungent. When the dry is transformed in the heavens but is reversely dominated by the heat, the disease can be treated with the pungent and the cold and assisted with the bitter and the sweet. When the cold is transformed in the heavens but is reversely dominated by the heat, the disease can be treated with the salty and the cold, and assisted with the bitter and the pungent.

Emperor: What are the situations about domination among six Qi in order?

Qibo: The domination of Jueyin leads to tinnitus, vertigo, and vexation with vomiting, and cold feeling in stomach and diaphragm; gales blow frequently and naked insects fail to breed; people then tend to have Qi accumulation of armpit and hypochondria turning into heat in the armpit and hypochondria, epigastric pain involving heart, sticking feeling over hypochondria, rumbling and diarrhea after indigestion, pain in the lower abdomen, diarrhea with mucus and blood, even vomiting, and obstruction of the chest and throat.

The domination of Shaoyin leads to feverish feeling below heart, Qi surging up from the navel and wandering in triple-Jiao; there comes the flaming summer when sap is exuded from the trees and grass is withering; people then tend to have vomiting, restlessness, abdominal fullness and pain, sloppy diarrhea and even bloody dysentery.

The domination of Taiyin leads to internal depression of the fire Qi; people then tend to have internal sore and ulcer, spreading externally with the disorders in the armpit and hypochondria, even heartache, dysphagia due to heat, headache, throat obstruction and stiff nape; the domination of the damp leads to internal depression of the damp Qi, cold evil oppressing lower Jiao, pain lingering in the vertex referred to both brows, and stomach fullness; there is frequent rain and dry transformation. People tend to have fullness in the lower abdomen, heaviness and stiffness of the waist and buttocks, sexual dysfunction, frequent watery diarrhea, warm feeling in the soles, heavy head, edema of shank and foot, fluid retention in the upper and edema in the lower.

The domination of Shaoyang leads to invasion of heat evil into stomach, vexation, heartache, red eyes, nausea, vomiting acid, frequent hunger, ear pain, dark urine, frequent fright and delirium; the climate suddenly becomes hot leading to exhaustion, withering grass and water drying up, and beetles shrinking; people tend to have pain in the lower abdomen and dysentery with mucus and blood.

The domination of Yangming leads to cool Qi rising from the interior; people then tend to have the pain in the left armpit and hypochondria, loose diarrhea, stuffy throat internally, and swollen scrotum externally; with the constriction and inhibition of severe cool Qi, there will appear discoloration of flowers over grass and trees and hairy insects will die. There is discomfort in the chest and throat obstruction with cough.

The domination of Taiyang leads to the arrival of congealing and chilly air, unexpected water freezing, and late breeding of winged insects. People then tend to have paroxysm of hemorrhoids and malaria, cold Qi invading stomach and turning into heartache internally, genital sores, sexual dysfunction, referred pain between the pubis and thigh, spasm of sinews and muscles, congealing and constriction of blood vessels, collateral fullness with the altered complexion or bloody stool, skin edema due to oppressive fullness, abdominal fullness and poor appetite, heat Qi surging reversely with the pain in the head, nape, fontanels, vertex and brain, and bulging eyes; the cold Qi invades the lower Jiao and turns into soggy diarrhea.

Emperor: How to treat them?
Qibo: The disease by domination of Jueyin can be treated with the sweet and the clear, assisted by the bitter and the pungent, and be purged with the sour. The disease by domination of Shaoyin can be treated with the pungent and the cold, assisted by the bitter and the salty, and be purged with the

sweet. The disease by domination of Taiyin can be treated with the salty and the heat, assisted by the pungent and the sweet, and be purged with the bitter. The disease by domination of Shaoyang can be treated with the pungent and the cold, assisted by the sweet and the salty, and be purged with the sweet. The disease by domination of Yangming can be treated with the sour and the warm, assisted by the pungent and the sweet, and be discharged with the bitter. The disease by domination of Taiyang can be treated with the sweet and the heat, assisted by the pungent and the sour, and be purged with the salty.

Emperor: What is situation about the retaliation of six-Qi?
Qibo: What a detailed question you have asked! The retaliation of Jueyin leads to hardness and fullness in the lower abdomen, internal straining and acute abdominal pain. Trees fall down, sand and dust are flying and naked worms cannot multiply. Then people tend to have angina pectoris, perspiration and vomiting, anorexia and vomiting immediately after eating, sinew spasm, vertigo, reversal cold of limbs; even evil Qi invades spleen leading to dysphagia and vomiting. Exhaustion of Chongyang meridian indicates incurable disease and death.

When Shaoyin retaliates, internal stuffy heat, restlessness, stuffy nose, sneeze, and colic in the lower abdomen can develop; with blazing fire spreading, dry throat can develop as can intermittent urination and defecation; with Qi starting from the left and ascending to the right, cough, skin pain, sudden dysphonia, heart pain and unconsciousness can be manifested; further manifestations include chill, fearing cold, shivering with teeth chattering, and delirium; with fever after cold subsiding, there develops thirst with desire to drink water, shortness of breath and bone flaccidity, obstruction of the intestines with constipation, external edema and hiccups. If the fire Qi is transformed later, flowing water won't freeze, heat Qi will spread and then beetles won't multiply; then people tend to have miliaria, rash, sore, ulcer, carbuncles, acnes and hemorrhoids. With heat evil invading lung, cough and chronic rhinitis can develop. The exhaustion of Tianfu pulse indicates incurable disease and death.

When Taiyin retaliates, the damp Qi rises, leading to heavy body and middle fullness and dyspepsia; with Yin Qi ascending reversely, there develops discomfort in the chest, internal fluid retention in the middle, cough and panting with hoarseness. With heavy rain falling frequently, there develops vertex pain especially with vertigo and convulsion, vomiting and indifference, spitting clear saliva; with damp evil invading kidney orifices, there develops incessant urination and defection. The exhaustion of Taixi pulse indicates incurable disease and death.

When Shaoyang retaliates, great heat is arriving with dryness and blazing heat and beetles are reduced. Then people tend to have fright, convulsion, cough and bleeding, heart heat, dysphoria, frequent defecation, and fearing wind; with reversal Qi ascending, people develop dusty complexion and eye twitching; with internal emergence of fire Qi, oral erosion, vomiting and hiccup, hemorrhage and hematochezia can develop; with paroxysm of malaria, the patient will fear cold and chill and teeth chattering; with extreme cold turning into heat, dryness of throat collateral, thirst with desire to drink water and yellowish and reddish complexion, shortness of breath and weak pulse can be seen; with turning into water, there develops edema and the water can even invade the lung with cough and hematochezia. The exhaustion of Chize pulse indicates incurable disease and death.

When Yangming retaliates, the cool Qi rises greatly, the trees are withering away and caterpillars die of epidemics; then people tend to have disorders in the armpit and hypochondria; with Qi remaining in the left side, frequent sighing and even heart pain, oppressive distension with diarrhea, vomiting bitter water, cough, hiccup and dysphoria can develop; with disorder in diaphragm, there develops headache, and even with evil Qi invading liver, there develops fright and sinew spasm. The exhaustion of Taichong pulse indicates incurable disease and death.

When Taiyang retaliates, the cold Qi ascends, water turns into rain and ice and winged insects die. Then people tend to have cold in heart and stomach, discomfort in the chest and diaphragm, heartache and oppressive distension, headache with frequent sorrow, intermittent vertigo and syncope with poor appetite, pain of the waist and buttocks with inflexibility; while the earth is split, ice is hard, and sunshine is weak, people tend to have the pain in lower abdomen involving the scrotum, referred to the waist and spine, Qi surges up to heart leading to spitting of clear saliva and hiccups, and evil Qi invades heart leading to amnesia and frequent sorrow. The exhaustion of Shenmen pulse indicates incurable disease and death.

Emperor: Good. How to treat them?

Qibo: The disease by retaliation of Jueyin can be treated with the sour and the cold, assisted with the sweet and the pungent, purged with the sour, and be moderated with the sweet. The disease by retaliation of Shaoyin can be treated with the salty and the cold, assisted with the bitter and the pungent, purged by the sweet, astringed by the sour, dispersed with the bitter and the pungent, and be softened by the salty. The disease by retaliation of Taiyin can be treated with the bitter and the heat, assisted with the sour and the pungent, and be purged and dried by the bitter. The disease by retaliation of Shaoyang can be treated with the salty and the cold, assisted with the bitter and the pungent, softened with the salty, and be astringed with the sour and dispersed with the pungent; the dispersing treatment doesn't avoid the heat but does not violate the warm and the cool. That of Shaoyin is the same as Shaoyang. The disease by retaliation of Yangming can be treated with the pungent and the warm, assisted with the bitter and the sweet, purged with the bitter and supplemented with the sour. The disease by retaliation of Taiyang can be treated with the salty and the heat, assisted with the sweet and the pungent, and be hardened with the bitter.

For any disease caused by retaliation, the cold one can be treated with the heat, the heat with the cold, the warm with the cool, the cool with the warm, the scattered with the astringent, the inhibited with the dispersed, the dry with the moist, the drastic with the moderate, the hard with the soft, the fragile with the hard, the decline with supplement, and the hyperactive with the purgative, in order to calm the Qi accordingly, clearly and peacefully, so that the disease Qi can be declined and the original Qi can return to its own position, which is the general regulation.

Emperor: Good. Qi has the division of the upper or lower, and how about it?

Qibo: Qi in the upper body has three divisions corresponding to the heavens, which is dominated by heaven-governing Qi;

Qi in the lower body has three divisions corresponding to the earth, which is dominated by earth-governing Qi. Qi is named by the upper or lower body, and the focus of diseases is named by the Qi; as to the name of "half", it is so called heaven-pivot. Thus domination in the upper leads to disease in the lower, which is named by the earth, and domination in the lower leads to disease in the upper, which is named by the heavens. As to domination arriving above, it indicates that retaliating Qi is inhibited with no surging. The retaliating Qi arrival isn't differentiated by either the heavens or the earth, which is named by its own way.

Emperor: Is there any constant phase about the movement of dominating Qi and retaliating Qi? Does six-Qi have the necessary phase?
Qibo: The seasons have constant phase, but the movement of six-Qi has no necessary phase.

Emperor: I'd like to know the reason.
Qibo: From the primary Qi to the third Qi, the heavenly Qi governs, which is the constant of dominating Qi; from the fourth to the final Qi, the earthly Qi governs, which is constant of retaliating Qi. There is dominating Qi which must be followed by retaliating Qi, there is no dominating Qi, which means there must be no retaliating Qi.

Emperor: Good. After the retaliating Qi has subsided, the dominating Qi returns. How is this so?
Qibo: The arrival of dominating Qi is followed by retaliating Qi that has no constant number, which will subside till decline of Qi. The retaliating Qi has subsided, the dominating Qi

returns, as otherwise there will be harm, due to which the vitality is damaged.

Emperor: There comes the retaliating Qi to cause diseases instead, why?
Qibo: Because the retaliating Qi doesn't come at the due phase, it isn't harmonized with the host Qi. When the retaliating Qi overcomes the dominating Qi, the host Qi will dominate to cause disease instead, which pertains to the fire, dry and heat.

Emperor: How about the treatment?
Qibo: Among the diseases caused by the domination of six-Qi, the mild form can be observed and the severe one can be inhibited; for the disease by retaliating Qi, the moderate form can be balanced and the violent one can be deprived. Whatever is done, the treatment should comply with the dominating Qi and calm the inhibited Qi with no limitation of the times, which aims at balancing the Qi, and this is also the principle of the treatment.

Emperor: Good. How about the domination or retaliation between guest Qi and host Qi?
Qibo: Guest Qi and host Qi have only domination but no retaliation.

Emperor: How about the reversal and compliance?
Qibo: Host Qi dominating is associated with the reversal, while guest Qi with compliance, which is the law of nature.

Emperor: How about the pathogenesis of the diseases caused?
Qibo: When Jueyin governs the heavens, the domination of guest Qi leads to tinnitus and vertigo, even cough if severe, while the domination of host Qi leads to pain in the chest and

hypochondriac pain and stiff tongue with difficulty in speaking.

When Shaoyin dominates the heavens, the domination of guest Qi leads to stuffy nose, sneeze, stiff neck and nape, feverish feeling in the shoulders and back, headache, shortness of breath, fever, deafness, blurred vision, even edema, hemorrhage, sores, cough and panting; the dominating of guest Qi leads to heart heat, vexation, even pain and sticking fullness of hypochondria if severe.

When Taiyin governs the heavens, the domination of guest Qi leads to edema of head and face and panting; the domination of host Qi leads to fullness of the chest and abdomen, and mental confusion after eating.

When Shaoyang governs the heavens, the domination of guest Qi leads to red eruption, erysipelas, sores, vomiting, throat obstruction, headache, swollen pharynx, deafness, hemorrhage and convulsion; the domination of host Qi leads to chest fullness, cough, nodding respiration, even hemoptysis and hand heat.

When Yangming governs the earth, the domination of guest Qi leads to cooling Qi redominating and remaining inside, even cough, nosebleed, pharyngeal obstruction, feverish feeling in the heart and diaphragm, lingering cough, and death if vomiting pale blood can be seen.

When Taiyang dominates the heavens, the domination of guest Qi leads to discomfort of the chest, clear nasal discharge and cough if affected by cold; the domination of host Qi leads to stridor in the throat.

When Jueyin governs the earth, the domination of guest Qi leads to stiff large joints, spasm and cramp internally, and difficulty in movement externally; the domination of host Qi leads to shaking and constriction of sinews and bones, and frequent pain of the waist and abdomen.

When Shaoyin governs the earth, the domination of guest Qi leads to lumbago, diseases involving the buttocks, thighs, knees, calf, tibia and feet with hot and sour feeling, edema and inability to stand for a long time, changes in urination and defecation; the domination of host Qi leads to reversal Qi surging up, heart pain, fever, oppression of diaphragm, paroxysm of various Bi syndromes in armpit and hypochondria, incessant sweating and coldness of the four limbs.

When Taiyin governs the earth, the domination of guest Qi leads to flaccidity and heaviness of feet, frequent defecation and urination, retention of dampness in lower Jiao, diarrhea, edema and genital diseases; the domination of host Qi leads to reversal and full cold Qi, anorexia, and even hernia.

When Shaoyang governs the earth, the domination of guest Qi leads to pain of the waist and abdomen, fearing cold, and even frothy urine and stool; the domination of host Qi leads to reversal heat Qi ascending involving heart with heart pain, fever, dysphagia and vomiting; the manifestation of Shaoyin is the same.

When Yangming governs the earth, the domination of guest Qi leads to cool Qi activating in the lower, lower abdominal hardness and fullness, frequent defecation and diarrhea; the domination of host Qi leads to heavy waist, abdominal pain, cold feeling in lower abdominal region, sloppy diarrhea, reversal cold in the intestines surging up to the chest, even panting and inability to stand for a long time.

When Taiyang governs the earth, the domination of guest Qi leads to cold Qi redominating and remaining inside, pain of the waist and buttocks, inflexibility of the extremities, and pain of the thigh, shank, feet and knees.

Emperor: Good. How to treat them?
Qibo: The upsurging should be inhibited, the descending be lifted, the excess be reduced, the insufficient be supplemented, assisted with benefit Qi and regulated with the proper medication and diet; the host Qi and guest Qi can be harmonized peacefully; according to the adaptation to the cold and heat, the identified should be treated with reversal therapy while the opposite should be treated with compliance therapy.

Emperor: The cold disease should be treated with the heat therapy while the heat be treated with the cold therapy; if host Qi and guest Qi are identified, the reversal should be applied, while if host Qi and guest Qi aren't identified, the compliance be applied; I know this. How to correct selection of medical flavors?
Qibo: At the stage of Jueyin-wind-wood as host Qi, the disease should be treated with the sour for purgation and with the pungent for supplement; at the stage of fire of Shaoyin and Shaoyang as host Qi, the disease should be treated with the sweet for purgation and with the salty for supplement; at the stage of Taiyin-damp-earth as host Qi, the disease be treated with the bitter for purgation and with the sweet for supplement. At the stage of Yangming-dry-metal as host Qi, the disease should be treated with the pungent for purgation and with the sour for supplement. At the stage of Taiyang-damp-earth as host Qi, the disease should be treated with salty for purgation and with the bitter for supplement.

At the stage of Jueyin as guest Qi, the disease should be treated with the pungent for supplement, with the sour for purgation and with the sweet for moderation. At the stage of Shaoyin as guest Qi, the disease should be treated with the salty for supplement, with the sweet for purgation and with the salty for astringency. At the stage of Taiyin as guest Qi, the disease should be treated with the sweet for supplement, with the bitter for purgation and with the sweet for moderation. At the stage of Shaoyang as guest Qi, the disease should be treated with the salty for supplement, with the sweet for purgation and with the salty for softening. At the stage of Yangming as guest Qi, the disease should be treated with the sour for supplement, with the pungent for purgation and with the bitter for discharging. At the stage of Taiyang as guest Qi, the disease should be treated with the bitter for supplement, with the salty for purgation and with the bitter for hardening, and with the pungent for moistening, in order to open interstitial striae and promote the Qi communication of liquid and fluid.

Emperor: Good. I'd like to know what the three divisions of Yin and Yang are.
Qibo: There are different proportions and functions between Qi of Yin and Yang.

Emperor: What does Yangming mean?
Qibo: It means the brightness evolved from both Taiyang and Shaoyang.

Emperor: What does Jueyin mean?
Qibo: It means the end evolved from Taiyin and Shaoyin.

Emperor: Qi will be more or less, disease serious or mild, treatment drastic or moderate, and formula large or small; I'd like to know the guidance.

Qibo: Since Qi will be high or low, disease can be distal or proximal, syndrome internal or external, and treatment moderate or drastic, which is determined by the medicinal Qi to take effect adequately. It's said in *The Chief Essentials* that there is one chief ingredient and two subordinate ingredients, which is called odd formula in regulation; there are two chiefs and four subordinates, which is called even formula; there are two chiefs and three subordinates, which is called odd formula; and there are two chiefs and six subordinates, which is called even formula. It's believed that the proximal disease should be treated with odd formula while the distal disease should be treated with even formula; odd formula cannot be applied to promote sweating and even formula cannot be applied for purgation; moderate formula should be applied to supplement and treat the upper, while the drastic formula should be applied to supplement and treat the lower; the thick flavor should be selected for the drastic, while the thin flavor should be selected for the moderate, which is determined by the medicinal Qi to take effect; this is the information concerned. If the focus is distal while the ingredient acts on the way, the medication can be taken before or after meal, in order have an effect on the focus of the disease, the guidance of which shouldn't be violated. Hence the principle for regulating Qi is that the proximal disease should be treated first with odd and then even formula with small dosage of ingredients, while the distal disease should be treated first with odd and then even formula with large dosage of ingredients; large formula contains fewer ingredients while small formula more ingredients; there are as many as nine ingredients or as few as two ingredients in the formula. If odd formula cannot cure the disease, even formula can be applied instead, which is called compound formula; if even formula cannot cure the disease, ingredients with different properties from the disease can be selected, that is to say, the properties cold, heat, warm or cool of the medicinal are selected differently from that of disease.

Emperor: Good. Some diseases are caused by the root, and I know this. Some diseases are caused by the branch, and how to treat them?
Qibo: The disease opposite to the root is caused by the branch and the treatment also opposite for the root is the therapy for the branch.

Emperor: Good. How to observe the domination of six-Qi?
Qibo: It can be observed when six-Qi arrives. When cool Qi arrives excessively, the dry is in domination, wind-wood is affected by evil and liver disease is caused. When heat Qi arrives excessively, fire is in domination, metal-dry is affected and lung disease is caused. When cold Qi arrives excessively, water is in domination, the fire is affected and heart disease is caused. When damp Qi arrives excessively, the earth is in domination, the cold water is affected and kidney disease is caused. When wind Qi arrives excessively, the wood is in domination, the damp-earth is affected and spleen disease is caused. This is the effect of evil that leads to disease. If Qi of the year phase is deficient, the evil is more serious. If seasonal Qi is in disharmony, evil is also more serious. If the moon is waning, the evil is more serious. Being affected by evil repeatedly causes the disease to be critical. If there is dominating Qi, there must be retaliating Qi that comes.

Emperor: How about the pulse coming when six-Qi is coming?
Qibo: If Jueyin is coming, the pulse appears stringy; if Shaoyin is coming, the pulse appears hooky; if Taiyin is coming, the pulse appears deep; if Shaoyang is coming, the pulse appears large and floating; if Yangming is coming, the pulse appears short and unsmooth; if Taiyang is coming, the pulse appears large and long. When Qi arrives with the moderate pulse, it is normal; when Qi arrives and the pulse is drastic, it is abnormal; when Qi arrives and the pulse is opposite, it is abnormal; when Qi arrives with no pulse to come, it is abnormal; if Qi doesn't arrive but the pulse has come, it is abnormal. If Yin pulse and Yang pulse interchange their positions, it indicates crisis.

Emperor: Six-Qi tends to branch and root in different ways, why?
Qibo: Qi can tend to the root, or to the branch and root, or not to the branch and root.

Emperor: I'd like to know why.
Qibo: Shaoyang and Taiyin tend to the root, Shaoyin and Taiyang tend to branch and root, Yangming and Jueyin don't tend to branch and root but to the middle. So, Qi tending to the root can be transformed in the root, Qi tending to the branch and root can be transformed in the branch and root, and Qi tending to the middle can be transformed in the middle.

Emperor: The pulse seemingly is consistent with the disease, but in fact is opposite to it; so, how to make a diagnosis and schedule treatment?
Qibo: The pulse appears to be consistent with the disease but doesn't beat forcefully, as it is for the false Yang syndromes.

Emperor: How is the pulse for the false Yin syndrome?

Qibo: The pulse appears to be consistent with the disease but beats forcefully and in a drum-like way.

As to the pathogenesis of all diseases, some originate from the root, some from the branch, or some from the middle Qi; as to the treatment, some can be cured by treating the root, some by treating the branch, some by treating the middle Qi, some by treating the branch and root; some can be cured by the reversal therapy while some by compliance therapy. The so-called reversal therapy actually refers to normal treatment while the so-called compliance therapy actually means the complying treatment. So, it's believed that knowing branch and root ensures successful treatment, and understanding the reversal therapy and compliance therapy ensures correct treatment, which is the rule. If not knowing the rule, then diagnosis and treatment violate the medical classics. Hence, it's said in *The Chief Essentials* that the careless doctors tend to be self-satisfied and flatter themselves on understanding all diseases; actually, there appears cold manifestation again before they finish discussion on heat syndrome; the same Qi also has different manifestations, which can confuse and disturb the diagnosis and treatment, which are the rules concerned. Therefore, the theory of branch–root is concise and comprehensive, and cover from small to large application; analysis of one example can disclose the essential pathogenesis of all diseases, discussion of branch–root can help one master the rules thus leading no harm, observation of root–branch can regulate the Qi of diseases, and identification of dominating and retaliating Qi can help set up a model for people to follow, which are all the laws of nature.

Emperor: There are changes of dominating Qi and retaliating Qi; how is the early or late occurrence?

Qibo: In terms of domination, when the dominating Qi arrives, the disease then occurs, and when the disease Qi is accumulated, the retaliating Qi is stirring. In terms of retaliation, the retaliating Qi emerges in the end of dominating Qi and is exuberant in due position; since there are mild or severe dominating Qi, there can be more or less retaliating Qi; the moderate dominating Qi leads to moderate retaliating Qi, and the deficient dominating Qi leads to deficient retaliating Qi, which is the constant of nature.

Emperor: When the dominating Qi and the retaliating Qi emerge, they will act in the improper position or arrive later than the due time, and what is the cause of this?
Qibo: The generation and transformation of Qi are characterized by decline and exuberance. The effects of the cold, heat, warm, cool, decline and exuberance are all manifested in late months; thus, the action of Yang starts from the warm and exuberates in the summer-heat; the action of Yin starts from the cool and exuberates in the cold; there is some difference among spring, summer, autumn and winter in order. Hence, it's said in *The Chief Essentials* that the warm of spring turns into the heat of summer, the cool depression of autumn turns into cold anger of winter. With careful observation of the four late months and expectation of climatic Qi in position, the termination can be observed and the initiation can be expected, which are the details concerned.

Emperor: Is there any time length for the difference?
Qibo: In total 3 days.

Emperor: How is the reflection on the pulse?

Qibo: The pulse reflection of the difference is the same as the normal, and it will disappear as time passes by. It's said in *The Essentials of Pulse* 'Pulse in spring isn't sunken, pulse in summer isn't stringy, pulse in winter isn't unsmooth, and pulse in autumn isn't rapid, which are called Four Stagnation of pulse'. Too sunken pulse is abnormal, so is too stringy pulse, too unsmooth pulse, and too rapid pulse; irregular pulse is abnormal, so is the repeated irregular pulse, pulse going with no Qi going, and pulse not going with Qi going; the contradictory pulse indicates death. Hence, the collaboration of Qi and pulse is the governing, just like scale and weight with no loss of balance. It's believed that, if the Qi of Yin and Yang is clear, there is generation and transformation, while if there is disturbance, the diseases arise, and this is the information concerned.

Emperor: What do the darkness and the brightness mean?
Qibo: At the end of convergence between two Yin, there is darkness, while in the combination of two Yang, there is brightness. By the combination of darkness and brightness, there is difference of the cold and the heat.

Emperor: What about the point of equinox and solstice?
Qibo: The arrival of Qi is called solstice term, while the separation of Qi is called equinox term. When arriving, Qi is the same while when separating, Qi is different, which is the normal rule for transformation of the heavens and the earth.

Emperor: You've said that Qi of spring and autumn starts early and Qi of winter and summer starts late, which I have understood. However, six climatic Qi rotates alternatively and Qi of year phase isn't constant; how about the therapy of supplementation and purgation?

Qibo: When the upper and the lower dominates, respectively, varying according to the property, the correct selection of the ingredient is the key point. The interval Qi on the left or the right is the same. It's said in *The Chief Essentials* that on Shaoyang dominating, the sweet is selected first and then the salty; on Yangming dominating, the pungent is selected first and then the sour; on Taiyang dominating, the salty is selected first and then the bitter; on Jueyin dominating, the sour is selected first and then the pungent; on Shaoyin dominating, the sweet is selected first and then the salty; and on Taiyin dominating, the bitter is selected first and then the sweet. Assisting with the proper ingredient and promoting the source of Qi, it is called mastering Qi.

Emperor: Good. All diseases are caused by wind, cold, heat, damp, dryness and fire, which are transformed into various conditions. It's said in the medical classics that the excess should be treated with purgation while the deficiency should be treated with supplementation; I have given this information it to the doctors but they haven't obtained the perfect therapeutic effect. I hope that the essential methods can be effective in practice, like the sound created when drumsticks beat on a drum, or like drawing out the thorn and cleaning the stain; there are inspection, inquiry, listening and smelling, and palpation; can I know about this?
Qibo: The pathogenesis should be observed carefully without loss of proper Qi, which is the principle.

Emperor: I'd like to know what the pathogenesis is.
Qibo: Any wind disease with vertigo and tremor is attributed to liver; any cold disease with constriction is attributed to kidney; any Qi disease with full depression is attributed to lung; any

damp disease with edema and fullness is attributed to spleen; any heat disease with dizziness and convulsion is attributed to fire; any sore disease with pain and itch is attributed to heart; any reversal disease with critical Qi reversal with excretory obstruction and incontinence is attributed to the lower Jiao; any disease with flaccidity, panting and vomiting is attributed to the upper Jiao; any disease with lockjaw, shivering and chattering is attributed to fire; any disease with convulsion and stiff nape is attributed to damp; any reversal disease with surging upward is attributed to fire; any disease with distension and big abdomen is attributed to heat; any disease with restlessness and mania is attributed to fire; any sudden disease with body rigidity is attributed to wind; any disease with noise or drum-like sounds by palpation is attributed to heat; any edema disease with ache, pain, and fright is attributed to fire; any disease with spasm, opisthotonos and turbid excretory fluid is attributed to heat; any disease with clear and cold excretory fluid is attributed to cold; and any disease with vomiting acid, explosive diarrhea and tenesmus is attributed to heat.

Therefore, it is said in *The Chief Essentials* that the pathogenesis should be observed carefully and the respective attributes should be identified; the cause should be found for the manifestation and also for cases with no obvious manifestation; the exuberance should be analyzed carefully and the deficiency should also be analyzed carefully; the domination of five elements should be differentiated, and the blood and Qi should be soothed and regulated for distribution and harmony; this is pathogenesis.

Emperor: Good. What is the action of the five flavors with Yin or Yang?

Qibo: The pungent and sweet flavors with dispersing action correspond to Yang, the sour and bitter with action of vomiting and excretion to Yin, the salty with action of vomiting and excretion to Yin, and the bland with action of drainage and diarrhea to Yang. These six have actions of astringing or dispersing, moderate or drastic, drying or moistening, and softening or hardening, which can be applied aiming at improvement in order to regulate and harmonize the Qi.

Emperor: Some diseases can be cured not by regulating Qi; how to treat them? How are toxic or non-toxic drugs applied, and how is the time order? I'd like to know its principle.
Qibo: The application of toxic or non-toxic drugs depends on the conditions, and the dose should be determined according to the formula regulation.

Emperor: Please introduce the formula regulation.
Qibo: There is one chief ingredient, two subordinates and five assistants in a small formula; one chief and three subordinates in a middle formula; and one chief, three subordinates and nine assistants in a large formula. The cold should be treated with the heat method, the heat with the cold, the mild with reversal, the severe with compliance, the hard with breaking, the invading with elimination, the exertion with the warm, the binding with the dispersing, the retention with attacking, the dry with the moistening, the acute with the moderate, the diffusive with the astringent, the damage with the warm, the flaccid with the activation, and the fright with the calming; other methods include the ascending, descending, massage, bathing, reducing, removing, opening and dissipating, which are applied based on the pathologic conditions.

Emperor: What are the reversal and compliance treatments?
Qibo: The reversal method is the ordinary treatment, while the non-contrary method is the extraordinary treatment; the extent of the extraordinary treatment depends on the pathologic conditions.

Emperor: What is the contrary treatment?
Qibo: That includes treating the disease due to heat with the cold, treating the disease due to cold with the heat, treating the obstructive with the tonic, and treating diarrhea with the purgation. In order to control the root of the diseases, the original cause should be identified first; at the very beginning, the property of medication is similar to the disease, but the outcome can show that they are different; thus, the contrary method can be applied to break the mass, erode the hard, harmonize the Qi and cure the disease in the end.

Emperor: Good. How to treat the disease that can be cured by regulating Qi?
Qibo: That is the reversal or compliance method, or the reversal first and then the compliance, or the compliance first and then the reversal, which can soothe and distribute Qi and further regulate Qi.

Emperor: Good. The disease has internal and external aspects, and how to treat them?
Qibo: Any disease from the internal to the external can be treated with internal regulation, any disease from the external to the internal can be treated with external regulation, any disease from the internal to the external with external exuberance can be treated by internal regulation and then external treatment, and any disease from the external to the internal can be treated with

external treatment and then internal regulation, and if the internal and external aspects of the disease are independent of each other, the main aspect of the disease can be treated.

Emperor: Good. When the disease with fire-heat recurs, there will be fearing cold and fever, and some of these aspects are similar to malaria occurring every day or every few days; what is the cause for this?
Qibo: When dominating Qi and retaliating Qi meet, there is a difference in the proportion of Yin and Yang. If there is more Yin Qi and less Yang Qi, the attack occurs for a longer time; while there is more Yang Qi and less Yin Qi, the attack occurs for a shorter time. It is the result of struggle between dominating Qi and retaliating Qi as well as the key of exuberance and decline, which is the same as in malaria.

Emperor: It is said in the medical classics to treat the cold with the heat and to treat the heat with the cold, and that no doctor should ignore the principle and change the convention. If the case with heat still has the heat after cold-treatment, the case with cold still has the cold after heat-treatment, or the case has both the diseases that are further complicated by new disease, how to treat them?
Qibo: If any patient develops the heat after cold-treatment, the treatment should be directed to Yin, while if there is development of cold after heat-treatment, the treatment should be directed to Yang, which is the selective treatment based on the attribute.

Emperor: Good. There develops the heat after the cold medications while the cold after heat medications, and what is the cause?

Qibo: It is the treatment only for the most exuberant Qi that causes the reversal outcome.

Emperor: What is the cause for the similar outcome after treatment not for the most exuberant Qi?
Qibo: What a detailed question Your Majesty has asked! That is caused by the treatment not being directed to the attributes of five flavors. After they are taken into stomach, the five flavors enter the viscera which correspond to the soild viscus, respectively. So, the sour firstly enters liver, the bitter firstly enters heart, the sweet firstly enters spleen, the pungent firstly enters lung, and the salty firstly enters kidney; after a long time, the five flavors can increase visceral Qi, which is the convention of material transformation. However, if visceral Qi is increased for too long, it may be the cause of death.

Emperor: Good. The ingredients in the formula are categorized into the monarch and the minister, and what is their mechanism?
Qibo: The ingredients for main aspects of disease are called the monarch, the ones assisting the monarch are called the minister, and the ones guiding are called guide, which are different from the three grades of medicinal properties.

Emperor: What are the three-grade of medicinal properties?
Qibo answered: This is the classification for distinguishing the good and bad property of medicinals.

Emperor: Good. How to treat internal and external aspects of the disease?
Qibo: The principle for correcting the Qi of diseases necessarily depends on distinguishing Yin from Yang, differentiating

internal from external aspects of the disease, and following the respective treatment for the different locations. The internal should be treated internally, the external treated externally, the mild treated with adjustment, the severe treated with inhibition, the hyperactive treated with extinguishment, and the sweating treated with purgation; according to the property of cold, heat, warm and cool, the Qi of diseases can be decreased specifically, varying with the conditions. If these principles are observed carefully, it will ensure effectiveness of therapies, harmony of Qi-blood and a longer life-span.

Emperor: Good.

Chapter 75

Elucidation of Perfect Teaching

When Yellow Emperor sat in the bright hall, he summoned Leigong and asked him: Do you understand the fundamentals of medicine?
Leigong answered: I have read the books about it, but I can hardly understand it. Even though I can elucidate it, I can hardly analyze it; even though I can analyze it, I can hardly understand it; even though I can know it, I can hardly apply it. Hence, with my knowledge available, I can only treat my common officials but I am not qualified to treat the kings and the nobles. I hope I can be taught about the measurements of celestial motion, comprehension of four seasons and Yin–Yang, and differentiation of stars, the sun and the moon, by which the medical theory and practice can be developed and become perfect in the later generations. Thus, the medicine can tally with Shennong and reach the level it was during the reign of the two emperors (Fuxi and Shennong) in ancient times.

Emperor said: Good. These fundamentals mustn't be lost because they are the collaboration among Yin and Yang, exterior and interior, ups and downs, or males and females. Moreover, if astronomy in the upper, geography in the lower and the human

affairs in the middle can be mastered, the medical knowledge can last long and be taught to common people without any puzzles. Thus, the medical principles and theories can be passed down to the generations to come as treasures.
Leigong said: Please instruct me on the medical principles, and let me read and understand them well.

Emperor: Haven't you heard of the book *Transmission of Yin–Yang*?
Leigong: No.

Emperor: The third Yang (Taiyang) will follow the law of heavens, and if it moves up and down irregularly and is combined leading to diseases, they will cause the unbalance of Yin and Yang harmfully.
Leigong: The arrival of third Yang (Taiyang) cannot be halted; I'd like to know the explanation behind this.

Emperor: The third Yang (Taiyang) arrives alone, which is actually the simultaneous arrival of third Yang (Taiyang), just like wind and rain. They cause head diseases in the upper and incontinence in the lower. Because this kind of disease has no external signs, no internal regular changes and no compliance with transmission rule, there is no definite diagnosis for the upper or lower location. Thus, the disease can be differentiated according to the details given in the medical book.
Leigong: I treated this kind of disease with few cures, which is caused by my rough understanding of the medicine after all.

Emperor: The third Yang (Taiyang) is the extreme Yang. Their accumulation and combination can cause the frightening disease. The onset of the disease is like a swift wind while the

peak is like a thunderbolt, accompanied by nine blocked orifices and overflowing Yang to cause dry larynx and obstructed throat. If evil is combined with Yin, there will develop diseases irregularly both up and down, and if attacked in the lower, there will be dysentery. The so-called third Yang (Taiyang) surging to heart leads to the failure of standing up after sitting and not feeling comfortable after lying down. Yet in order to know nature and human, one should know the difference between Yin and Yang, the compliance with four seasons and combination of five elements.
Leigong: I cannot differentiate it when you instruct me plainly and cannot comprehend it when you instruct me cryptically. So, please allow me to stand up to listen to you and understand the supreme principle.

Emperor: If you have received an instruction but cannot know how to integrate it with the supreme principle, you might doubt the teaching. Hence I'd like to tell you the supreme fundamentals: There is the instance that five solid viscera are impaired by the disease and then sinews and bones are consumed. If you cannot understand and differentiate them, the ancestral medicine will have been lost. For example, if kidney-pulse Qi is exhausted, the patient will feel depressive and become worse at dusk, be unwilling to go out due to lassitude and even be reluctant to meet people.

Chapter 76

Administration of Reasonable Analysis

Yellow Emperor was sitting greatly and summoned Leigong and asked him: You have learnt medicine, recited the medical books and even read comprehensive books, so that you can draw analogies and give an overall consideration; please tell me your medical expertise on five solid viscera and six hollow viscera like gallbladder, stomach, small or large intestine, spleen, womb and bladder as well as brain, marrow, snivel and saliva, emotions like crying, weeping, sadness and sorrow, and the fluid circulation in the body. All of them are factors for all human beings to live by, and the doctors can easily make mistakes in these conditions. You must fully understand the knowledge to make your medical practice perfect, as otherwise you will receive complaints from patients in the world.

Leigong said: Though your humble servant has recited many chapters in *The Upper and Lower Volume of The Pulse Classics*, I haven't applied the method through drawing the analogy perfectly, let alone fully understand all the medical theory.

Emperor: Please tell me the knowledge about, beyond what is given in the upper and lower volume of *The Pulse Classics*, the pathology of five solid viscera, disharmony of six hollow viscera, side effect of acupuncture therapy, indication of poisonous drug, and property and flavor of thin and thick medical wine. Please state the details in a concrete manner and give the answers to the questions in detail, and also tell me something you don't know.
Leigong: The deficiencies of liver, kidney and spleen can all cause heavy body and vexation, and the diseases can be medicated with drugs, acupuncture, moxibustion, stone needles, and thin medical wine, by which some can be cured but some not; I want to know the solution.

Emperor: You became a minister at a certain age but ask such inferior questions. Maybe the real question I asked isn't suitable for you. After I ask you the quite profound questions, you can only answer me with the knowledge from the upper and lower volume of *The Pulse Classics*, why is this so? The case with spleen disease has deficient and floating pulse like lung pulse, the case with kidney disease has small and floating pulse like spleen pulse, and the case with liver disease has the deficient and floating pulse like kidney pulse, all of which the doctor tends to make errors in looking at and so should be analyzed reasonably. As to the three solid viscera, spleen, liver and kidney, they are located near together; this is known even to kids, why do you ask about this?
Leigong: There is the patient with headache, sinew spasm, heavy bone, timidity, less Qi, belching, abdominal fullness, usual fright and failing to sleep. Which solid organ is involved in these disorders? The pulse was floating and stringy and firm

as stone under heavy pressure. I cannot understand the mechanism, and so I asked the questions concerned with the three solid viscera again in order to know the differentiation by comparison.

Emperor: It just requires consideration through unhurried and reasonable discussion. For the elderly, the treatment focuses on hollow viscera; for the young, on the meridians; and for adults, on the solid viscera. Now what you have said is all wrong. It is associated with stagnated heat of eight winds, which damages the functions of five solid viscera and can be transmitted in the body. Here, the floating and stringy pulse is due to kidney deficiency, sunken and stone-like pulse is due to internal stagnated kidney Qi, timidity with less Qi is due to blockage of water way and dispersed physique Qi, and cough with vexation is due to reversal kidney Qi. The morbid Qi of the body is just rooted in sole solid viscus. If it's said that the disease is associated with the three solid viscera, it doesn't tally with the medical principle.

Leigong: There is another case where the patient has four heavy and flaccid limbs, panting, cough and bloody stool, which was wrongly diagnosed by me as lung damage with floating, large and deficient pulse. I didn't dare to treat for the case. But an inferior doctor instead gave the stone needle treatment for it, and finally the disease was actually cured after some more bloody stool was passed, and later the patient was relaxed after bleeding stopped. What is the disease?

Emperor: You could have treated the disease and have gained much knowledge, but you failed in treating the disease. It's like wild geese flying with slowly beating wings and also can hover high in the sky. The doctor as the saint can follow the principles and accord the measurement, have differentiation by comparison, and make analysis and apply principles broadly; observing the upper can actually help in knowing the lower. And you needn't consider the meridians Qi in a mechanical way. Now the floating, large and deficient pulse indicates the external exhaustion of spleen Qi that leaves stomach to be combined into Yangming. Since stomach fire cannot dominate spleen water, the pulse becomes disordered leading to loss of the routine pulsation. The four heavy and flaccid limbs indicate dysfunction of spleen essence. Panting and cough indicate water Qi combined into Yangming meridian. Bloody stool indicates the vessel spasm, and blood has no normal way to flow. If you diagnosed it as lung damage, it's a mistake that will result in serious outcome. There is no differentiation by comparison, which is in fact due to being blind to the truth. However lung damage manifests in dysfunction of spleen Qi, turbidity of stomach Qi, abnormality of meridians, damage of genuine solid viscera, exhaustion of meridian Qi, leakage of five solid viscera Qi, and there will be either nose bleeding or vomiting blood, which is obviously distinguished from spleen damage. It's just like the heavens having no shape and the earth having no borderline as well as inverting black and white. It's my fault that I thought you had known it and so I needn't instruct you. The analogous and logic differentiation cited from *Unhurried Reasonable Analysis* is the classic text for diagnosis, and it is an absolutely essential medical principle.

Chapter 77

Listing and Analysis of Five Diagnostic Errors

Yellow Emperor asked: Oh! How profound the medical theory is! It's so subtle as if gazing down into the abyss or looking up to the floating clouds. The abyss can be measured, while it is impossible to know the limit of floating clouds. The medical technique of the Sage is the model to serve the people. All their clinical analysis and judgment will follow the principles, refer to the classics and abide by the regulation, in order to perform medical practice and bring benefit for the people. Thus, there are regulations of five faults and four virtues in medicine. Have you heard of this?
Leigong moved back and kowtowed once and again to say: I'm rather young, ignorant and puzzled, so I haven't heard of five faults and four virtues. Though I can categorize the diseases according to their symptoms and terms, I tend to cite the evidence from the classics aimlessly and actually haven't got any idea on how to answer your question.

Emperor said: Prior to diagnosis, a doctor should inquire about the history of the patient. If the patient used to be noble and is now humble, though without being attacked by evil, he will have got the disease from the internal, termed loss of nourishment; if he used to be rich and is now poor, the disease is termed loss of essence. The Qi of five solid viscera is stagnated so that there will be complicated occurrence of disease. When the doctor is going to diagnose the disease that has no involvement of the viscera and no manifestations in the physique, he remains uncertain about diagnosis and cannot define what the disease is. The patient will lose weight day by day, suffer from Qi deficiency with no essence, and severe disease with no Qi, and develop continuous chill and fright. The reason for the deterioration of the disease is due to the external exhaustion of the defense Qi and internal depletion of the nutrition Qi. The doctor's neglect is that he doesn't inquire about the condition of the disease adequately. This is the first fault of the diagnosis and treatment.

When diagnosing the disease, the doctor should inquire about the diet, housing and other life conditions; any sudden joys and bitterness or joy followed by bitterness can all damage and even exhaust the essence Qi completely, leading to deterioration of the physique. Sudden rage can impair Yin, while sudden joy can impair Yang; and the consequent Qi reversal will ascend and overfill the meridians while the spirit leaves the physique. When an unqualified doctor treats the disease, he is unable to select the proper supplement or purging method as well as know the pathologic conditions, so the patient will suffer loss of essential Qi day by day, causing evil Qi to accumulate. This is the second fault of diagnosis and treatment.

A doctor good at pulse-taking should categorize symptoms, distinguish the common and uncommon ones and know the conditions by logic analysis. If any doctor fails to know the rules, his diagnosis or treatment has no value certainly. This is the third fault of diagnosis and treatment.

There are three routines for diagnosis including inquiries about the noble or humble rank, official promotion or demotion, and whether he possesses ambition for a duke or a king. So, a noble person who loses the power and influence, though not being attacked by evil, will have internal emotional damage and his general health must be deteriorated. Any person experiencing wealth and consequent poverty, though not damaged by evil, can also develop withering skin, sinew spasm, flaccid leg and even contracture. If the doctor cannot advice the patient strictly and change their mind, and just yields to the patient's preference, it will cause the condition to worsen, so that the disease cannot be relieved and the treatment has no effect. This is the fourth fault of diagnosis and treatment.

Whenever diagnosing the diseases, the doctor should know the onset and end of the disease as well as the other factors concerned with the disease. When inquiring into the history and taking pulse, the different features of male or female patients should also be taken into consideration. Separation from friends and family and endless memory will cause disturbance of anxiety, fear, joy and anger, deficiency of five solid viscera, and depletion of blood and Qi. If a doctor doesn't know them, what is the point in his medical technique? Anyone who was once rich will have severe impairment of spirit, causing damage to the sinews and meridians. Though the patient can still walk about, there will be no production of body fluid; so, the old impairment and stagnation will cause Qi-blood to be retained in Yang aspect leading to pus accumulation and the intermittent attack of heat and cold. When an unskillful doctor treats this kind of disease, he will needle Yin–Yang meridians time after time, resulting in body collapse and spasm of four limbs and hastening of death. For this disease, the doctor can neither understand the condition nor inquire about the cause of disease, and he can only predicate the date of death. He is really a kind of quack doctor. This is the fifth fault in diagnosis and treatment.

All the five faults above are caused by careless learning of medical technique and unawareness of social and personal life. It's believed that when the sage treats diseases, he should be familiar with Yin–Yang of the heavens and the earth, orders of four-season, five solid viscera and six hollow viscera, Yin–Yang and exterior–interior of meridians, and indications of acupuncture, moxibustion, stone needle and indication of drugs. He must also have enough social experience to understand the classical principles, distinguish the features of the noble or humble and poor or rich to differentiate the nature of diseases, and inquire the age of the young or the old patient to know the condition of being strong or weak. He should observe the part of the abnormal complexion and know the onset and end of the disease combined with information of eight winds and nine pulse-taking locations, so his diagnosis and treatment will be relatively perfect.

The key principle of treatment is to emphasize the Qi status in the body and hence seek the root of the disease; if this fails, its pathological changes are located between the exterior and interior. The doctor should apply the treatment based on the condition of blood and Qi and stick to the principles of acupuncture. In this way, the doctor shall make no mistakes in his medical career. If not knowing the principle of acupuncture, it will cause heat stagnation and accumulation in the five solid viscera and carbuncles in the six hollow viscera. Diagnosing carelessly is called loss of routine. The doctor should cautiously follow the principles is in accordance with principles in the classics: *The Upper Set of Classics* and *The Lower Set of Classics*. If a doctor can ponder Yin and Yang, differentiate common and uncommon diseases as well as the changes of the five solid viscera, judge complexion on Mingtang (nasal region), and integrate the onset and end, he can practice medicine in an invincible manner.

Chapter 78

Precautions for Four Diagnostic Faults

Yellow Emperor was sitting in the bright hall with Leigong beside him. Yellow Emperor said: You are proficient in many books and have undergone many practices. Please introduce your experience about the success and failure, and explain why it is successful and why it failed.

Leigong answered: I learned the specialty from the classical books and former teachers. Though they are known for perfect knowledge, they still make some faults and errors clinically. Please explain the reason behind this for me.

Emperor said: Is it because you are young and your intelligence hasn't matured? Is the classical analysis interfered by incorrect view of crowd? There are twelve meridians and 365 collaterals, which are known to all and applied by all doctors. The so-called imperfect effect is attributed to no concentration, no regular thinking and no harmony between the external and the internal, leading to puzzles and errors.

The doctors don't know the reversal and compliance of Yin and Yang in diagnostics, which is the first cause of failure in the treatment. The student is not proficient in the teacher's instruction and becomes infatuated with informal techniques, takes the wrong as the right, concocts various excuses with self-content, and wrongly uses stone needles leading to sequelae, which is the second cause of failure in the treatment. The doctor does not know the difference between house condition and life status among the poor or rich, noble or humble as well as physical cold or warm, he cannot distinguish the proper diet for patients, nor identify individual braveness and timidity, and he does not know the analogy comparison, so this can disturb his medical thinking and reasonable analysis in clinical practice, which is the third cause of failure in the treatment. When diagnosing the disease, the doctor ignores the onset of the disease, ill emotion and improper diet, indulgence of daily life or impairment due to toxin during history-taking, which is preceded by examination including palpating Cunkou. Thus, how can the correct diagnosis be made? So instead, the wrong diagnosis and the related terms are given carelessly, which is the fourth cause of failure in the treatment.

Therefore, some doctors at present are content to talk freely and endlessly, but in fact they have no elucidation about Chi and Cun and no consideration about human affairs closely. The principle for clinical treatment is to concentrate attention calmly and firmly. If the doctor feels the Cunkou pulse hastily after sitting, he can be blind to five pulses and the various causes of different cases. Then he begins to blame himself, and even attributes this failure to his teachers. Hence, his treatment cannot follow the proper principle and so will be distrusted by the mass of patients. However, he will be satisfied with his occasional success in his careless clinical treatment. Ah! How mysterious and delicate the medical knowledge is! Who can really master its truth?! The law of medicine is comprehensive, which can be compared to the heavens and the earth as well as four seas. If you don't realize it, I can tell you the truth so that you can be enlightened from the blurred world.

Chapter 79

Categorization of Yin and Yang

On the first day of spring, Yellow Emperor was sitting in great state to observe the eight directions and inspect eight winds.

Emperor asked Leigong: In terms of categorization of Yin and Yang and the fundamental of meridians, which one is the most important among five solid viscera?
Leigong answered: Spring is categorized as the first and second in heavenly stem, as well as wood element in green, which corresponds to liver and governs 72 days in spring. Then liver pulse is the main manifestation. So, I think liver is the most important.
Emperor said: Through reading *The Upper Set of Classics* and *The Lower Set of Classics* involving Yin–Yang and reasonable analysis, the most important one that you regard is actually the most inferior.

After fasting for seven days, Leigong sat beside the Emperor again in the morning.

Emperor said: The third Yang (Taiyang) is the cardinal meridian, the second Yang (Yangming) is the linking meridian and the first Yang (Shaoyang) is the free meridian, by which the start and termination of Qi from five solid viscera can be informed. The third Yin (Taiyin) is the exterior meridian, the second Yin (Shaoyin) is the interior meridian and the first Yin (Jueyin) is the start and termination of meridian like moon waxing and waning, which reflects the moving phase of Yin and Yang.

Leigong said: I still do not understand it.

Emperor said: The so-called third Yang is Taiyang as cardinal meridian. The pulse of third Yang terminates at hand-Taiyin, and it is stringy and floating but not sunken, which should be judged with measurement and observed attentively in terms of the theory of Yin–Yang. The so-called second Yang is Yangming. The pulse of second Yang terminates at hand-Taiyin and it is stringy, sunken and rapid but not tympanic. For the disease with high fever, the corresponding pulse indicates death. The first Yang is Shaoyang. The pulse of Shaoyang terminates at hand Taiyin and connects upward with Renying region. The pulse of Shaoyang is stringy, rapid, suspending but not expired and indicates the disease of Shaoyang. The solitary Yin pulse indicates doomed death.

The third Yin refers to the Taiyin meridian and governs the six meridians to connect the lung meridian of hand-Taiyin, which has the deep and bouncing but not floating pulse and indicates heart spirit deficiency. The second Yin refers to the Shaoyin meridian and extends to lung. Its pulse Qi flows to the bladder and is connected with spleen and stomach. The first Yin, i.e., Jueyin meridian moves solitarily to Cunkou of hand-Taiyin meridian, and meridian-Qi is exhausted under such a condition. Its pulse is floating but not bouncing, hooky and slippery. The pulses of the six meridians appear alternatively, like alternation of Yin and Yang. They are interlaced, connected with the five solid viscera and synthesized to Yin–Yang. The single pulse toward Cunkou is regarded as the host pulse and the following pulse as the guest pulse.

Leigong: I understood what Your Majesty has said, and with the theory of meridians that you instructed me and the way mentioned in *Reasonable Analysis* I learned that knowledge can be integrated reasonably. However, I still don't understand the relationship between Yin and Yang as well as male and female.

Emperor: The third Yang (Taiyang) serves as father, the second Yang (Yangming) as defense and the first Yang (Shaoyang) as pivot. The third Yin (Taiyin) serves as mother, the second Yin (Shaoyin) as female and the first Yin (Jueyin) as solitary envoy.

With the second Yang (Yangming) and the first Yin (Jueyin) involved, Yangming mainly governs disease, which cannot dominate the first Yin and has soft and stirring pulse and sinking Qi of the nine orifices. With the third Yang (Taiyang) and the first Yin (Jueyin) involved, Taiyang meridian governs the disease. And the first Yin (liver Qi) cannot stop cold-water (Jueyin), leading to disturbance of five solid viscera internally and fright externally. With the second Yin (Shaoyin) and the second Yang (Yangming) involved, the disease occurs in lung. The pulse of Shaoyin is sunken, and its Qi dominates lung to damage spleen internally and to impair the four limbs externally. With the second Yin (Shaoyin) and the second Yang (Yangming) involved, the disease occurs in kidney and has incoherent scolding, frantic behavior and head disease as mania. With the second Yin (Shaoyin) and the first Yang (Shaoyang) involved, the diseases occur in kidney, in which Yin evil lingers in the heart freely, the cavity below epigastrium is obstructed as if being embanked, and the four limbs are flaccid as if falling apart. With the first Yin (jueyin) and the first Yang (Shaoyang) involved and exhausted, Yin Qi invades heart and moves up and down irregularly with anorexia, incontinence of excretion and dry throat, leading to the disease in spleen. With the second Yang (Yangming) and the third Yin (Taiyin) involved, all the extreme Yin are included, in which Yin Qi fails to come through Yang, Yang Qi fails to inhibit Yin or both Yin and Yang are confined and exhausted; with Yang Qi floating, blood lump can develop; with Yin Qi sinking, abscess will develop. If both Yin and Yang are hyperactive, the diseases will involve the genitals of the males and females. Analysis of the bright heavens in the upper combined with profound earth in the lower can help anticipate the date of death through consideration of the yearly Qi as the primary factor.

Leigong: I'd like to ask how to anticipate the date of death.
Yellow Emperor gave no response. Leigong asked again.
Yellow Emperor: It's stated in the classics.

Leigong: I'd like to know about the date of death.
Yellow Emperor: For the diseases occurring in winter, if manifestation is associated with Yang hyperactivity, there will appear dead sign of pulse in the first month of spring and death will occur at the end of spring. For the diseases occurring in winter, if the normal functions are exhausted, just like grass and salix leaves being killed, there will be exhaustion of both Yin and Yang in spring and the death will occur in the first month of spring. The diseases occurring in spring are Yang-killing; if both Yang and Yin are exhausted, death will occur on the date when grass turns dry. For the diseases occurring in

summer, the death date will be within ten days. If Yin and Yang are intercrossed, death will occur on the date when thin ice is formed. For the diseases occurring in autumn, if triple Yang meridians are involved, the diseases will be cured automatically. If Yin and Yang are intercrossing, the patient finds it difficult to sit down after standing and difficult to stand after sitting down. If the third Yang (Taiyang) is coming alone, the death will occur on the date when water is frozen thick. If the second Yang (Shaoyin) is coming alone, the death will occur in solar term of Rain-water.

Chapter 80

Measurement of Exuberance and Exhaustion

Leigong asked: Qi can be exuberant or deficient. And what is the reversal? What is the compliance?
Yellow Emperor answered: Yang Qi tends to run from the left while Yin Qi from the right. Qi of the aged declines from the upper and Qi of the young exuberates from the lower. Therefore, the diseases in spring and summer have the returning Yang, indicating life, while the diseases in autumn and winter have returning Yang, indicating death. Conversely, the diseases in autumn and winter have the nature of Yin, which indicates life. Therefore no matter how strong Qi is, any Qi reversal contributes to critical syndrome.

Leigong asked again: Does the excess contribute to crisis?
Emperor answered: As soon as it ascends, Yang Qi fails to descend and severe cold comes down to the knees. It indicates death in autumn and winter for the young, while for the aged it indicates life in autumn and winter. After ascending Qi fails to descend, vertex diseases are caused, which can neither be attributed to Yang nor Yin. Since Qi in five solid viscera is isolated without any obvious features that are observed, like

staying in the wild or living in an empty room till his last breath, the patient can survive no more than one day.

Therefore, the critical reversal due to less Qi makes the patient have absurd dreams and even nightmares in extreme cases. The pulses of triple Yang are critically depleted and the pulses of triple Yin are faint, all indicating less Qi. Therefore, deficiency of lung Qi makes the patient dream of miserable events, seeing bloody corpses everywhere, or at the dominating time of battlefield scenery. The deficiency of kidney Qi makes the patient dream of shipwreck and drowning people, or at the dominating time of diving into water as fearing something. The deficiency of liver Qi makes the patient dream of aromatic mushroom and green herbs, or at the dominating time of hiding under trees and not daring to stand. The deficiency of heart Qi makes the patient dream of firefighting and something burning or at the dominating time of a big fire flaring. The deficiency of spleen Qi makes the patient dream of food deficiency, or at the dominating time of building a wall and roof. All these changes are associated with Qi deficiency of five solid viscera with excessive Yang Qi and deficient Yin Qi. Five examinations are comprehended and Yin and Yang are regulated based on *Medirians*.

Examinations and diagnosis have five measurements of human body, including that of pulse, solid viscera, muscles, sinews and acupoints of Yin or Yang. Yin Qi and Yang Qi are observed completely, whereby human disease must be identified. Because the pulsation is not constant as usual, sometimes Yin pulse is disordered, Yang pulse is hyperactive and pulse is missed, so the examination and diagnosis don't have an invariable method. When examining and diagnosing, the social position of the patient should be identified to distinguish the ordinary from the notable people. If a doctor cannot comprehend his teacher's instruction, his medical technique cannot be excellent; so, he cannot distinguish the reversal and compliance. He will have inappropriate practice by caring this and ignoring that and follow Yang instead of Yin, and also fail to integrate everything. Finally his examination and diagnosis cannot be reasonable, and this will be passed down, misguiding the generations and exposing the mistakes of violating the ancient methods.

When extreme Yin deficiency is reached, the heavenly Qi is exhausted, while when Yang exuberance is reached, the earthly Qi is deficient. To combine Yin and Yang is the principle that the superior doctors should follow. When Yin and Yang are combined together, Yang Qi arrives earlier and Yin Qi arrives later. Hence, any saint doctor should uphold the regulation of examination and diagnosis, including differentiating the priority of Yin or Yang, with reference of *Ordinary and Extraordinary Manifestations* as well as *Diagnostic Sixty Poems*, synthesizing the detailed clinical information, taking the history of Yin and Yang variation, and analyzing the status of five emotions. After that, the judgment can be made to define the key of excess and deficiency and findings of five measurements, by which the doctor can confidently make a diagnosis. Thus, the diagnosis is impossible if looking at Yin but ignoring Yang. The medical personnel is not qualified if observing Yang but neglecting Yin. His medical practice cannot last long if he knows only the left but not the right, the right but not the left, the upper but not the lower, or knowing the first but not the later. The doctor should know ugliness and kindness, illness and health, high and low, sitting and rising, and acting and resting. Only in this way can the diagnosis be made perfect, which has been proven to be correct from generation to generation.

When the excess is seen at onset, the deficiency should be considered. The doctor should examine the upper and lower part of the body and the conditions of pulses to find out the pathologic mechanism. Notably, the weak physique and deficient Qi indicate death; the excessive physique and Qi with deficient pulse Qi indicate death; excessive pulse Qi and deficient physique Qi indicate life. Hence, the medical consultation has rigid regulations, the doctor should follow the proper living manner and behave in good and moral way to embody God's will with a clear and pure mind. The details include observation of the upper and lower, identification of the evils in four seasons and eight solar terms, differentiation of the affected region in five solid viscera, palpation of the dynamic pulse, examination of the smooth, unsmooth, cold or warm profiles of Chi-skin, and inspection of stool and urine together with the tendency of reversal or compliance. By these methods, the disease can be confirmed and the diagnosis can also be perfect. Hence when examining or diagnosing, either respiration or mind should be observed, nothing can be out of order, and the medical behavior should be qualified, by which the practice of medicine can be continued for a long time. Otherwise, the principles will be violated and morals will be lost.

Chapter 81

Explanation of Subtleties of Essence

When Yellow Emperor was sitting in the bright hall, Leigong asked: I learn medicine from Your Majesty and will pass it on, and these teachings are based on the medical classics, including human behavior, physique and functions, theory of Yin and Yang, acupuncture and moxibustion, and decoction and nourishment. However, clinical practice varies from wisdom to indifference, which is not always perfect. If the primary knowledge is instructed first, like emotion of sadness, sorrow, joy and anger, climatic factors of the dry, damp, cold and summer-heat, the difference of Yin and Yang as well as female health, students will inquire about their fundamentals. Then the information of the noble or humble, the rich or poor, and strong or weak physique of human is introduced and the students are required to master and apply properly according to the clinical situation, which I have learnt carefully. Now I have some silly and simple questions, which have not been addressed in the medical classics, and I will like to know their answers.
Emperor said: It's really a big problem.

Leigong asked: When crying, there is less shedding or even no shedding of tears or there is shedding of tears with less snivel; what is the reason for this?
Emperor answered: It is recorded in the medical classics.

Leigong asked again: Where does tear come from and where does snivel come from?
Emperor answered: Though the question you've asked isn't significant to the treatment, doctors should know it, which is also a phenomenon of natural law. Heart is the organ responsible for the essence among the five solid viscera, while the eyes are the orifices of heart and the complexion is the expressive luxury of heart. Hence when a person is in good health, the harmony is expressed in the eyes, while when he is in poor health, the depression is expressed in the eyes. Therefore when a person is sad or sorrowful, tears run down his eyes, which are produced from water. Water originates from the stored fluid that originates from the extreme Yin that originates from the essence of kidney. The reason why the water from the kidney essence doesn't flow out usually is that the water is controlled, restrained and hidden by the kidney essence, which makes the water not flow without control.

The essence from water forms the mind and the essence from the fire forms the spirit. When water and fire interact with each other and are both in sorrow, the tears then are produced. As the saying goes, 'If the sorrow in heart is actually the sorrow in mind, the mind essence and heart essence will converge in the eyes.' When heart and kidney are both in sorrow, spiritual Qi will be transmitted to heart-essence. However if not to the mind (kidney), the mind (kidney) will be alone in sorrow so that the tears will run out of the eyes. The tears and snivel both originate from the brain. The brain corresponds to Yin while the marrow is the filling of the cavity of the bone, so water seeping out of the brain turns into snivel. Kidney (mind) governs the bones and hence tears come out followed by snivel, because both of them pertain to the same element. In fact, the snivel is related to tears, as if they are brothers, and they will die together under critical condition and live together under normal condition. If the mind (kidney) is in sorrow first, then both tears and snivel come out together and weep bitterly. Tears and snivel fall down at the same time just because they belong to the same category.

Leigong: Great. When a person is crying, they shed no tears or shed only a few tears with no snivel, and why?

Emperor: They shed no tears when crying just because there is no sorrow when crying. There is no weeping because the person has no sympathy and does not feel sadness. If having no sympathy, the mind (kidney) is not in sorrow and Yin–Yang fails to be maintained mutually. So, how can tears be shed alone? Hence, if mind is in sorrow, it leads to depression that surges to Yin (brain), which makes mind leave the eyes and then the spirit cannot protect the essence; when both the essence and the spirit leave the eyes, the tears and snivel will be shed.

Moreover, don't you read and recite the quotation from the medical classics? With the reversal, the eyes fail to see anything. When a person is ill with Qi reversal, Yang Qi will be confined to the upper while Yin-Qi is confined to the lower. With Yang-Qi confined in the upper, the fire Qi is flaming up alone; with Yin Qi confined in the lower, the feet become cold, which leads to distension. Since solitary water cannot dominate the fire of five solid viscera, the eyes fail to see. Therefore, when facing wind, tears are shed ceaselessly. Because the wind attacks the eyes, in which Yang Qi is kept in the essence and then fire Qi is flaming in the eyes, tears will be shed when facing wind. It could be used as a metaphor that rapid fire causes the wind that causes the rain, which shares the similar mechanism.

Appendix A

Acupuncture Therapy for Abnormal Qi-Phase*

Yellow Emperor asked: The interval Qi fails to ascend and descend in the current year with changed Qi-shifting, leading to fulminant depression, which I already know. However, is there any solution to get rid of it for prevention and for saving creatures?

Qibo kowtowed and bowed again to answer: What a clever question! I was taught by the Master that, if having understood the motion of primordial six-Qi, one should be versed in methods of acupuncture in order to reduce depression, promote motion of six-Qi, reinforce weakness, maintain genuine-Qi, purge exuberance and eliminate excess, and finally get rid of the suffering.

Emperor: I'd like to know the details.

Qibo: The interval Qi fails to ascend, indicating crisis. Wood Qi is going to ascend, which is inhibited by Tianzhu Star of metal. If the depression of wood Qi wants to be dispersed, it

---

* The content was probably added by anonymous authors after the middle of the 8th Century as the original text has been lost.

has to wait for the time on the throne, when the well acupoint of foot-Jueyin meridian should be needled. Fire Qi is going to ascend, which is inhibited by Tianpeng Star of water. If the depression of fire Qi wants to be dispersed, it has to wait for the time on the throne, when the creek acupoint of pericardium meridian for both monarch-fire and minister-fire should be needled. Earth Qi is going to ascend, which is inhibited by Tianchong Star of wood. If the depression of earth Qi wants to be dispersed, it has to wait for the time on the throne, when the creek acupoint of foot Taiyin meridian should be needled. Metal Qi is going to ascend, which is inhibited by Tianying Star of fire. If the depression of metal Qi wants to be dispersed, it has to wait for the time on the throne, when river acupoint of hand Taiyin meridian should be needled. Water Qi is going to ascend, which is inhibited by Tianrui Star of earth. If the depression of water Qi wants to be dispersed, it has to wait for the time on the throne, when estuary acupoint of foot Shaoyin meridian should be needled.

Emperor: The interval Qi fails to ascend with no advancement, which can be prevented; I'd like to know the descent of interval Qi so that the failure of descending can be prevented.
Qibo: If the ascent of interval Qi is understood, it may help us understand well the descent, and so the failure of ascending or descending can be all prevented. Wood Qi is going to descend but is inhibited by Dihao Star (earth-white), so it is descending in vain. Wood Qi is depressed due to inhibition and can be dispersed to reach the position. The descending Qi in depression bursts out violently just as ascending Qi is waiting for the position. Wood Qi is descending in vain, so its depression is formed more quickly. After having descended, its exuberant Qi

can be reduced. To this end, the exit accupoint of hand-Taiyin and entry acupoint should be needled. Fire Qi is going to descend but is inhibited by Dixuan Star (earth-black), so it is descending in vain. Fire Qi is depressed due to inhibition and can reach the position after the depression is inhibited. Then the dominating Qi should be reduced and the depression be dispersed. For this, the exit acupoint of foot Shaoyin and the entry acupoint of Taiyang should be needled. Earth Qi is going to descend but is inhibited by Dicang Star (earth-green), so it is descending in vain. Earth Qi is depressed due to inhibition, and after depression is dispersed, it can reach the position. To this end, the exit acupoint of foot Jueyin and the entry acupoint of foot Shaoyang should be needled. Metal Qi is going to descend but is inhibited by Ditong Star (earth-red), so it is descending in vain and is depressed due to inhibition. After the depression is inhibited, it can reach the position. Then its exuberant Qi should be reduced and its depression should be dispersed. For this, the exit acupoint of pericardium meridian and the entry acupoint of hand Shaoyang should be needled. Water Qi is going to descend but is inhibited by Difu Star (earth-hill), so it is descending in vain. Water Qi is depressed due to inhibition, and after the depression is dispersed, water Qi can reach the position. Then the exuberant Qi of water should be reduced and its depression be dispersed. For this, the exit acupoints of foot Taiyin and the entry acupoint of foot Yangming should be needled.

Emperor: The five-phase arrives early or late and six-Qi ascends or descends alternatively with mutual acception or non-acceptance; can I know the acupuncture method concerned?

Qibo: The treatment should be based on the source of the transformation. The excess should be purged, while the insufficiency should be supplemented. So-called reducing the excess means to inhibit the depression according to the order of six-Qi, and to reduce the depressive Qi by regulating the transformative source of five-phase; so-called supplementing the insufficiency means to support the phase-Qi and avoid deficiency evil. Both reducing and supplementing methods are drawn from *The Secrete Analects*.

Yellow Emperor: As regards the needling for the disease concerned with ascending and descending, I've already understood the key. Now I know that the heaven-governing Qi isn't promoted and then loses its normal administration, which makes all the transformation disturbed and even abnormal and then people suffer from diseases. Can we prevent it to protect the health of people? I'd like to know the explanation for this. **Qibo kowtowed and bowed again to answer**: What a detailed question! Your Majesty has mentioned the superior principle that shows your sagely notion and great sympathy for saving the people, so I will make a full statement to help clarify the complex situation. If Taiyang continues to govern the throne, Jueyin cannot be promoted, and it makes Jueyin Qi obstructed in the upper, for which the creek (Xingjian, LR02) acupoint of foot-Jueyin should be purged. If Jueyin continues to govern the throne, Shaoyin cannot be promoted, and it makes Shaoyin Qi obstructed in the upper, for which the creek (Laogong, PC08) acupoint of pericardium meridian should be needled. If Shaoyin continues to govern the throne, Taiyin cannot be promoted, and it makes Taiyin Qi obstructed in the upper, for which the creek (Dadu, SP02) acupoint of foot-Taiyin should be needled. If Taiyin continues to govern the throne, Shaoyang cannot be promoted, and it makes Shaoyang Qi obstructed with no communication, for which the creek acupoint (Yemen, TE02) of hand-Shaoyang should be needled. If Shaoyang continues to govern the throne, Yangming cannot be promoted, and it makes Shaoyang-Qi obstructed with no communication to the upper, for which the creek acupoint (Yuji, LU10) of hand-Taiyin should be needled. If Yangming continues to govern the throne, Taiyang cannot be promoted, and it makes Taiyang Qi still obstructed, for which the creek acupoint (Rangu, KI02) of foot-Shaoyin should be needled.

Emperor: As to yearly Qi failing to be promoted, I know the key. Now I'd like to know the unabdication so as to reduce the excess and avoid its harmful effects; can I understand it?
Qibo: If yearly Qi is excessive and continues to administer the throne, it is called unabdication. It makes earth-governing Qi fail to come back as interval Qi and makes new heaven-governing Qi be promoted, so that the yearly Qi continues to administer as in the previous year. In the year of the 6th and 12th, the yearly Qi has excess so that Jueyin won't abdicate with wind prevailing in the upper and wood transformation being distributed in the heavens, for which the entry acupoint (Ququan, LR08) of foot-Jueyin should be needled. In the year of 1st and 7th, the yearly Qi has excess so that Jueyin won't abdicate with heat prevailing in the upper and fire transformation being distributed in the heavens, for which the entry acupoint (Quze, PC03) of hand-Jueyin should be needled. In the year of 2nd and 8th, the yearly Qi has excess so that Taiyin won't abdicate with the damp prevailing in the upper and rain transformation being distributed in the heavens, for which the entry

acupoint (Yinlingquan, SP09) of foot-Taiyin should be needled. In the year of 3rd and 9th, the yearly Qi has excess so that Shaoyang won't abdicate with heat prevailing in the upper and fire transformation being distributed in the heavens, for which the entry acupoint (Tianjing, TE10) of hand-Taiyin should be needled. In the year of 4th and 10th, the yearly Qi has excess so that Yangming won't abdicate with metal prevailing in the upper and dry transformation being distributed in the heavens, for which the entry acupoint (Chize, LU05) of hand-Taiyin should be needled. In the year of 5th and 11th, the yearly Qi has excess so that Taiyang won't abdicate with cold prevailing in the upper and transformation of fierce cold being distributed in the heavens, for which the entry acupoint (Yingu, KI10) of foot-Shaoyin should be needled. The Qi reversal of the heavens and earth will be expressed in the human diseases, and by the same needling method these diseases can be treated or be prevented.

Yellow Emperor: The stiff or soft heavenly stem loses the position, and can it make Qi of both year phase and six-position deficient? It can be expressed in the human diseases, and can they be calmed down?

Qibo: What a profound question! The profound principle should be understood as the abnormal Qi shifting of the heaven-governing and earth-governing accumulating for three years and turning into pestilence; if the root can be identified, the pestilence will be avoided.

Supposing in the year of the first-1st if stiff or soft heavenly stem loses the positions, the stiff Qi of heaven-governing cannot be promoted, the soft Qi of solitary earth-governing will be deficient, and the orders of four seasons are deranged to which the tonality cannot comply. Thus after three years, it will turn into pestilence, and its severity should be analyzed while its depth should be observed. With the pestilence coming, needling should be given; when needling, the kidney acupoint (Shenshu, BL23) is needled first, and in three days the stream acupoint (Taibai, SP03) of foot Taiyin. Also if the Qi in the lower of the sixth-4th cannot be promoted, the Qi in the heavens of the first-1st will become isolated, which will turn into the earth-pestilence in three years. Its treatment with supplementing and reducing methods are just the same as that in the first-1st year. After acupuncture, the patient is not allowed to take a night walk or a long journey and must also keep clean and quiet and practice abstinence, so that the healthy Qi will be restored. Those with chronic kidney diseases should face the south at the third watch-time, clear the mind and settle the disordered brain as well as hold their breath after inhalation and stretch the neck to swallow down saliva, imagined as a hard thing, seven times, during which much saliva underneath the tongue is swallowed.

Supposing in the year of the third-3rd if stiff or soft heavenly stem loses the position, in this case the stiff heavenly stem in the upper loses its position while the soft earthly branch in the lower cannot administer alone. Then the yearly Qi of water phase isn't too excessive and cannot execute and control the climatic Qi. The heaven-governing Qi is excessive but fails to be promoted in the upper, which results in disharmony between the heavens and the earth, leading to the abnormal note in tonality. Thus Qi of the heaven-governing and five-phase are discordant and will turn into pestilence in three years. Since there are various severities and differences, the pestilence will emerge in the later three years if slow, but in the first three years if severe. The heart-acupoint (Xinshu, BL15) should be supplemented first and, the next five days, then the entry-acupoint (Yingu, KI10) of kidney meridian. Also in the year of the first-1st or the eighth-6th, the soft heavenly stem cannot be promoted in accordance with the stiff heavenly stem, which is also called missing position. That is, Qi of both the earth-governing and year phase are deficient and in three years turns into water pestilence, whose acupuncture treatment is the same as the mentioned above. After acupuncture, the patient should avoid great joy with a sentimental quality, otherwise his Qi will be scattered again. The patient is required to keep quiet for seven days, calm down the mind and avoid contemplation.

Supposing in the year of the seventh-5th, if stiff or soft heavenly stem loses the position, the heaven-governing Qi in the upper will lose its position while the earth-governing Qi in the lower will have no cooperation. Since the year of the second or seventh corresponds to the metal phase, the upper and lower cannot cooperate mutually, the previous heaven-governing Qi fails to abdicate, and the dominant Qi of current year phase is coming, leading to the discordance between the upper and lower, which is called missing position and non-response of Shang note in tonality of Guxi and Linzhong. Thus the celestial motion becomes abnormal, which then turns into great pestilence in three years. Then the changes of celestial motion should be observed, and there are various differences; mild difference will result in mild pestilence in three years, while the severe difference will result in the severe pestilence. For treatment, the liver-acupoint (Ganshu, BL18) should be supplemented and in three days the current-acupoint (Jingqu, LU08) should be needled. After acupuncture, the patient should tranquilize the spirit for seven days, that is, avoid raging, as otherwise the genuine Qi will be scattered. Also in the year of the first-1st, the lower earth-governing Qi in the year of the first-1st or the second-7th loses the positions, when the earthly branch of the second is soft while the heavenly stem of the 7th administers alone, which is also called missing position. That is, when the Qi of climatic positions and year phases administer alone, it will turn into pestilence till the metal phase is coming. The various differences of earthly Qi should be analyzed, and after considering the degrees of differences, the emerging speed of the pestilence can be anticipated. For any positions lost in the year of the second or the seventh, the acupuncture methods are the same, during which liver Qi should be kept smooth and anger should be avoided.

Supposing in the year of the ninth-7th, if stiff or soft heavenly stem loses the position, the upper Qi of the ninth year fails to be promoted as heaven-governing while the lower Qi of the fourth year administers alone. Though the ninth year pertains to Yang, there is still insufficiency, abnormality, and missing position of the upper and the lower, but both upper and lower will collaborate one day. Between the two there appears mild or severe difference with respective definite changes, which is similar to the fact that the two discarded Jues in Yang and Yin aspects will have the chord one day. There is mild or severe difference to be observed, which will turn into great pestilence in three years. The spleen-acupoint (Pishu, BL20) should be needled and in three days the well-acupoint (Dadun, LR01) of liver meridian should be needled. After acupuncture, the patient is required to calm down the spirit for seven days, avoid indulgence in drinking and singing, to prevent no Qi scattering, avoid overeating and raw food to keep spleen Qi replete with no congestion and Qi stagnation, and avoid sitting for a long time, too sour food and all raw food. The patient had better take the sweet and plain food. Also in the year of the first-1st or the fourth-10th, the lower Qi loses the position without coordination with the heaven-governing Qi; that is, Qi is not in the due position and Qi in the lower cannot cooperate with the upper Qi of the ninth year, which is also called missing position, but there exists disharmony between nature and human. Hence, the soft heavenly stem cannot coordinate with the stiff heavenly stem, and then earthly Qi and year phase fail to coordinate, which then turns into pestilence in three years; the acupuncture treatments are the same as that for wood-pestilence.

Supposing in the year of the fifth-9th, if stiff or soft heavenly stem loses the position, though the year of the fifth or tenth pertains to fire phase, this Yang year isn't too excessive, in which the upper Qi fails to be promoted as stiff heaven-governing Qi while the lower soft Qi administers alone at the earth-governing throne, so that the Qi isn't normal and the evil Qi appears. When overlapping and shifting the positions, there are various differences between the upper and the lower, which is going to coordinate with each other, just like the tonality firstly being cord. Thus the yearly phase loses its due time, and the fire pestilence will come in three years, and at this time the lung-acupoint (Feishu, BL13) should be needled. After acupuncture, the patient should calm down the mind for seven days and avoid great sorrow, which will otherwise stir lung to scatter the genuine Qi. If the patient wants to replete his lung Qi, the key is to perform breath exercise. Also in the year of the first-1st or tenth-12th, so-called missing throne is that the soft heavenly stem loses the throne in the lower, which has no coordination with the stiff heavenly stem in the upper. It is also called no harmony between the years of the fifth or tenth, leading to deficiency of both the year phase and earth-governing Qi. After three years, it will turn into pestilence termed fire-pestilence.

Therefore, the five phases are applied to distinguish the five successive years, define the missing throne and elucidate the acupuncture therapy. Then, both epidemic and pestilence are defined based on missing throne of the stiff heavenly stem in the upper and the soft heavenly term in the lower, which are of the same entity. With regard to acupuncture for pestilence, there are only five therapies, all of which can direct every type of missing throne and also be generalized into the theory of five elements.

Yellow Emperor: I've heard that five kinds of pestilence can all be spread among people from adults to children with the similar manifestations. If the therapies are not applied, how to prevent the infection?
Qibo: If one isn't infected, there will be healthy Qi inside the body so that the evil Qi cannot invade. In addition, one should avoid the toxic Qi, which can be inhaled and exhaled through the nose. If the healthy Qi flows out of the brain continuously, the evil Qi cannot invade. So-called healthy Qi originating from the brain just concentrates the mind in the room and imagines that heart is as bright as the sun.

Before entering a pestilence room, one can imagine that the blue Qi comes out of liver, runs to the east and transforms into woods. Then one can imagine that the white Qi comes out of lung, runs to the west and transforms into metal spear and armor. Then one can imagine that the red Qi comes out of heart, runs to the south and transforms into bright flame.

Then one can imagine that the black Qi comes out of kidney, runs to the north and transforms into water. Then one can imagine that the yellow Qi comes out of spleen, remains in the central region and transforms into earth. Once the imagination of protecting the body by five-Qi is clear, one should also imagine that there is shining Big Dipper over the head and then can enter the pestilence room. The next method is to apply emetic therapy on the Spring Equinox before the sunrise.

The next method is to induce sweating with medicated bathing three times the day after the Rain Water term. The next method is to use the formula Small Gold Bolus, composed of 2 liang of cinnabar, 1 liang of water grinding realer, 1 liang of lamellar orpiment and half liang of purple gold, which are put into one box and then sealed tightly. Then a one-chi pit is dug and rammed with no stove and processing, which is calcined with 20 jin of fuel for seven days. After cooling for another seven days, the box is taken out; the next day the drugs are taken out of the box and buried into the ground. In seven days, the drugs will be taken out and ground for three days, then mixed with fined white sandy honey and made into pills the size of Chinese parasol seeds. Every morning, one should face the east to inhale solar essence, take one pill with ice water and swallow it along with the inhaled air; taking ten pills can prevent the epidemic infection.

Yellow Emperor asked: When one is in poor health, the spirit will be wandering and lose its position, which makes ghost evil invade externally, leading to early death; so, how to maintain the genuine Qi? I'd like to know the acupuncture therapy concerned.

Qibo again kowtowed and answered: What a meaningful question! Though wandering and losing its position, the spirit is inside the body so as not to cause death. However, if there is evil that invades, it will result in early death. Specifically when Qi of Jueyin loses its position with deficient heavenly Qi and one is ill with innate deficiency of liver Qi, the patient will suffer from double Qi deficiency. That is, when the soul is wandering in the upper, the evil will invade the body, leading to great Qi reversal. If the body is warm, the needling therapy can be applied, in which the original acupoint Qiuxu (GB40) can be needled first for inhibition followed by liver-acupoint (Ganshu, BL18). If one is ill with innate heart deficiency in the year when both monarch-fire and minister-fire lose their positions as heaven-governing, the patient will suffer from triple Qi deficiency. When the patient has insufficient fire Qi, the black ghost pestilence will invade the body and make him suddenly die. Then the acupoints (Yangchi, TE04) of hand-Shaoyang can be needled and then heart-acupoint (Xinshu, BL15) can be needled repeatedly. If one is ill with innate spleen deficiency in the year when Taiyin loses the position as heaven-governing, the patient will suffer from triple Qi deficiency. When there is insufficient earth Qi, the green ghost pestilence will invade the body and make him suddenly die. Then the original acupoint (Chongyang, ST42) of foot-Yangming can be needled and then spleen-acupoint (Pishu, BL20) can be needled repeatedly. If one is ill with innate lung deficiency in the year when Yangming loses the position as heaven-governing, the patient will suffer from triple Qi deficiency; when with insufficient metal Qi, the red ghost pestilence will invade the body and make him suddenly die; then the acupoints of hand-Yangming can be needled and then lung-acupoint (Feishu, Bl13) can be needled repeatedly. If one is ill with innate kidney deficiency in the year when Taiyang loses the position as heaven-governing, the patient will suffer from triple Qi deficiency. When the patient has insufficient Qi of water phase, the yellow ghost pestilence will affect the healthy Qi of the body, destroy his spirit and soul, and make him suddenly die. Then the acupoints (Hegu, LI04) of foot-Taiyang can be needled and then kidney-acupoint (Shenshu, BL23) can be needled repeatedly.

Yellow Emperor asked: The twelve viscera promote their functions mutually, and if the spirit loses its position, it will make the spirit and vitality imperfect, and this when the evil will take the opportunity to invade the body. Is it possible for acupuncture to treat this? I'd like to know the key.
Qibo kowtowed and bowed again to answer: What a detailed question! These are called the superior theory and genuine principle, and if not for the saint emperors, who can explore these basic questions? Heart is an organ serving as monarch, which is responsible for spirit and mind; for the treatment concerned, the original acupoint (Shenmen, HT07) of hand-Shaoyin meridian can be needled. Lung is an organ serving as prime minister, which is responsible for administration and regulation; for the treatment concerned, the original acupoint (Taiyuan, LU09) of hand-Taiyin meridian can be needled. Liver is an organ serving as general, which is responsible for consideration; for the treatment concerned, the original acupoint (Taichong, LR03) of foot-Jueyin meridian can be needled. Gallbladder is an organ serving as judger, which is responsible for decision; for the treatment concerned, the original acupoint (Qiuxu, GB40) of foot-Shaoyang meridian

can be needled. Pericaridium is an organ serving as envoy, which is responsible for happiness and joy; for the treatment concerned, the creek acupoint (Laogong, PC08) of pericardium meridian can be needled. Spleen is an organ serving as expostulator, which is responsible for wisdom and comprehension; for the treatment concerned, the original acupoint (Taibai, SP03) of spleen meridian can be needled. Stomach is an organ serving as granary official, which is responsible for five flavors; for the treatment concerned, the original acupoint (Chongyang, ST42) of stomach meridian can be needled. Large intestine is an organ serving as transportation official, which is responsible for five changes; for the treatment concerned, the original acupoint (Hegu, LI04) of large intestine meridian can be needled. Small intestine is an organ serving as reception official, which is responsible for transformation; for the treatment concerned, the original acupoint (Wangu, SI04) of small intestine meridian can be needled. Kidney is an organ serving as powerful actor, which is responsible for elaborate functions; for the treatment concerned, the original acupoint (Taixi, KI03) of kidney meridian can be needled. Triple-Jiao is an organ serving as transference dredging official, which is responsible for water passage; for the treatment concerned, the original acupoint (Yangchi, SJ04) of triple-Jiao meridian can be needled. Bladder is an organ serving as reservoir official, which is responsible for storing essence liquid and discharging after Qi transformation; for the treatment concerned, the original acupoint (Jinggu, BL64) of bladder meridian can be needled. The twelve viscera mentioned above cannot lose the collaboration of their functions. Hence, acupuncture therapy has significant functions for maintaining spirit and genuine origin and also for cultivating the genuine Qi, not only for treating disease, so that the spirit Qi should be cultivated and regulated. The most important thing is perseverance, for which the spirit should be supplemented and root of health be strengthened, so that the essence Qi cannot be scattered and the spirit can be kept without separation. Only if the spirit can be kept, so that it does not leave, can the genuine Qi can be intact. If the spirit and physique are separated, it is impossible to reach the genuine realm. The key of genuine realm is closely associated with the natural law, and if the spirit can keep consistent with the natural vitality, the Qi of primordial origin can be restored, which is called primordial returning.

Appendix B

Root of Diseases*

Emperor: The movement of yearly-phase Qi has nine kinds of inhibition, which I already know. Now I'd like to know the details about the shifting and integration of six-Qi. What does position-missing mean?

Qibo: It is associated with ascending to the upper and descending to the lower as well as promotion and abdication, which are stated in the medical classics, respectively. The failure of advancement to the upper or to the lower is termed position-missing. Thus, Qi-shifting fails to interchange position and then has disorders, so that the position-interchanging is in abnormal sequence, i.e., the disorders of four seasons, which finally causes the disturbance of the transformation of everything and leads to human diseases.

Emperor: Six-Qi fails to ascend and descend, I'd like to know the reason for this; there is also the disorder of Qi shifting, and how to understand it?

---

* The content was probably added by anonymous authors after the middle of the 8th Century as the original text has been lost.

Qibo: What a meaningful question you've asked and what a bright principle you've inquired about. The Qi-shifting has some disorders which are associated with the moving mechanism of the heavens and the earth. However, the Qi that should have descended fails to descend, which is blocked by earthly Qi. Moreover the excessive five-phase comes earlier than the due time, which causes the failure of advancement. The Qi that should have descended fails to descend, which is inhibited by yearly-phase while the Qi that should have ascended fails to ascend, which is inhibited by yearly-phase. Then, there is the ascending with no advancement while there is descending with no comedown, the descending with no comedown but ascending to the heavens, or both failure of ascending and descending, which should be differentiated to show disorders of Qi-shifting. The disorders of Qi-shifting often vary with respective differences and accordingly lead to either mild or severe disasters.

Emperor: I'd like to know the reason for meeting the Qi-shifting as well as their domination and inhibition, and how do they turn into human diseases and how are their severities?

Qibo: When Qi-shifting meets with its dominating Qi, inhibition takes center stage. Thus in the year with record of the 5th or 11th, when ascending, wood Qi meets inhibitive Tianzhu Star with excessive metal Qi and is prevented from advancing. Concisely, in the year of Seventh-11th, metal phase comes earlier and this year phase dominates, when wood Qi suddenly fails to advance. That is, when ascending, Qi of wood phase is prevented from ascending. Hence, there is cool air with less wind to constrict and conquer in spring, falling dew and fog again, and withering grass and trees. People then tend to get epidemic diseases earlier, dry throat, fullness of four limbs, and pain of limbs and joints. With prolonged transformation into depression, the big gales are pulling up, breaking and blowing down things with noisy whistling sound. People tend to have stroke, hemiplegia and numbness of hands and feet.

So, in the year marked with 6th or 12th, when ascending to the heavens, monarch-fire meets inhibitive Tianpeng Star with excessive wood Qi and is prevented from advancing. Concisely when Jueyin hasn't been promoted, Shaoyin cannot ascend to the heavens, and when water-phase hasn't ascended to the heavens and Qi of water phase comes into it, monarch-fire is ascending but is prevented by water phase-Qi from advancing, leading to the cool emerging again and the cold rising at dawn and at dusk. People then tend to have hidden Yang turning into vexation internally, fright and palpitation, and intermittent chill and fever. After the prolonging fire Qi culminates in depression, it causes arrival of fulminant heat with reddish wind and atmosphere, transmission of epidemic diseases, the intermittent warm infectious diseases under the warm climate, and even diffusive reddish Qi turning into fire-pestilence. People tend to have heart vexation, agitation and thirst, and if severe the disease can be cured by discharging the heat.

In the year marked with the 1st or 7th, when ascending to the heavens, Taiyin meets inhibitive Tianchong Star with excessive wood Qi and is prevented from advancing. Concisely in the year marked with the Ninth-1st, Qi of wood-phase comes earlier and is prevented from advancing, which causes wind and dust spreading to four directions, frequent rising of gloomy air and no transformation of rain and damp. People then tend to have reversal syndrome due to wind and frequent drooling, hemiplegia with rigidity, distension and fullness. Earthly Qi culminates in depression leading to yellow dust to turn into epidemic diseases. People tend to have illness and die early, and have jaundice on face, limbs and six hollow viscera with fullness and blockage. There is no damp distribution and less rain transformation.

In the year marked with the 2nd or 8th, when ascending to the heavens, Shaoyang meets inhibitive Tianpeng Star with excessive water Qi and is prevented from advancing. Concisely in the year when Taiyin hasn't been promoted, Shaoyin hasn't ascended to the heavens; and when water-phase Qi comes into it, Shaoyin is prevented from advancing, which causes reversal distribution of cold ice with biting cold air like being in winter, water drying up and freezing again, intermittent heat, distributive cold air in summer and intermittent cold. People then tend to have hidden Yang internally, vexing heat rising in the middle, fright and palpitation, and struggle between cold and heat. After prolonged accumulation of fire Qi into depression, there appears rise of sudden heat, reddish wind and diffusive atmosphere, which is transformed into pestilence or hidden heat with internal vexation, impediment syndrome and even reversal syndrome, and bleeding if severe.

In the year marked with the 3rd or 9th, when ascending to the heavens, Yangming meets inhibitive Tianying Star with excessive fire Qi and is prevented from advancing. Concisely in the year marked with the Fifth-9th or Fifth-3rd, when fire-phase Qi comes earlier, metal-Qi is ascending to the heavens but is prevented by fire-phase from advancing, in which no rain falls, west wind frequently blows, and salt and dryness concentrate in nature. People then tend to have heat surging up with panting, cough and bleeding; after prolonged accumulation of metal Qi into depression, there appears white dusty fog and rise of conquering cool Qi. People tend to have hypochondriac fullness, sorrow, cold nasal obstruction, sneeze, dry pharynx, chapped hands and dry skin.

In the year marked with the 4th or 10th, when ascending to the heavens, Taiyang meets inhibitive Tianrui Star with the excessive earthly Qi and is prevented from advancing. Concisely in the year when Yangming hasn't be promoted and Taiyang cannot ascend to the heavens, the earthly phase Qi comes and water-phase Qi is ascending but is prevented from advancing, in which the damp and heat are evaporating and cold Qi is emerging between the heavens and the earth. People then tend to have diarrhea and dyspepsia after prolonged accumulation of water Qi into depression, the cold is coming and overcomes the heat, and hailstones suddenly fall. People then tend to have critical reversal and hiccup, rising internal heat, external Qi impediment, ache of feet and shank, palpitation, vexing heat, sudden anxiety and repeated reversal.

Yellow Emperor: Ascending Qi is prevented from advancing, and I know this. Now I'd like to know how six-Qi is prevented from descending, can I understand it?

Qibo: What a detailed question you've asked! It is just the subtle mechanism of the heavens and the earth, which I can explain in detail. The so-called complete ascending necessarily followed by descending is that, after lasting for three years, any Qi has to descend to the earth as the left interval Qi. Thus, ascending and descending as going and coming is termed rotation of six-phase.

So, in the year marked with the 2nd or 8th, when descending to the earth, Jueyin meets inhibitive Dixiao Star with excessive metal Qi and is prevented from advancing. Concisely in the year when Shaoyin hasn't abdicated and Jueyin cannot descend, metal-phase Qi comes and wood Qi is prevented from descending and inhibited into depression, in which wood Qi is descending while metal Qi prevents it from descending, leading to dark dusts seen in the distance, wind rising with obscure dusts, cool and dry conquering Qi, frost and dew falling again, and distribution of conquering Qi. After prolonged failure of descending and depression into wood Qi, the wind and dryness are hidden, the warm climate is soon overcome by cool Qi, grass and trees are agitating, conquering frost falls, hibernating insects fail to emerge, and people fear the cold as damaging the solid viscera.

In the year marked with the 3rd or 9th, when descending to the earth, Shaoyin meets inhibitive Dixuan Star with excessive water Qi and is prevented from descending. Concisely in the year marked with Third-9th or Third-3rd, when Qi of water-phase is excessive and comes earlier, monarch-fire is descending but is prevented by water-phase Qi from descending, in which reddish clouds are emerging, black Qi is soon rising unexpectedly, and the comfort in warm climate is overcome by falling snow in cold weather with biting icy air and chilly cloud. After prolonged failure of descending and depression into fire Qi, there appears cold domination soon followed by heat, and reddish wind turning into pestilence. People then tend to have reddish complexion, heart vexation, headache and vertigo, and fire Qi is spreading and warm diseases may break out.

In the 4th or 10th year, when descending to the earth, Taiyin meets inhibitive Dicang Star with excessive wood Qi and is prevented from descending; concisely, Shaoyang hasn't abdicated while Taiyin cannot descend. Concisely, Qi of wood-phase comes and prevents Taiyin from descending; then there appear yellow clouds with bluish glow, depressive evaporation with great gales, fog spreading with more atmospheric dusts and plants can be broken and pulled down. After prolonged failure of descending and depression into damp earth, there appear yellow dusts in the sky and distribution of steaming damp over the earth. People then tend to have flaccid limbs, vertigo, limbs and joint pain, abdominal fullness and chest bloating.

In the year marked with the 5th or 11th, when descending to the earth, Shaoyang meets Dixuan Star and is prevented from descending. Concisely in the year when Qi of water phase is excessive and comes earlier, the summer fire is prevented by water Qi from descending, leading to reddish cloud emerging soon followed by the black Qi rising unexpectedly. The warm Qi is about to rise while the cold Qi suddenly falls, even with hailstones falling. After prolonged failure of descending and depression into fire Qi, icy air is overcome by the heat and reddish wind turns into pestilence. People then tend to have red complexion, heart vexation, headache and vertigo; reddish Qi is diffusing and the heat disease develops.

In the year marked with the 6th or 12th, when descending to the earth, Yangming meets Ditong Star with excessive fire Qi but is prevented from descending. Concisely in the year when Taiyang hasn't abdicated, Yangming cannot descend, in which Qi of fire-phase comes and prevents fire Qi from descending, leading to the cool sky and constriction, diffusion of the reddish air and paroxysm of heat Qi. People then tend to have lassitude, restless sleeping, dry throat with desire for water, vexing heat and internal dysphoria, cool sky in the morning and in the evening, and returning warmth; after prolonged failure of descending and depression into metal Qi, there appears cool sky with cold air and rising white air in the distance. People then tend to have spasm and vertigo, rigidity of hand and feet with numbness, hypochondriac pain and blurred vision in both eyes.

In the year marked with the 1st or 7th, when descending to the earth, Taiyang meets the inhibitive Difu Star with excessive earth Qi and is prevented from descending; concisely in the year, when Qi of earth phase is excessive, earth phase comes earlier, its Qi prevents the water Qi from descending, leading to diffusion of black air, gloomy chill in the sky, the yellow dusting soon followed by damp transformation and repeated distribution of steam and damp. After prolonged failure of descending and depression into earth-phase Qi, people tend to have stroke, heavy and flaccid limbs, impotence and weakness; there appear heavy clouds in the sky and intermittent steam and damp.

Emperor: There is failure of ascending or descending, and I've understood the original cause clearly; now I'd like to know the promotion of six-Qi; shall I understand it?
Qibo: The yearly Qi takes the middle position, which is called promotion to the right position; the heaven-governing Qi cannot be promoted to the right position while the previous heaven-governing Qi exceeds due time; that is, after meeting the previous heaven-governing Qi with the excess Qi that still governs the natural changes, the new heaven-governing Qi hasn't be promoted to the right position. When current Jueyin cannot be promoted, there is no warm wind in due time with fading and withering flowers. People then tend to have stranguria, rapid oscillation of eyeballs, frequent anger and cramp and dark urine. Wind Qi is executing its role while the

previous cold Qi doesn't recede, so that the warm climate cannot come in due time and the spring loses its proper climate. When current Shaoyin cannot be promoted, that is, the cold Qi doesn't recede, there comes cold spring followed by cold climate, and there is no warm transformation in due time. People then tend to have chill-fever, vexation and pain of limbs, and rigid waist and spine. Though excessive, the previous wood Qi cannot overcome monarch fire as host Qi. When current Taiyin cannot be promoted, and the cloud and rain lose the due time, everything is withering and the growing is halted. People then tend to have swelling and fullness of hands, feet and joints, bulging belly and edema, chest bloating with anorexia, diarrhea after indigestion, hypochondriac fullness, and flaccid limbs. The rain is going to fall but is prevented by the heat domination, and there is the hyperactive warmth in the air with less rain and moisture. When current Shaoyang cannot be promoted, it will execute its role of hot climate, leading to failure of plants to sprout and flourish, intense heat lingering into autumn, constriction and conquering Qi arriving late and frost and dew failing to fall in due time. People then tend to have tertian malaria, bone-heat, palpitation, fright and bleeding if severe. When current Yangming cannot be promoted, the transformation of summer heat is followed by late constriction and conquering Qi, leading to unexpected flourishing of grass and trees. People then tend to have chill-fever, nasal obstruction and sneeze, brittle hair and dry skin, withered nails; if severe, they will have panting, cough and dyspnea, and sorrow. Heat transformation is distributing, dry transformation fails to execute, vigorous cool air fails to prevail and lung is susceptible to diseases. When current Taiyang cannot be promoted, cold Qi in winter is abnormally prevalent in the coming spring and killing frost precedes cold ice; when sunshine dominates again, the biting cold air disappears and the white fog and clouds will appear in due time. People then tend to have warm diseases, stuffy throat and dry pharynx, vexation and thirst, and panting with wheeze. The cold transformation is waiting for dry Qi to subside so as to govern heavenly Qi, and otherwise the order will be disturbed and bring disasters to people.

Emperor: With regard to the early and late promotion, you've explained them; now, I'd like to know about abdication, and shall I understand it?
Qibo: The so-called unabdication means that, the days for heavenly Qi to govern have not yet expired, i.e., having its residual days, called as re-administration or as governing heavens again, in which the Qi governs the heavens as before and won't abdicate. When Jueyin doesn't abdicate, big gales come early, there is no falling of the due rain and no damp transformation. People then tend to have epidemic diseases, disability, wind diseases, pain of all limbs and joints, headache, eye pain, hidden heat with internal vexation, and dry throat with desire for water. When Shaoyin doesn't abdicate, warm Qi will appear in transition between winter and spring, insects will emerge early from hibernation and there will be early growth of grass and trees. People then tend to have heat in diaphragm, dry pharynx, bleeding, fright, reddish and dripping urine, blood tumor, sores and lingering toxin. When Taiyin doesn't abdicate, irregular cold and heat, dust spreading dimly and damp transformation lingering will be seen. People then tend to have flaccidity of four limbs, anorexia, acute diarrhea, stranguria, abdominal fullness, cold feet and shank, impotence, constipation, urinary

incontinence or frequent urination. When Shaoyang doesn't abdicate, there will appear heat rising in spring, late summer-heat transformation, no freezing in warm winter, no freezing of flowing water, and insects emerging from hibernation. People then tend to have short breath, alternative chill and fever, blood stool, feverish feeling in the upper, hard fullness in the lower abdomen, and reddish urine and bleeding if severe. When Yangming doesn't abdicate, there will appear cool Qi in spring, later flourishing of grass and trees, and intermittent chill and fever. People then tend to have vomiting, acute diarrhea, anorexia, dry feces, flaccidity of four limbs, blurred vision and vertigo. When Taiyang doesn't abdicate, there will be cool Qi of the spring appearing in the summer, cold hailstones falling, heavy and dim atmosphere and lingering cold in the second position. People then tend to have impediment and reversal syndromes, impotence, urinary incontinence, pain of the waist and knees and later prevalence of the warm diseases.

Emperor: There is early or later heaven-governing Qi, and I know them now; I'd like to know the change of earth-governing Qi, and shall I understand it?
Qibo: If there is no advancement of promotion, ascending and abdication among three earth-governing Qi, it will correspond to earth-governing transformation with loss of due transformation of all the things.

Emperor: I have heard that there are two First-1st systems of the heavens and the earth as well as 10 heavenly stems and 12 earthly branches, in which the upper and lower integrate mutually to administer nature, shifting the position and losing the due position, and shall I understand them?

Qibo: Through overlapping the due position, the six-Qi reaches the right position but cannot execute its normal role, leading to disorder in four seasons and great pestilence. It's said in *Secrete Words as Mysterious Pearls* that in the thirty Yang years, except for six years with mutual restraining, there are 24 remaining excessive years, that is, except for the six years, the other years are all regarded as excessive ones. Otherwise the current shifting Qi into the due position is all regarded as deficient years.

Supposing in the year of the First-1st as Yang, earth-phase Qi is inhibited severely; if the previous year marked with the Tenth-12th has more days to govern, the current year has reached the position with the First-1st but Jueyin is still governing the heavens, so that earthly Qi has been promoted and Yangming is at the position of the earth with previous Shaoyang as right interval Qi. Then, Jueyin lingers in the heavens while Yangming is in the earth, both of which will be not in harmony. When the Tenth meets the Sixth, the earth phase should have excessive, but it is dominated by the wood and isn't excessive; so, how can it be regarded as too excessive earthly phase. Moreover the greater Gong shouldn't be inhibited too much, so that when the wood phase dominates the earth, the metal phase will retaliate, followed by Shaoyin. Thus wood domination like fire and metal retaliation is mild, and finally the year of First and Sixth lose the role, which will turn into the earth-pestilence later in the year of Fourth-4th or sooner in the year of Third-3rd. The earth-pestilence will come, the scale and severity of which depend on the heavens and the earth as well as the universe. Concisely supposing in the year of the First-1st, since the First is harmonized with the 1st, it can shift and govern the heavens. Then Yangming in the current year of the Sixth-4th hasn't been promoted while Shaoyang in the previous year of the Fifth-3rd hasn't abdicated, leading to disharmony between the First and the 6th and no excess of the earth phase. Moreover, wood Qi seizes the opportunity to dominate the earth while the metal Qi again retaliates, turning into the evil Qi contrarily. Therefore, there is great difference of Yin–Yang changes between the heavens and the earth, whose scale and severity are determined by the law of the nature as usual.

Supposing in the Yang year of the Third-3rd with excess if the previous year of the Second-2nd has more days to govern, the current year has reached the phase of Third-3rd but Taiyin is still governing the heavens. Earthly Qi has been promoted with Jueyin at earth-governing position and with Taiyang as right interval Qi, so that Taiyin lingers in the heavens while Jueyin is in the earth, in which the earth doesn't respect the transformation of heavens. Thus, the Second meets the Eighth, the water phase is too deficient and dominated by the earth reversely, which isn't excessive; equally, the tone of greater Yu is in discord with Taizu. Hence, the domination of the earth results in the rain transformation with wood retaliation as wind, in which the Third and the Eighth lose the due position and harmony, which will turn into water-pestilence emerging in three years, later in the year of the Sixth-6th or sooner in the year of the Fifth-5th, and even its emergence is rapid if severe and slow if mild, and its scale and severity depend on the heavens and the earth as well as the universe. Concisely supposing in the year of the Third-3rd, the Third meets the 3rd to shift and govern the heavens, then the Eighth-6th hasn't been promoted while the Seventh-5th as Taiyang hasn't abdicated, leading to disharmony of the Third and the Eighth. That is, the water phase is less deficient but has slight domination or some retaliation, which will turn into the epidemic diseases termed as water-leprosy, whose manifestation is similar to the water pestilence; its treatment is the same as the above.

Supposing in the Yang year of the Seventh-5th with excess if the previous year of the Sixth-4th has more days to govern, the current year has reached the position of the Seventh-5th but Yangming is still governing the heavens. Earthly Qi has been promoted but Taiyin lingers in the earth with Shaoyin as right interval Qi. Then Yangming lingers in the heavens but Taiyin is in the earth, in which the earth doesn't respect the heavens. When the Second meets the Sixth, the metal phase is too deficient so as to be dominated by the earth reversely, which isn't excessive; equally, the tone of greater Shang is in discord with Guxi. The fire domination results in heat transformation that triggers the retaliation of cold water, in which the year of the Second and Seventh lose their functions and in three years turn into metal-pestilence; the pestilence will emerge sooner in the year of the Ninth-7th and later in the Tenth-8th, and the scale and severity depend on the heavens and the earth as well as the universe. Concisely supposing in the year of the Seventh-5th, the Seventh meet the 5th to shift and govern the heavens, then in the earth the Second-8th hasn't been promoted while Shaoyin in the previous year of the First-7th hasn't abdicated, in which the Second and the Seventh aren't in harmony. That is, in the Second-8th, the soft Qi in the earth isn't harmonized with the hard Qi in the heavens, leading to slight deficiency and finally slight domination or no retaliation afterwards. In three years, it turns into the epidemic diseases termed metal-pestilence, and its manifestation is similar to the metal-pandemic diseases; its treatment is the same as above.

Supposing in the Yang year of the Ninth-7th with excess if the previous year of the Eighth-6th has more days to govern, the current year has reached the phase of the Ninth-7th but Jueyin is still governing the heavens, in which earthly Qi has been promoted as Yangming in the earth with Shaoyin in the year of the Third-9th as the right interval Qi. Then, Jueying lingers in the heavens while Yangming is in the earth, in which the earth doesn't respect the heavens. When the Fourth meets the Eighth, the wood-phase is too deficient so as to be dominated by the metal earth reversely, which isn't too excessive. Equally, the tone of Ruibin is in discord with greater Jue. The domination of the dry metal results in the fire transformation with heat retaliation, which occurs sooner if severe, and more slowly if mild. The scale and severity of the pestilence depend on the heavens and the earth as well as the universe. Concisely supposing in the Ninth-7th year, it shifts and governs the heavens; then earthly Qi in the Fourth-10th year hasn't been promoted while in the earth the Third-9th Shaoyang hasn't abdicated, indicating disharmony between the Fourth and Ninth. That is, the soft earthly branch loses the hardness from the heavenly stem, leading to slight deficiency of wood phase with slight domination and slight retaliation. In three years, it turns into the epidemic diseases termed wood pestilence, whose manifestation is similar to the wind-pestilence; its treatment is the same as above.

Supposing in the Yang year of the Fifth-9th with excess if the previous year of the Fourth-8th is too excessive, the current year reaches the phase of Fifth-9th, but Taiyin is lingering in the position of heaven-governing while earthly Qi has been promoted as Jueyin in the earth, and the previous year of Ninth-11th as Taiyang abdicates to the right interval. That is, the Fourth-8th is in the heavens while the Tenth-12th is in the earth, in which the earth doesn't respect the heavens. When the Fourth meets the Tenth, the fire phase is too deficient so as to be dominated by the water, indicating not too excessive; equally, the tone of Yize is in discord with greater Zhi, indicating that the Fifth and Tenth lose their functions in the due position; in three years, it turns into pestilence and will emerge sooner in the Fifth or Tenth year; the scale and severity of the pestilence depend on the heavens and the earth as well as the universe. Concisely supposing in the Fifth-9th year, when the Fifth meets the 9th to shift and govern, the Tenth-12th hasn't been promoted in the earth while in the earth the Ninth-11th Taiyang hasn't abdicated, indicating the disharmony between Fifth and Tenth. That is, the soft heavenly stem of the Tenth loses the hardness, by which the fire phase is slightly deficient with slight domination or has no retaliation. In three years, it turns into the epidemic diseases termed the fire-pestilence; the treatment is the same as above, and the diseases can be treated with cold and discharging therapy.

Yellow Emperor: For anyone with deficient healthy Qi, when heavenly Qi is insufficient, the human body will lose mental Qi and the spirit is scattered, while the evil Qi can invade the body leading to sudden death; shall I know about it?

Qibo: Human body has five solid viscera, and if any one of them is insufficient and coincides with heavens deficiency, it will cause evil to come. It coincides with Shaoyin governing the heavens with its insufficient heavenly Qi and then Taiyin as the interval Qi comes. It indicates the deficiency of heavenly Qi and is summed up as both human Qi and heavenly Qi deficiency. Concisely with fright and being deprived of the essence, sweat is produced from heart to develop triple deficiency, indicating that spirit loses its place. Heart is an organ serving as the chief of all, from which the spirit originates. If losing its place, the spirit will be wandering between the two brows and the brain. Since the spirit loses its place, the mental light is scattering, and if meeting insufficient fire, there appears black-ghost (water) pestilence causing sudden death. Improper diet and overstrain will damage spleen, which happens in the year when Taiyin governs the heavens with insufficient Qi, in which Shaoyang comes as interval Qi, indicating the deficiency, and this is summed up as deficiency of both human and the heavens. Concisely with much satiety, sweat originates from stomach, and with intercourse after being drunk, sweat originates from spleen, which pertains to triple deficiency and causes loss of spleen spirit. Spleen is an organ serving as remonstrator, from which the thoughtful wisdom comes. The spirit loses its place and the mental light loses its position and is scattered, which meets the insufficiency in the year of the Sixth or the First or in the year of Taiyin deficiency. There appears green ghost (wood) pestilence causing sudden death. Sitting on wet ground for long or overstraining in water will damage kidney. Kidney serves as an organ for powerful action, from which the elaborate functions come. Due to triple deficiency, the kidney spirit loses its place, the mind loses its function and metal light is scattered, which meets the insufficiency in the year of the Eighth with neither yearly identification nor heavens identification, nor in the year of the Third with losing the place, and nor in the year of deficiency of Taiyang heavens-governing. There will be the yellow ghost (earth) pestilence causing sudden death. When a man is angry, Qi will ascend reversely and cannot descend, which can damage liver. Concisely happening in the year of Jueyin heaven-governing with insufficient heavenly Qi and with Shaoyin arrival as interval Qi, it is called deficiency of heavenly Qi, summed up as deficiency of both the heavens and human. Concisely with scurrying away and a feeling of horror, sweat originates from liver. Liver is an organ serving as general, from which the deliberation comes. If the spirit loses its place, the mental light is scattered. If concisely in the year of wood insufficiency, or with the Fourth stem having no identification, or with the Ninth stem losing the place or with the deficiency of Jueyin heaven-governing, there will be white ghost (metal) pestilence causing sudden death. The five types of spirit-losing mentioned above are caused by deficiency of both heavenly Qi and human Qi, and as a result their organ-spirit will wander and lose its place. Then there will be five deadly ghost-pestilence to attack people and cause sudden death, termed sudden reversal death. If a human violates the five solid viscera with their positions, the spirit light cannot be perfect. Under this condition, not only ghost-pestilence but all evils attacking people are caused by the spirit-losing. It is believed that spirit keeping its place results in survival, while spirit losing its place results in death. Equally, maintaining spirit results in vitality while losing spirit results in death.

About the Editor

Jinghua Fu is a research scientist at China Academy of Chinese Medical Sciences. He graduated from Inner Mongolia Medical College, China, in 1968 and received his graduate degree in 1980 from China Academy of Chinese Medical Sciences. He was the Editor-in-Chief of Traditional Chinese Medicine Classics Publishing House. He is also an adjunct researcher at Cui Yueli Traditional Medicine Research Center.

List of Translators

Translator-in-Chief:	Mingshan Yang
Associate Translators-in-Chief:	Yong Jin
	Cui Zhu
Translators:	Changxiang Li
	Yi Li
	Ding Sun

Mingshan Yang, Professor of Shanghai University of Traditional Chinese Medicine, is engaged in the research and practice of Pediatrics (Western Medicine), pedagogy, medical English and TCM English. He has written or edited ten books, including *Essential Chinese–English TCM Dictionary*, *Concise Quotations from Clinical TCM Classics (Chinese–English)*, *New Course for Medical English*, *Course of Medical English Terminology*, *Modern Medical Bedside Teaching in English.*

www.ingramcontent.com/pod-product-compliance
Ingram Content Group UK Ltd.
Pitfield, Milton Keynes, MK11 3LW, UK
UKHW020404150926
8624IPUK00004B/342

9 789813 273573